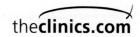
theclinics.com

HEMATOLOGY/ ONCOLOGY CLINICS OF NORTH AMERICA

Immunotherapy of Cancer

GUEST EDITOR
Madhav V. Dhodapkar, MD

June 2006 • Volume 20 • Number 3

SAUNDERS
An Imprint of Elsevier, Inc.
PHILADELPHIA   LONDON   TORONTO   MONTREAL   SYDNEY   TOKYO

W.B. SAUNDERS COMPANY
A Division of Elsevier Inc.

Elsevier Inc. · 1600 John F. Kennedy Boulevard · Suite 1800 · Philadelphia, Pennsylvania 19103-2899

http://www.hemonc.theclinics.com

HEMATOLOGY/ONCOLOGY CLINICS
OF NORTH AMERICA   Volume 20, Number 3
June 2006   ISSN 0889-8588
Editor: Kerry Holland   ISBN 1-4160-3905-8

Reprints. For copies of 100 or more, of articles in this publication, please contact the Commercial Reprints Department, Elsevier Inc., 360 Park Avenue South, New York, New York 10010-1710. Tel. (212) 633-3813; Fax: (212) 462-1935; email: reprints@elsevier.com.

The ideas and opinions expressed in *Hematology/Oncology Clinics of North America* do not necessarily reflect those of the Publisher. The Publisher does not assume any responsibility for any injury and/or damage to persons or property arising out of or related to any use of the material contained in this periodical. The reader is advised to check the appropriate medical literature and the product information currently provided by the manufacturer of each drug to be administered to verify the dosage, the method and duration of administration, or contraindications. It is the responsibility of the treating physician or other health care professional, relying on independent experience and knowledge of the patient, to determine drug dosages and the best treatment for the patient. Mention of any product in this issue should not be construed as endorsement by the contributors, editors, or the Publisher of the product or manufacturers' claims.

The Hematology/Oncology Clinics of North America (ISSN 0889-8588) is published bimonthly by W.B. Saunders, 360 Park Avenue South, New York, NY 10010-1710. Months of publication are February, April, June, August, October, and December. Business and Editorial Offices: 1600 John F. Kennedy Boulevard, Suite 1800, Philadelphia, PA 19103-2899. Accounting and Circulation Offices: 6277 Sea Harbor Drive, Orlando, FL 32887-4800. Periodicals postage paid at New York, NY and additional mailing offices. Subscription prices are $220.00 per year (US individuals), $330.00 per year (US institutions), $110.00 per year (US students), $250.00 per year (Canadian individuals), $395.00 per year (Canadian institutions), $140.00 per year (Canadian students), $280.00 per year (international individuals), $395.00 per year (international institutions), $140.00 per year (international students). International air speed delivery is included in all *Clinics* subscription prices. All prices are subject to change without notice. **POSTMASTER:** Send address changes to *The Hematology/Oncology Clinics of North America*, Elsevier Periodicals Customer Service, 6277 Sea Harbor Drive, Orlando, FL 32887-4800. Customer Service: 1-800-654-2452 (US). From outside of the US, call 1-407-345-4000.

Hematology/Oncology Clinics of North America is covered in *Index Medicus, EMBASE/Excerpta Medica,* and *BIOSIS.*

Printed in the United States of America.

ELSEVIER
SAUNDERS

HEMATOLOGY/ONCOLOGY CLINICS
OF NORTH AMERICA

Immunotherapy of Cancer

GUEST EDITOR

MADHAV V. DHODAPKAR, MD, Irene Diamond Associate Professor and Head
of Laboratory, Laboratory of Tumor Immunology and Immunotherapy,
The Rockefeller University; and Hematology Service, Memorial Sloan-Kettering
Cancer Center, New York, New York

CONTRIBUTORS

PAUL B. CHAPMAN, MD, Associate Chairman, Department of Medicine,
and the Melanoma/Sarcoma Service, Memorial Sloan-Kettering Cancer Center,
New York, New York

RAPHAEL CLYNES, MD, PhD, Departments of Medicine and Microbiology,
Columbia University, College of Physicians and Surgeons, New York, New York

ADAM D. COHEN, MD, Department of Medicine, Memorial Sloan-Kettering
Cancer Center, New York; Weill Medical College of Cornell University,
New York, New York

MADHAV V. DHODAPKAR, MD, Irene Diamond Associate Professor and Head
of Laboratory, Laboratory of Tumor Immunology and Immunotherapy,
The Rockefeller University; and Hematology Service, Memorial Sloan-Kettering
Cancer Center, New York, New York

PETER DUBSKY, MD, Baylor Institute for Immunology Research, Dallas, Texas

ANDREW EISENBERGER, Division of Medical Oncology, Columbia University,
New York, New York

BRIAN M. ELLIOTT, The Tumor Immunology Laboratory, Department of Surgery,
Columbia University, New York, New York

DAVOR FRLETA, PhD, Baylor Institute for Immunology Research, Dallas, Texas

HOWARD L. KAUFMAN, MD, Divisions of Surgical Oncology and The Tumor
Immunology Laboratory, Department of Surgery, Columbia University,
New York, New York

KELVIN P. LEE, MD, Department of Microbiology, Immunology and Division of
Hematology and Oncology, Department of Medicine, University of Miami Miller
School of Medicine, Miami, Florida

A. KAROLINA PALUCKA, MD, PhD, Baylor Institute for Immunology Research, Dallas, Texas

ECKHARD R. PODACK, MD, PhD, Department of Microbiology and Immunology, University of Miami Miller School of Medicine, Miami, Florida

LUIS E. RAEZ, MD, Division of Hematology and Oncology, Department of Medicine, University of Miami Miller School of Medicine, Miami, Florida

GERT RIETHMÜLLER, Institut fuer Immunologie, Ludwig-Maximilian Universitaet, Muenchen, Germany

PETRA RIETSCHEL, MD, Department of Medicine, and the Melanoma/Sarcoma Service, Memorial Sloan-Kettering Cancer Center, New York, New York

DONALD A. ROWLEY, MD, The Committee on Immunology, Department of Pathology, The University of Chicago, Chicago, Illinois

HIROAKI SAITO, MD, PhD, Baylor Institute for Immunology Research, Dallas, Texas

HANS SCHREIBER, MD, PhD, The Committee on Immunology and Committee on Cancer Biology, Department of Pathology, The University of Chicago Cancer Center, The University of Chicago, Chicago, Illinois

KARIN SCHREIBER, BS, Department of Pathology, The University of Chicago, Chicago, Illinois

RADEK SPISEK, MD, PhD, Laboratory of Tumor Immunology and Immunotherapy, The Rockefeller University, New York, New York

RODICA STAN, PhD, Department of Medicine, Memorial Sloan-Kettering Cancer Center, New York, New York

JEDD D. WOLCHOK, MD, PhD, Department of Medicine, Memorial Sloan-Kettering Cancer Center, New York; Weill Medical College of Cornell University, New York, New York

CASSIAN YEE, MD, Clinical Research Division, Fred Hutchinson Cancer Research Center; and Department of Medicine, University of Washington Medical Center, Seattle, Washington

HEMATOLOGY/ONCOLOGY CLINICS
OF NORTH AMERICA

Immunotherapy of Cancer

CONTENTS   VOLUME 20 · NUMBER 3 · JUNE 2006

Preface   **xi**
Madhav V. Dhodapkar

**Cancer Immunotherapy and Preclinical Studies:
Why We Are Not Wasting Our Time with
Animal Experiments**   **567**
Karin Schreiber, Donald A. Rowley, Gert Riethmüller,
and Hans Schreiber

> Experimental research on the immune response to transplanted tumors
> has led to pioneering discoveries that laid many of the foundations for the
> current field of immunology. Experimental research in oncology has
> proven that murine and human tumors have antigens that are truly cancer
> specific. This article discusses research investigating how can antigens on
> cancer cells be used to help eradicate cancer.

**Antitumor Antibodies in the Treatment of Cancer:
Fc Receptors Link Opsonic Antibody with
Cellular Immunity**   **585**
Raphael Clynes

> Engineered antibody therapeutics have provided new treatment options
> in cancer. Genetic evidence in man and in the mouse suggests that Fc
> receptor (FcR) engagement contributes mechanistically to the therapeutic
> activity of naked antibodies. Preferential activation of activating FcRs
> and limited engagement of inhibitory FcRs enhance tumor responses in
> mouse models. Thus, engineered Fc domains with favorable affinities for
> specific FcR types may prove to be clinically superior.

DNA Vaccines Against Cancer   **613**
Rodica Stan, Jedd D. Wolchok, and Adam D. Cohen

> Significant progress made in the field of tumor immunology by the
> characterization of a large number of tumor antigens, and the better
> understanding of the mechanisms preventing immune responses to
> malignancies has led to the extensive study of cancer immunization

approaches such as DNA vaccines encoding tumor antigens. This article reviews major aspects of DNA immunization in cancer. It gives a brief history and then discusses the proposed mechanism of action, preclinical and clinical studies, and methods of enhancing the immune responses induced by DNA vaccines.

Heat Shock Protein–Based Cancer Vaccines   637
Kelvin P. Lee, Luis E. Raez, and Eckhard R. Podack

The ability to duplicate the remarkable success of infectious disease vaccines in cancer, with durably robust and highly specific antitumor immune responses, has been long held as one of the keys in developing true "magic bullet" cancer therapies. This article attempts to explain why cancer vaccines have failed (so far), delineates the increasingly complex barriers that prevent the eliciting of effective antitumor immunity, and examines the ability of heat shock protein–based vaccines to overcome these barriers. This article is not a definitive compendium of the huge body of relevant literature but rather focuses on the major concepts underlying active specific immunotherapy in general and heat shock protein vaccines in particular.

Viral Vaccines for Cancer Immunotherapy   661
Andrew Eisenberger, Brian M. Elliott, and Howard L. Kaufman

The understanding that tumor cells can be recognized and eliminated by the immune system has led to intense interest in the development of cancer vaccines. Viruses are naturally occurring agents that cause human disease but have the potential to prevent disease when attenuated forms or subunits are used as vaccines before exposure. A large number of viruses have been engineered as attenuated vaccines for the expression of tumor antigens, immunomodulatory molecules, and as vehicles for direct destruction of tumor cells or expression of highly specific gene products. This article focuses on the major viruses that are under development as cancer vaccines, including the poxviruses, adenoviruses, adeno-associated viruses, herpesviruses, retroviruses, and lentiviruses. The biology supporting these viruses as vaccines is reviewed and clinical progress is reported.

Dendritic Cell–Based Vaccination Against Cancer   689
Hiroaki Saito, Davor Frleta, Peter Dubsky, and A. Karolina Palucka

Vaccination against infectious agents represents a success of immunology, although many infectious diseases still evade the immune system, including chronic infections, such as tuberculosis, malaria, and HIV. Further progress is expected through rational design based on increased understanding of how the immune system works, and how the induction of protective immunity is regulated. The same principle applies to cancer vaccines, particularly because cancer is a chronic disease. Owing to their capacity to regulate cellular and humoral immunity, dendritic cells are increasingly used as vaccines; the immunogenicity of antigens delivered on dendritic cells has been shown in cancer patients. A better understanding of how dendritic cells regulate immune responses would allow clinicians to exploit them better to induce effective immunity against cancer.

Adoptive T-Cell Therapy of Cancer 711
Cassian Yee

Adoptive therapy involves the transfer of ex vivo expanded immune effector cells to patients as a means of augmenting the antitumor immune response. In general, this transfer is accomplished by harvesting cells from the peripheral blood, tumor sites, or draining lymph nodes and expanding effector cells in a specific or nonspecific fashion for adoptive transfer. This article describes the rationale for adoptive T-cell therapy, the developments that have led to the translational application of this strategy for the treatment of cancer, the challenges that have been addressed, and future approaches to the development of adoptive therapy as a treatment modality.

Immunoprevention of Cancer 735
Radek Spisek and Madhav V. Dhodapkar

This article discusses the current understanding of the interactions between tumors and cells of the immune system, particularly at the early stages of carcinogenesis. A growing body of data suggests that these interactions help shape the eventual development of tumors. Inflammation is a common feature of several cancers, and the immune system can serve as a two-edged sword against cancer, capable of supporting and suppressing cancer. Data from human studies show that the immune system is capable of detecting the smallest expansions of transformed cells, well before the development of clinical cancer. These advances suggest a need to change the current emphasis for harnessing antitumor immunity from therapy to prevention of cancers.

Immunotherapy of Melanoma 751
Petra Rietschel and Paul B. Chapman

Melanoma has been widely studied as a target for immunotherapy because it has been considered more susceptible to immune attack than other tumors and because of the relative ease with which melanoma cells can be adapted to in vitro culture. The availability of hundreds of melanoma cell lines for study has led to the identification of tumor antigens and the development of monoclonal antibodies and T cells against these antigens, revolutionizing the understanding of how the immune system sees and reacts to cancer. This article reviews the recent clinical results of trials exploring different immunotherapy strategies against melanoma.

Index   *767*

ELSEVIER
SAUNDERS

HEMATOLOGY/ONCOLOGY CLINICS
OF NORTH AMERICA

FORTHCOMING ISSUES

August 2006

Prostate Cancer
William Oh, MD
Guest Editor

October 2006

Hairy Cell Leukemia
Alan Saven, MD
Guest Editor

December 2006

Advances in Neuro-oncology
Lisa DeAngelis, MD, and Jerome Posner, MD
Guest Editors

RECENT ISSUES

April 2006

Radiation Medicine Update for the Practicing Oncologist, Part II
Lisa A. Kachnic, MD, and Charles R. Thomas, Jr, MD
Guest Editors

February 2006

Radiation Medicine Update for the Practicing Oncologist, Part I
Lisa A. Kachnic, MD, and Charles R. Thomas, Jr, MD
Guest Editors

December 2005

Mesothelioma
Hedy Lee Kindler, MD
Guest Editor

PREFACE

Immunotherapy of Cancer

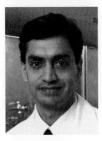

Madhav V. Dhodapkar, MD

Guest Editor

N early a century after Paul Ehrlich's prediction about the development of "magic bullets" against cancer, harnessing the specificity of the immune system against cancer is now rapidly becoming a reality. Biologics such as monoclonal antibodies now represent the biggest class of FDA-approved new therapies for human cancer in the last five years, and several vaccine-based approaches (including DNA and dendritic cell vaccines) are also showing promise. In this issue, we have brought together several thought leaders in this rapidly advancing field to present the current status as well as the near future of immunologic approaches against human cancer.

Schreiber discusses the lessons learned from preclinical studies, as well as the need to correctly interpret the data to facilitate realistic translation to the clinic. Clynes reviews the biology behind the application of monoclonal antibodies as immune therapeutics in cancer therapy. The importance of dendritic cells in anti-tumor immunity has led to approaches to target them, as explored by Palucka et al. Specific targeting of tumor antigens is also being attempted with DNA vaccines (presented by Wolchok), viral vectors (discussed by Kaufmann), and heat shock proteins (reviewed by Lee). Yee examines the technology of the adoptive transfer of T cells as an approach to boosting immunity against cancer and viral infections. Spisek et al. present the emerging data about immune prevention of cancer, which is already becoming a reality with the development of vaccines for the human papilloma virus. Finally, Chapman discusses the application of immune approaches in the context of a specific cancer, melanoma.

It has been a privilege to edit this issue of the *Hematology/Oncology Clinics of North America*, with contributions by many of the thought leaders in this field.

0889-8588/06/$ – see front matter
doi:10.1016/j.hoc.2006.02.012

I hope that these articles will convey both the challenge and the tremendous promise of harnessing the immune system not only to treat but also to prevent human cancer.

Madhav V. Dhodapkar, MD
The Rockefeller University
Laboratory of Tumor Immunology & Immunotherapy
1230 York Avenue #176
New York, NY 10021-6399, USA
E-mail address: dhodalpm@rockefeller.edu

Hematol Oncol Clin N Am 20 (2006) 567–584

HEMATOLOGY/ONCOLOGY CLINICS
OF NORTH AMERICA

Cancer Immunotherapy and Preclinical Studies: Why We Are Not Wasting Our Time with Animal Experiments

Karin Schreiber, BS[a], Donald A. Rowley, MD[a],
Gert Riethmüller, MD, DMSc[b], Hans Schreiber, MD, PhD[a],*

[a]Department of Pathology, The University of Chicago, Room G-308, MC 3008, 5841 South Maryland Avenue, Chicago, IL 60637, USA
[b]Institut fuer Immunologie, Ludwig-Maximilian Universitaet, Goethestrasse 31, 80336 Muenchen, Germany

Experimental research on the immune response to transplanted tumors has led to pioneering discoveries that laid many of the foundations for the current field of immunology. Examples are the discovery of the major histocompatibility complex (MHC) by Peter Gorer (for review see [1]), the development of inbred mouse strains, and the identification of T-cell subsets, natural killer cells, and tumor necrosis factor, to name only a few. Experimental research in oncology has proven that murine and human tumors have antigens that are truly cancer specific, but century-old questions have still not been answered [2]: (1) when and how does the immune system protect us against cancer development, and (2) how can antigens on cancer cells be used to help eradicate cancer? This article focuses on the second question.

From the beginning, the idea that immunologic tools or approaches can be used to fight cancer has been fraught with alternating cycles of enthusiasm and disillusionment. For example, on the basis of his experiments, Paul Ehrlich [2] believed that powerful immunity could be induced to diverse groups of cancers without affecting the normal tissues of the host. Gorer's work [1] showed that the success seen in Ehrlich's experiments was the result of responses to histocompatibility antigens on allogeneic tumor transplants. Ehrlich's idea of a "magic bullet" specific for virtually all cancers was completely unrealistic. Nevertheless, the idea persisted, and claims of success continued during the following decades. Typically, misleading terminology and sweeping conclu-

This work was supported by National Institutes of Health grants RO1-CA22677, RO1-CA37516, PO1-CA97296 and by the University of Chicago Cancer Research Center CA-14599.
* Corresponding author. Department of Pathology, The University of Chicago, Room G-308, MC 3008, 5841 South Maryland Avenue, Chicago, IL 60637. E-mail address: hszz@midway.uchicago.edu (H. Schreiber).

0889-8588/06/$ – see front matter
doi:10.1016/j.hoc.2006.03.001

sions fueled by wishful thinking and wording were published to impress and encourage other scientists, physicians, patients, laypersons, and stockholders. When these experimental findings were translated to the therapy of patients, the high hopes vanished. This cycle of unrealistic enthusiasm and resulting disappointment has led to a widespread impression that little real progress has been made and that animal experiments have been a waste of time. Researchers have failed to scrutinize the results of experimental research rigorously and have failed to accept and use the lessons of past experiments. The result has been unnecessary repetition. Careful analysis would have exposed the inappropriateness of certain animal models to answer the questions addressed. Closer examination of the results of animal experiments would have exposed the stumbling blocks and made clear why procedures based on animal experiments would fail in humans. Nevertheless, major progress is being made in cancer immunology. This article reviews the enormous value of past and present animal experimentation to help clinicians and experimental investigators focus on appropriate experimental settings that can be used to improve immunotherapy of cancer.

ANTIGENS ON MURINE OR HUMAN CANCERS TO BE TARGETED

Truly Tumor-Specific Antigens

One of the most important discoveries in tumor immunology following Gorer's [1] work was the identification of unique tumor-specific antigens [3–6]. For example, a landmark paper by Klein and colleagues [7] demonstrated that a host could be immunized to reject its own cancer cells. The elegant experimental design of this study proved that autologous T-cell responses destroy autologous cancer cells; the study excluded the possibility that the antigens were artificially caused by residual remaining or newly arising heterozygosity in inbred mouse strains. Importantly, the antigens were individually specific; that is, they were unique and did not cross-react with other cancers induced by the same carcinogen in other mice of the same inbred strain. More than 3 decades later it was finally proven, first in mice and then in humans, that these antigens were encoded by somatic tumor-specific mutations. These studies also excluded problems with residual heterozygosity because they used as controls autochthonous cells from the individual that developed the cancer [8–10]. In addition, these studies revealed that many of these antigenic mutant proteins seem to play a functional role in causing or supporting the malignant behavior of the cancer cells [11–15].

Because it was deemed impractical to immunize each patient to the unique antigen of the individual's tumor, extensive studies were undertaken to identify shared antigens that could elicit effective rejection of certain tumor types. No such antigens have been identified thus far, but the search for such antigens persists, and few questions in tumor immunology have been (and still are being) more hotly debated. Nevertheless, the experimental and clinical data of more than half a century confirm that unique truly tumor-specific (ie, altered-self) antigens are the most powerful targets to cause rejection of tumors. Altered-self antigens released from cancer cells and taken up by surrounding stroma cells can sensitize the tumor-supporting stroma for destruction [16,17]. Furthermore, unique tumor-specific antigens have been found on all spontaneous or induced cancers in humans and mice that have been carefully analyzed (for review, see [18]). Also, recent work suggests that responses of autologous T cells to a human melanoma can be dominated by mutated neoantigens [19]. Finally, individualized treatments using autologous tumor cell vaccines [20,21] or reinfusion of autologous expanded T cells in vitro [22,23] have shown promising results in patients who have aggressive cancers. These results are consistent with the results of genetic and pharmacologic studies suggesting the need for individualized cancer medicine [24].

Self-Antigens

Antigens that are not tumor-specific but are expressed on at least some normal host cells are commonly referred to as "tumor-associated antigens." Expression may be shared among many tissues or restricted to selective tissues or even to a single cell type. Most molecules expressed on cancer cell surfaces are probably normal self-antigens, but the frequent statement that most cancer antigens on human cancers are self-antigens unfortunately gives the erroneous impression that being an antigen on a cancer cell means being a useful target. This statement also evades the critical question of why the response to a self-antigen on a cancer cell should be more destructive than a response to the same normal-self molecule expressed by normal host cells. The mere fact that a self-antigen is molecularly defined, thereby allowing "molecularly targeted anti-cancer therapy," does not make it an appropriate target. Even Ehrlich postulated that his magic bullet had "no affinity to normal constituents of the body" to be successful [2]. Some of the confusion originates from the facts that CD8+ or CD4+ T cells can recognize normal self-molecules on cancer cells and that these T cells are derived from human or murine tumor-infiltrating or peripheral blood lymphocytes of the cancer-bearing host or even from healthy donors. Furthermore, testing sera from patients who have cancer revealed that by far the most frequent reactions to autologous tumor cells are those to normal cell-surface antigens widely distributed on normal and malignant cells [25]. Similar responses seem to trigger viral infections [26] and tissue destruction [27]. Thinking that these responses are beneficial is a great leap of faith. The biologic consequences of weak or strong responses to these antigens remain unclear.

Research has shown that the use of high-affinity antibodies or induction of powerful T-cell responses to self-antigens can lead to the destruction of the normal tissues expressing the same self-antigens [28]. Transcripts of most of the so-called "tumor-associated" antigens (differentiation antigens or onco-spermatogonal/cancer-testis antigens) are also expressed on thymic medullary epithelial cells [29]. The level of translation of these messages into proteins and antigens remains to be determined. The likely result of such expression would be the elimination of T cells with T-cell receptors (TCRs) having affinity to these self-peptide MHC complexes [30,31]. Such tolerance may create an important problem, because the destruction of well-established tumors may depend on high-affinity TCR:peptide-MHC interaction and peptides that form very stable complexes with the MHC class I molecule as target. Central tolerance usually does not affect responses to idiotypes of immunoglobulin, which are highly restricted to a particular B-cell clone. Differences in central tolerance may be one reason for the success of dendritic cell–based vaccination for induction of anti-idiotypic responses [32] and for the poor clinical success when other self-antigens are targeted by vaccine approaches [33]. High-affinity antibody and TCR reagents to self-antigen can be generated artificially by several methods that circumvent central tolerance, including molecular engineering or manipulation of the response [34–36]. Overcoming self-tolerance may only worsen the problems of self-reactivity, however.

Antibodies against growth factors or their receptors (eg, anti-vascular endothelial growth factor, anti-epidermal growth factor receptor, and anti-HER-2) on cancer cells are effective in some patients, and treatment may be tolerated relatively well because the most important effect may be growth inhibition by blocking signaling rather than destruction of cells. A major part of the in vivo efficacy of anti-HER-2 antibody, however, seems to depend on Fc and Fcγ receptors, strongly suggesting that immunologic mechanisms are also involved in the antitumor effect [37]. Engagement of Fc receptors leads to release of a variety of cytokines with pleotropic effects; blocking of signaling thus may synergize with immune effectors to cause growth arrest and possibly, but not necessarily, death of the cancer cells. All of these types of antibodies were first found to be effective in relevant animal experiments before clinical efficacy was shown [38–40]. Promising targets are also tissue- or clone-specific self-antigens for which immune destruction of the normal cells expressing the same antigen can be tolerated (eg, CD20 on malignant and normal B cells [41] or the idiotype of surface immunoglobulin on the B-cell malignancy and its normal B-cell precursor clone [32]). Unfortunately, few truly tissue-specific target antigens (eg, antigens selectively expressed on epithelial cells of the prostate, breast, or pancreas) have been identified.

Importance of the Amount of Target Antigen

The amount of target antigen on cancer cells is usually unknown, although the amount of target antigen expressed by cancer cells critically determines the outcome of an immune reaction to an established tumor. For example, solid tumors consisting of cancer cells expressing low levels of a target antigen tend to escape as antigen loss variants because the amount of antigen is insufficient to sensitize the surrounding tumor stroma for destruction by T cells [16,17]. In contrast, cure can be achieved if the antigen is tumor specific and is expressed at high levels, because of destruction of tumor stroma cross-presenting the tumor antigen. This bystander killing of the stroma apparently also results in the indirect killing of escape variants that have lost the antigen in the tumor.

Many molecularly defined normal self-molecules recognized by cytotoxic T lymphocytes are highly overexpressed on human tumors. Because cross-presentation does not distinguish between self- and nonself molecules, some peptides derived from these overexpressed self-proteins will be presented with high affinity by self-MHC on stromal cells, making them potential targets. T cells with TCRs having affinity to these self-peptide MHC complexes sufficient to cause damage may be deleted from the host repertoire during thymic evolution, however [31].

PROPER CHOICE OF ANIMAL MODEL

Almost all human tumors are established by the time they are recognized clinically. Therefore the main objective of the experimental immunologist is to select models that are relevant and have predictive value for patients who have established solid tumors, superficially spreading early-stage cancer or microdisseminated or dormant cancer cells. Furthermore, the experimental immunologist can address the problem of how to prevent some selected cancers. The main purpose of an animal model is to answer a specific question not answered readily in humans. It is also hoped that efficacy in preclinical models has some predictive value for efficacy in patients. Proper choice of the model therefore is determined by the question asked.

Transplantation of murine cancer cell lines remains a stronghold for experimental immunotherapy studies. It therefore is essential to realize the major biologic and immunologic differences between using this approach and using primary solid tumors. In 1929, in the pre-MHC era, Woglom [42] discussed 600 papers published since 1913 on immune responses to transplantable murine tumors and concluded "Immunity to transplantable tumours … is effective during the first few days following inoculation, but entirely powerless against an established tumour." Indeed, an additional 75 years of experimental research have only confirmed this general problem through publication of many more papers. Fig. 1 provides a schematic diagram of the general problem that can be confirmed readily by consulting most current and past literature on the subject.

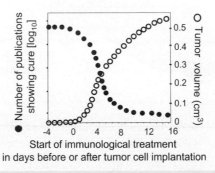

Fig. 1. Well-established solid tumors growing for 14 days or longer are rarely cured by experimental immunotherapy.

It probably understates the real problem because of what statisticians have called the "desk-drawer" phenomenon: failures of therapy are much less reported than successes. Fig. 1 also would predict immunotherapy as being most effective in eliminating recently disseminated cells.

During the first few days after tumor cell inoculation, a seemingly endless diversity of approaches is effective in causing immunologic rejection, but these procedures become entirely powerless against established tumors. Unfortunately, the words "established," "tumor," and "tumor-bearing" continue to be used inappropriately even for macroscopically undetectable or barely "palpable" lesions (usually those less than 1 mm in largest diameter). Histologic examination of lesions produced by injection of cancer cells (Fig. 2) may show "invasion" or early "vascularization" at the inoculum site within a few days, leading the investigator to call these lesions "established tumors." As can clearly be seen in Fig. 2, however, tumor cell inoculation causes remarkable artifacts during the first 10 days, including massive coagulation necrosis and acute inflammation. Only a thin rim of cancer cells survives next to pre-existent normal vasculature (H. Schreiber, unpublished data). Viable cancer and stromal cells usually replace these artifacts by about 2 weeks when most tumors have increased to about 1 cm in diameter. By this time, the acute inflammatory reaction and the coagulation necrosis have vanished, and the tumor becomes virtually indistinguishable from nontransplanted primary tumors, even to the trained eye of a

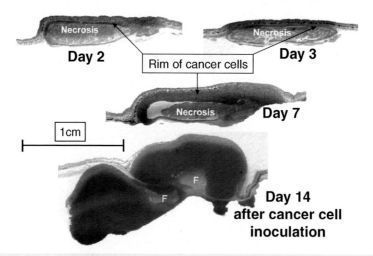

Fig. 2. Dramatic time-dependent changes in the microenvironment of the site of tumor cell inoculation. 10^7 murine methylcholanthrene-induced MC57 cancer cells were injected subcutaneously into a C57BL/6 RAG1$^{-/-}$ mouse. The cross-section of the site of inoculation is shown 2, 3, 7, and 14 days after the injection. At day 2 and 3, a rim of cancer cells (*arrows*) surrounds a large area of necrotic cancer cells and inflammatory cells (*Necrosis*). The rim thickens substantially by day 7, and the area of necrosis is being resorbed. By day 14, only a thin small fibrous remnant (*F*) remains surrounded by a homogenous viable tumor tissue. Slides were stained with hematoxylin and eosin.

pathologist. Unfortunately and importantly, most described immunotherapies become powerless for well-established experimental tumors that closely simulate clinically relevant solid cancers.

Cancer cells in well-established solid tumors are embedded in noninflammatory stroma that is essential for tumor growth and spread by providing growth factors, cytokines, and nutrition (for review, see [43,44]). The stroma in these tumors consists of extracellular matrix and a variety of nonmalignant cells comprising bone marrow–derived cells (mostly monocytes/macrophages but also some granulocytes and lymphocytes) and non–bone marrow–derived cells (such as endothelium and other cells of the vasculature and fibroblasts). The most frequent bone marrow–derived cells are CD11b+ cells, of which about one quarter are Gr-1+. There is overwhelming evidence that Gr-1+/CD11b+ bone marrow–derived cells [45,46] can promote tumor growth as well as angiogenesis [47]. They are also able to stimulate growth of cancer cells directly in vitro [48]. Progressively growing established tumors induce splenomegaly caused by increased number of Gr-1+/CD11b+ immature myeloid cells [49] (for review, also see [50,51]). Splenic Gr-1+ immature myeloid cells migrate to the tumor and differentiate there into tumor-associated macrophages [52]. Treatment of mice with anti-Gr-1 suppresses tumor growth in T-cell–deficient mice [45] and allows normal mice to reject otherwise lethal tumor challenge [53]. This treatment may reduce Gr-1+ splenic precursors of tumor-associated macrophages, abolish a neutrophil-dependent macrophage recruitment mechanism in the tumor by eliminating Gr-1+ granulocytes [54], or eliminate Gr-1+ tumor growth–promoting cells within the tumor microenvironment.

It is rare to observe an acute inflammatory stromal reaction in primary solid tumors or well-established transplanted cancers unless these tumors develop severe necrosis and become ulcerated and infected. As might be expected, cancer cells embedded in a noninflammatory tumor stroma as solid tumor fragment are 10 to 100 times more tumorigenic upon transplantation than an equal number of cancer cells injected as suspension [55–57]. Injection of cell suspensions is associated with artifacts of acute inflammation at the injection site (as discussed previously) and with much better cross-presentation leading to much better priming [58] and probably stromal targeting.

Eradication of Superficially Spreading or Early-stage Cancers

Some of the first successful attempts of immunotherapy of cancer by Fehleisen [59] more than 100 years ago in Germany involved intratumoral injection of live bacteria (also reviewed by Bruns [60]). Cultured bacteria from erysipelas were inoculated into cancers causing some amazing curative effects. A decade later, his work was acknowledged, confirmed, and extended by Coley [61]. Inoculation of live bacteria is still being used to treat superficial bladder cancer: live bacilli Calmette Guérin are instilled into the urinary bladder after surgical resection of the superficial lesions. The treatment effectively reduces local relapses [62]. The precise mechanisms are not understood, although there are a large number of suggested pathways. It is still not certain that antigen-specific

T cells are essential for the beneficial effect. Certainly many effectors of the innate and adaptive immune system are stimulated by the local cytokine storm associated with the acute infection.

Bacterial products activate Toll-like receptors (TLRs) on host cells as does topical imiquimod, a TLR-7 agonist ligand that displays substantial antineoplastic activity against localized skin cancers, intraepithelial neoplasias, and carcinomas in situ [63–66]. TLRs allow cells to recognize molecular structures and patterns associated with pathogens and to mount responses to fight the infection. Certain forms of acute inflammation favor immune-mediated rejection of malignant cells. For example, the immunotherapeutic procedures are most effective during the period of acute inflammation at the site of inoculation. The diversity of TLRs and their ligands provides a wealth of possibilities for immunotherapy, particularly of locally growing cancers, incipient cancers, and premalignant conditions.

TLR signaling plays a critical role in acute as well as chronic inflammation and also can favor tumor development [67]. It seems that, a very few days after inoculation of cancer cells, induction of TLR-8 signaling can prevent the development of regulatory T cells and thereby enhance the immune response of mice. In this study, however, the TLR-8 agonist, poly-G oligonucleotides, was applied on day 3 after cancer cell inoculation, before any measurable tumor grew [68]. Thus, the significance of this finding for hosts with true and well-established tumors is questionable.

There is one important caveat for using proinflammatory agents to treat incipient cancers: certain types of inflammation, particularly chronic inflammation, can be powerful promoters of cancer development and potentially tumor progression [69–73] and can suppress T-cell responses [74–77].

Eradication of Established Solid Tumors and Their Growth-promoting Stromal Microenvironment

Established solid tumors in humans have been growing for many months and often for years. Therefore, to study the immunotherapy of well-established solid tumors, the authors suggest using tumors that are at least 14 days old and more than 1 cm in average diameter, at which point the tumor becomes virtually indistinguishable from nontransplanted primary tumors. Because most current immunotherapies become powerless in animals with these tumors, finding effective ways to eliminate these tumors immunologically represents an important challenge. The growth curves of tumors have been analyzed carefully [78,79]. Obviously, tumors have volumes and cannot be properly described by area, because thickness and depth of invasion are critical [80]. Furthermore, transplanted tumors localized within the layers of the skin usually can be retracted from the body of the mouse and be measured in length (l), width (w), and height (h) to the nearest 0.5 mm with a caliper. The tumor volume is best approximated using the formula for hemi-ellipsoids: $V = (4\pi/3)\ (l/2)\ (w/2)\ (h/2) =$ approximately lwh (1/2) [78]. Thus, tumors averaging 1 cm in diameter have volumes of about 500 mm^3.

As mentioned previously, the acute inflammatory reaction and the coagulation necrosis at the site of injection of the cancer cells has vanished about 14 days after inoculation, and the tumor has developed assumes the appearance of nontransplanted primary tumors. There is good evidence that antigenic cancers may become well established without being recognized by the host. Introduction of lymphotoxin β signaling by artificially introducing LIGHT into the established tumor can create lymphoid tissue inside the tumor and thereby improve recognition [81,82]. Nevertheless, it would be naïve to assume that the host forgets the insult of tumor transplantation and resembles immunologically in every way a host developing a true primary cancer. Thus, ideally, a primary (ie, autochthonous) tumor model should confirm any result achieved with well-established transplanted solid tumors. Recently it has been shown that proinflammatory factors can render primary tumors permissive for infiltration and destruction [83].

Tumor stroma, although serving no beneficial purpose to the host, is essential for tumor growth, and its destruction leads to ablation of the tumor without recurrence. This point was highlighted by Spiotto and colleagues [16,17], who showed that targeting cancer cells as well as the tumor stroma is critical for eradicating well-established solid tumors by adoptively transferred CD8 T cells. When only the cancer cells, but not the stromal cells, were targeted, variant cancer cells resistant to the T cells escaped and killed the host. Curative adoptive T-cell therapy was associated with antigen-specific destruction of the tumor growth–promoting stromal CD11b+ cells; thus, the Gr-1+/CD11b+ immature myeloid cells did not interfere with the adoptive transfer of activated T cells. The bone marrow–derived as well as the non–bone marrow–derived components of the stroma needed to be targeted [16,17]. Others have studied extensively CD4+/CD25+/ Foxp3+ regulatory T cells, but it is not clear whether these T cells can interfere with tumor rejection in vivo if fully activated tumor-specific T cells are transferred. Certainly, much better evidence for the significance of suppressor/regulatory T cells in influencing the therapy of well-established cancers in mice and patients is needed. There is some suggestion, however, that anti-interleukin 10, anti-transforming growth factor-β1, or anti-CD4 antibodies injected into established solid tumors may counteract an immunosuppressive environment, unmask the immunogenicity, and assist tumor-specific T cells to reject well-established tumors [84].

Well-established solid tumors have been treated using adoptively transferred T cells, which, in contrast to the model described previously, were not directed against tumor-specific antigens but rather against a non–mutant differentiation antigen [85–88]. The tumor-bearing host needed additional treatment, such as repeated very high doses of interleukin 2. Usually, the cancer recurred after a temporary but potent anti-tumor effect, and it is tempting to speculate that a failure of the T cells to target the stroma cells also prevented cure. Differentiation and other self-antigens may bind poorly to the presenting MHC class I molecule [31] and therefore not sensitize stromal cells effectively even if the antigen is expressed at high levels in the cancer cells.

Eradication of Microdisseminated or Dormant Cancer Cells

One of the most important applications of cancer immunotherapy could be the elimination of microdisseminated cancer cells that often remain after removal of the primary tumor. In animals, curative therapies are effective before cancers are established as solid tumors. The question is whether active immunization can cause rejection of the residual cancer cells or whether adoptive or passive immunotherapy might be more effective. Published evidence indicates that tumor-specific active immunization is problematic. For example, it has been reported that immune suppression may be reversed after surgical removal of the transplanted "primary" tumor even though metastatic disease was present. There is no evidence, however, that these mice could mount responses to the rejection antigens on the residual metastatic cells [89]. In other circumstances, surgical tumor removal did not result in tumor-specific immunity, but immune suppression persisted [90] because micro-disseminated cancer cells persisted (R. North, personal communication, 1985). There is no question that complete tumor removal releases the generalized immune suppression and allows the host to reject re-challenge with the cancer cells from the tumor that had been removed [91,92]. These findings agree with a much earlier study by Klein and colleagues [7], who showed that it is possible to induce immunity in the autologous host against its own cancer. In this study, the host first had to be freed of its primary cancer cells completely before being vaccinated with irradiated cancer cell suspensions followed by re-challenge. Such a completely tumor-free interval is hardly a clinically realistic situation. Thus, it remains to be determined whether incomplete removal suffices to release the host from unresponsiveness caused by the disseminated antigen. Furthermore, it is not known how quickly after implantation cancer cells may become resistant to active immunotherapy. For example, some experimental cancer cell implants may remain visually undetectable for weeks before they grow out (for examples, see [93,94]). Nevertheless, these cancer cell deposits became resistant to active immunization weeks before becoming visible [93].

For patients who have micrometastatic disease, a major and important alternative to active immunization is treatment with antibodies that may lead to the destruction of the metastatic cells. One early approach that showed promise has been the passive antibody transfer using the epithelial cell adhesion molecule (EpCAM)-specific antibody 17-1A. This antibody seemed to prevent relapse caused by metastatic disease in a significant group of randomized patients and increased overall survival in a 7-year analysis [95,96]. This antibody had no effect on preventing local recurrences at the site of surgical tumor resection, however. This antibody had been shown to eliminate antigen-positive cancer cells in nude mice when given briefly after tumor cell inoculation [97]. The early concept that the adjuvant therapy setting may be the real domain of immunotherapy with antibodies was recently confirmed by a large trial in patients who had early-stage breast cancer. After adjuvant chemotherapy these patients, when treated with an anti-HER2 antibody for 12 months, experienced significantly fewer relapses than patients in the control group who received chemotherapy only [98,99]. Certainly, these important studies were stimulated by much earlier animal studies convincingly showing the therapeutic potential of anti-HER2-neu antibodies [38–40]. Great efforts are being made to produce new antibody-based reagents with clear-cut activity in preventing relapse of metastatic disease.

One of the major problems is the persistent lack of appropriate animal models for studying the effects of active or passive immunization on dormant micro-disseminated cancer cells. In humans, relapse from dormant cancer cells occurs many months to years after surgical tumor removal, and investigators are only beginning to understand the complexity of these dormant cells, some of which may become the source of the relapse [100–102]. In particular, more information is needed on how they relate genetically and biologically in stage and lineage to the cancer that had been removed surgically.

Immunoprevention of Cancer Development

Preventing infection with cancer-causing viruses by active immunization will, of course, be effective in preventing the cancer caused by that specific virus. For example, immunization against human papilloma virus (HPV) 16 or 18, the strains most commonly causing cervical cancer, may prevent the development of cancer caused by these strains of HPV. The immune system also prevents the development of cancer after infection with Epstein-Barr virus (EBV). Although most humans are latently infected with EBV, the immune system seems to eliminate any cells transformed by this virus because transformation results in expression of strong EBV-encoded rejection antigens. Only immunosuppressed patients (eg, transplant patients) develop B-cell malignancies expressing the full set of EBV rejection antigens. It is conceivable, therefore, that the earliest stage of the carcinogenic process may be treated effectively by active immunization when the relevant antigen on the initiated cells is known. In analogy to rabies infection, active immunization during the latency phase can prevent or at least greatly reduce later development of malignant growth. Several models have given similar results: neonatal infection of hamsters with SV40 causes the development of primary tumors many months later [103–105]. Immunization more than 3 months before the latency period ended gave the animals 100% protection, but there was no protection when immunization was delayed until 2 weeks before termination of the minimal latent period. Similarly, primary tumors in mice caused by sporadic activation of a dormant SV40 T oncogene are prevented if the animals are immunized before tumor development [106].

In several other primary tumor models there is a tissue-specific transgenic expression of an oncogene. Although cancers in these models may mimic closely the stages of development of certain cancers (eg, breast or prostate) in humans [107–109], the time of appearance of oncogene expression rarely simulates that of natural oncogene expression. For example, xenogeneic Her2/neu expressed under control of the murine mammary tumor virus (MMTV) promoter differs significantly in time of appearance and types of tissues expressed from that of self-Her-2 to which the host is tolerant. Furthermore, the broad tissue-wide expression of the oncogenes differs significantly from the pathogenesis of most human cancers that are caused by somatic mutations and result in sporadic, clonal initiation affecting relatively few cells. These problems reduce the likelihood that active immunization will have beneficial effects and counteract cancer development in humans. In any case, the major effects of active immunization in the current transgenic tumor models typically are restricted to the interval before the oncogene is expressed and only delay but do not prevent tumor development. The host does not ignore a sudden, widespread, or continually increasing expression on the initiating transgenic oncogene. The result may be CD4+ T-cell–dependent antibody production [72,110] and peripheral tolerance of CD8+ T cells. This response impedes effective protective immunization and may enhance tumor promotion. Such promoting immune responses may be prominent in cancers induced by hepatitis B or C virus and in cancers associated with *Helicobacter pylori* infection, inflammatory bowel disease, and other inflammatory conditions. For example, although immunization to prevent HPV infection may well prevent cancer [111], once the oncogene has inserted in the target cells or the carcinogen has caused the initiating mutation, immune responses by the host to the incipient cancer may promote cancer development [72]. A particularly interesting human model is monoclonal gammopathy, a precancerous condition associated with a significantly increased risk of contracting multiple myeloma [112,113]. In mice, there is clear evidence that inflammatory responses by the host promote the development of plasmacytoma [114], but this tumor model does not really simulate human myeloma. It therefore is unclear whether active vaccination of patients who have monoclonal gammopathy would promote or prevent cancer. There is overwhelming evidence that chronic inflammation can promote cancer development, and researchers must make certain that attempts to vaccinate against the developing malignant cell do not promote cancer development [110].

In principle, adoptive/passive immunotherapy could be used to eliminate premalignant or initiated cells from which cancer arises, for example the B-cell clone which causes the monoclonal gammopathy and from which myeloma may eventually develop. Similarly, eliminating initiated, mutant ras-expressing epithelial cells in the pancreas would reduce later development of pancreatic cancer, presently a virtually incurable disease. Cellular or antibody-based reagents eliminating premalignant cells with such selectivity are not yet available.

SUMMARY

Experiments using tumor transplantation have laid major foundations for immunology and cancer immunotherapy. Much evidence indicates that unique truly tumor-specific antigens are the most effective tumor-rejection antigens, and these antigens clearly occur on human tumors. Autologous tumor cell vaccination or autologous T-cell transfer allows T-cell responses to these antigens and opens the way to individualized cancer immunotherapy. Other promising targets are growth factors, growth factor receptors over-expressed on cancer cells, other self-antigens for which expression is restricted to normal cells or tissues whose immune destruction can be tolerated, or growth factors or their receptors targeted by antibodies.

Animal experiments properly interpreted often predict the stumbling blocks encountered when comparable approaches are translated to clinical treatment. A persistent problem in experimental models, however, is overinterpreting the success of eradication during the first few days after tumor inoculation, Histopathologic examination reveals massive acute inflammation at the site of implantation. Two weeks later, this transplantation artifact vanishes when the cancers are virtually indistinguishable from primary tumors of man or mouse. Using transplanted tumors at this time may be more clinically relevant for developing immunotherapy of established solid tumors. Curative treatment of these tumors in animals may well depend on immune destruction of the tumor stroma to avoid tumor escape.

Animal experiments have stimulated the development of extremely important novel approaches to human cancer therapy that use antibodies to eliminate dormant cancer cells remaining in the host after surgical excision of the primary tumor. There is a need to develop tumor dormancy models for further studies. Similarly, investigators seek to learn how to prevent cancer development by eliminating premalignant cells immunologically. To do so, they need models of sporadic and focal tumor induction, avoiding tissue-wide expression of oncogenes and multifocal cancer development.

Active antigen-specific immunization can be preventive by preempting infection with oncogenic viruses. More convincing evidence is needed that active immunization can be therapeutic and eliminate truly established cancers, dormant microdisseminated cancer cells, or premalignant lesions or help the induction and expansion in vitro of tumor-specific T cells for adoptive transfer. Despite all the hurdles mentioned, major accomplishments have been made, and further major success in cancer immunotherapy is only a question of time. It is highly likely that most, if not all, human cancer express truly tumor-specific antigens and other important immunologic targets. Antibody- and T-cell–based therapy can have enormous, specific, destructive or growth-inhibitory power.

Acknowledgments

The authors thank Dr. Thomas N. Krausz for helping with the examination of the histologic specimens.

References

[1] Gorer PA. Some recent work on tumor immunity. Adv Cancer Res 1956;4:149–86.

[2] Ehrlich P. Experimentelle Carcinomstudien an Mäusen. Arbeiten aus dem Königlichen Institut für Experimentelle Therapy zu Frankfurt a.M 1906;1:76–102.

[3] Gross L. Intradermal immunization of C3H mice against a sarcoma that originated in an animal of the same line. Cancer Res 1943;3:326–33.

[4] Foley EJ. Antigenic properties of methylcholanthrene-induced tumors in mice of the strain of origin. Cancer Res 1953;13:835–7.

[5] Baldwin RW. Immunity to methylcholanthrene-induced tumors-inbred rats following atrophy and regression of implanted tumors. Br J Cancer 1955;9:652–65.

[6] Prehn RT, Main JM. Immunity to methylcholanthrene-induced sarcomas. J Natl Cancer Inst 1957;18:769–78.

[7] Klein G, Sögren HO, Klein E, et al. Demonstration of resistance against methylcholanthrene-induced sarcomas in the primary autochthonous host. Cancer Res 1960;20:1561–72.

[8] Monach PA, Meredith SC, Siegel CT, et al. A unique tumor antigen produced by a single amino acid substitution. Immunity 1995;2:45–59.

[9] Coulie PG, Lehmann F, Lethe B, et al. A mutated intron sequence codes for an antigenic peptide recognized by cytolytic T lymphocytes on a human melanoma. Proc Natl Acad Sci U S A 1995;92:7976–80.

[10] Wölfel T, Hauer M, Schneider J, et al. A p16INK4a-insensitive CDK4 mutant targeted by cytolytic T lymphocytes in a human melanoma. Science 1995;269:1281–4.

[11] Zuo L, Weger J, Yang Q, et al. Germline mutations in the p16INK4a binding domain of CDK4 in familial melanoma. Nat Genet 1996;12:97–9.

[12] Robbins PF, El-Gamil M, Li YF, et al. A mutated beta-catenin gene encodes a melanoma-specific antigen recognized by tumor infiltrating lymphocytes. J Exp Med 1996;183:1185–92.

[13] Dubey P, Hendrickson RC, Meredith SC, et al. The immunodominant antigen of an ultraviolet-induced regressor tumor is generated by a somatic point mutation in the DEAD box helicase p68. J Exp Med 1997;185:695–705.

[14] Beck-Engeser GB, Monach PA, Mumberg D, et al. Point mutation in essential genes with loss or mutation of the second allele: relevance to the retention of tumor-specific antigens. J Exp Med 2001;194:285–300.

[15] Karanikas V, Colau D, Baurain JF, et al. High frequency of cytolytic T lymphocytes directed against a tumor-specific mutated antigen detectable with HLA tetramers in the blood of a lung carcinoma patient with long survival. Cancer Res 2001;61(9):3718–24.

[16] Spiotto MT, Rowley DA, Schreiber H. Bystander elimination of antigen loss variants in established tumors. Nat Med 2004;10(3):294–8.

[17] Spiotto MT, Schreiber H. Rapid destruction of the tumor microenvironment by CTLs recognizing cancer-specific antigens cross-presented by stromal cells. Cancer Immun 2005;5:8.

[18] Schreiber H. Tumor immunology. In: Paul W, editor. Fundamental immunology. 5th edition. Philadelphia: Lippincott Williams & Wilkins; 2003. p. 1557–92.

[19] Lennerz V, Fatho M, Gentilini C, et al. The response of T cells to a human melanoma is dominated by mutated neoantigens. Proc Natl Acad Sci U S A 2005;102(44):16013–8.

[20] O'Rourke MG, Johnson M, Lanagan C, et al. Durable complete clinical responses in a phase I/II trial using an autologous melanoma cell/dendritic cell vaccine. Cancer Immunol Immunother 2003;52(6):387–95.

[21] Schirrmacher V. Clinical trials of antitumor vaccination with an autologous tumor cell vaccine modified by virus infection: improvement of patient survival based on improved antitumor immune memory. Cancer Immunol Immunother 2005;54(6):587–98.

[22] Dudley ME, Wunderlich JR, Robbins PF, et al. Cancer regression and autoimmunity in patients after clonal repopulation with antitumor lymphocytes. Science 2002;298(5594):850–4.

[23] Dudley ME, Wunderlich JR, Yang JC, et al. Adoptive cell transfer therapy following non-myeloablative but lymphodepleting chemotherapy for the treatment of patients with refractory metastatic melanoma. J Clin Oncol 2005;23(10):2346–57.

[24] Weinshilboum R, Wang L. Pharmacogenomics: bench to bedside. Nat Rev Drug Discov 2004;3(9):739–48.

[25] Oettgen HF, Rettig WJ, Lloyd KO, et al. Serologic analysis of human cancer. Immunol Allergy Clin North Am 1990;10(4):607–37.

[26] Ludewig B, Krebs P, Metters H, et al. Molecular characterization of virus-induced auto-antibody responses. J Exp Med 2004;200(5):637–46.

[27] Preiss S, Kammertoens T, Lampert C, et al. Tumor-induced antibodies resemble the response to tissue damage. Int J Cancer 2005;115(3):456–62.

[28] Ludewig B, Ochsenbein AF, Odermatt B, et al. Immunotherapy with dendritic cells directed against tumor antigens shared with normal host cells results in severe autoimmune disease. J Exp Med 2000;191(5):795–804.
[29] Gotter J, Brors B, Hergenhahn M, et al. Medullary epithelial cells of the human thymus express a highly diverse selection of tissue-specific genes colocalized in chromosomal clusters. J Exp Med 2004;199(2):155–66.
[30] Coulie PG. Cancer immunotherapy with MAGE antigens. Suppl Tumori 2002;1(4): S63–5.
[31] Yu Z, Theoret MR, Touloukian CE, et al. Poor immunogenicity of a self/tumor antigen derives from peptide-MHC-I instability and is independent of tolerance. J Clin Invest 2004;114(4):551–9.
[32] Timmerman JM, Czerwinski DK, Davis TA, et al. Idiotype-pulsed dendritic cell vaccination for B-cell lymphoma: clinical and immune responses in 35 patients. Blood 2002; 99(5):1517–26.
[33] Rosenberg SA, Yang JC, Restifo NP. Cancer immunotherapy: moving beyond current vaccines. Nat Med 2004;10(9):909–15.
[34] Morris EC, Bendle GM, Stauss HJ. Prospects for immunotherapy of malignant disease. Clin Exp Immunol 2003;131(1):1–7.
[35] Chlewicki LK, Holler PD, Monti BC, et al. High-affinity, peptide-specific T cell receptors can be generated by mutations in CDR1, CDR2 or CDR3. J Mol Biol 2005;346(1):223–39.
[36] Kuball J, Schmitz FW, Voss RH, et al. Cooperation of human tumor-reactive CD4 + and CD8 + T cells after redirection of their specificity by a high-affinity p53A2.1-specific TCR. Immunity 2005;22(1):117–29.
[37] Clynes RA, Towers TL, Presta LG, et al. Inhibitory Fc receptors modulate in vivo cytotoxicity against tumor targets. Nat Med 2000;6(4):443–6.
[38] Drebin JA, Link VC, Stern DF, et al. Down-modulation of an oncogene protein product and reversion of the transformed phenotype by monoclonal antibodies. Cell 1985;41(3): 697–706.
[39] Drebin JA, Link VC, Weinberg RA, et al. Inhibition of tumor growth by a monoclonal antibody reactive with an oncogene-encoded tumor antigen. Proc Natl Acad Sci U S A 1986;83(23):9129–33.
[40] Kim KJ, Li B, Winer J, et al. Inhibition of vascular endothelial growth factor-induced angiogenesis suppresses tumor growth in vivo. Nature 1993;362:841–4.
[41] Maloney DG. Immunotherapy for non-Hodgkin's lymphoma: monoclonal antibodies and vaccines. J Clin Oncol 2005;23(26):6421–8.
[42] Woglom WH. Immunity to transplantable tumors. Cancer Rev 1929;4:129–214.
[43] Mueller MM, Fusenig NE. Friends or foes—bipolar effects of the tumour stroma in cancer. Nat Rev Cancer 2004;4(11):839–49.
[44] Bhowmick NA, Moses HL. Tumor-stroma interactions. Curr Opin Genet Dev 2005;15(1): 97–101.
[45] Pekarek LA, Starr BA, Toledano AY, et al. Inhibition of tumor growth by elimination of granulocytes. J Exp Med 1995;181:435–40.
[46] Bronte V, Wang M, Overwijk WW, et al. Apoptotic death of CD8 + T lymphocytes after immunization: induction of a suppressive population of Mac-1 + /Gr-1 + cells. J Immunol 1998;161:5313–20.
[47] Yang L, DeBusk LM, Fukuda K, et al. Expansion of myeloid immune suppressor Gr + CD11b + cells in tumor-bearing host directly promotes tumor angiogenesis. Cancer Cell 2004;6(4):409–21.
[48] Seung LP, Seung SK, Schreiber H. Antigenic cancer cells that escape immune destruction are stimulated by host cells. Cancer Res 1995;55:5094–100.
[49] Li Q, Pan PY, Gu P, et al. Role of immature myeloid Gr-1 + cells in the development of antitumor immunity. Cancer Res 2004;64(3):1130–9.
[50] Kusmartsev S, Gabrilovich DI. Role of immature myeloid cells in mechanisms of immune evasion in cancer. Cancer Immunol Immunother 2006;55(3):237–45.

[51] Serafini P, Borello I, Bronte V. Myeloid suppressor cells in cancer: recruitment, phenotype, properties, and mechanisms of suppression. Semin Cancer Biol 2006;16:53–65.

[52] Kusmartsev S, Gabrilovich DI. STAT1 signaling regulates tumor-associated macrophage-mediated T cell deletion. J Immunol 2005;174(8):4880–91.

[53] Seung LP, Rowley DA, Dubey P, et al. Synergy between T-cell immunity and inhibition of paracrine stimulation causes tumor rejection. Proc Natl Acad Sci U S A 1995;92: 6254–8.

[54] Conlan JW, North RJ. Neutrophils are essential for early anti-Listeria defense in the liver, but not in the spleen or peritoneal cavity, as revealed by a granulocyte-depleting mono-clonal antibody. J Exp Med 1994;179:259–68.

[55] Singh S, Ross SR, Acena M, et al. Stroma is critical for preventing or permitting immu-nological destruction of antigenic cancer cells. J Exp Med 1992;175:139–46.

[56] Ochsenbein AF, Klenerman P, Karrer U, et al. Immune surveillance against a solid tumor fails because of immunological ignorance. Proc Natl Acad Sci U S A 1999;96: 2233–8.

[57] Ochsenbein AF, Sierro S, Odermatt B, et al. Roles of tumour localization, second signals and cross priming in cytotoxic T-cell induction. Nature 2001;411:1058–64.

[58] Spiotto MT, Yu P, Rowley DA, et al. Increasing tumor antigen expression overcomes "ignorance" to solid tumors via crosspresentation by bone marrow-derived stromal cells. Immunity 2002;17(6):737–47.

[59] Fehleisen F. Über die Züchtung der Erysipel-Kokken auf künstlichen Nährböden und die Übertragbarkeit auf den Menschen. Deutsche Med Wochenschr 1882;8:553–4.

[60] Bruns P. Die Heilwirkung des Erysipels auf Geschwülste. Beitr Klin Chir 1887–1888;3: 443–66.

[61] Coley WB. The treatment of malignant tumors by repeated inoculations of erysipelas: with a report of ten original cases. Am J Med Sci 1893;105:487–511.

[62] Morales A, Eidinger D, Bruce AW. Intracavitary Bacillus Calmette-Guerin in the treat-ment of superficial bladder tumors. J Urol 1976;116:180–3.

[63] Villa AM, Berman B. Immunomodulators for skin cancer. J Drugs Dermatol 2004;3(5): 533–9.

[64] Ray CM, Kluk M, Grin CM, et al. Successful treatment of malignant melanoma in situ with topical 5% imiquimod cream. Int J Dermatol 2005;44(5):428–34.

[65] Vender RB, Goldberg O. Innovative uses of imiquimod. J Drugs Dermatol 2005;4(1): 58–63.

[66] Hengge UR, Roth S, Tannapfel A. Topical imiquimod to treat recurrent breast cancer. Breast Cancer Res Treat 2005;94(1):93–4.

[67] Tsan MF. Toll-like receptors, inflammation and cancer. Semin Cancer Biol 2006;16:32–7.

[68] Peng G, Guo Z, Kiniwa Y, et al. Toll-like receptor 8-mediated reversal of CD4 + regulatory T cell function. Science 2005;309(5739):1380–4.

[69] Schreiber H, Rowley DA. Inflammation and cancer. In: Gallin JI, Snyderman R, editors. Inflammation: basic principles and clinical correlates. 3rd edition. Philadelphia: Lippincott Williams & Wilkins; 1999. p. 1117–29.

[70] Philip M, Rowley DA, Schreiber H. Inflammation as a tumor promoter in cancer induction. Semin Cancer Biol 2004;14(6):433–9.

[71] Karin M, Greten FR. NF-kappaB: linking inflammation and immunity to cancer devel-opment and progression. Nat Rev Immunol 2005;5(10):749–59.

[72] de Visser KE, Korets LV, Coussens LM. De novo carcinogenesis promoted by chronic inflammation is B lymphocyte dependent. Cancer Cell 2005;7(5):411–23.

[73] de Visser KE, Eichten A, Coussens LM. Paradoxical roles of the immune system during cancer development. Nat Rev Cancer 2006;6(1):24–37.

[74] Baniyash M. The inflammation-cancer linkage: a double-edged sword? Semin Cancer Biol 2006;(Jan):14.

[75] Baniyash M. TCR zeta-chain downregulation: curtailing an excessive inflammatory im-mune response. Nat Rev Immunol 2004;4(9):675–87.

[76] Baniyash M. Chronic inflammation, immunosuppression and cancer: new insights and outlook. Semin Cancer Biol 2006;16:80–8.

[77] Rodriguez PC, Ochoa AC. T cell dysfunction in cancer: role of myeloid cells and tumor cells regulating amino acid availability and oxidative stress. Semin Cancer Biol 2006; 16:66–72.

[78] Dethlefsen LA, Prewitt JM, Mendelsohn ML. Analysis of tumor growth curves. J Natl Cancer Inst 1968;40(2):389–405.

[79] Rockwell SC, Kallman RF, Fajardo LF. Characteristics of a serially transplanted mouse mammary tumor and its tissue-culture-adapted derivative. J Natl Cancer Inst 1972;49(3): 735–49.

[80] Breslow A. Thickness, cross-sectional areas and depth of invasion in the prognosis of cutaneous melanoma. Ann Surg 1970;172(5):902–8.

[81] Yu P, Lee Y, Liu W, et al. Priming of naive T cells inside tumors leads to eradication of established tumors. Nat Immunol 2004;5(2):141–9.

[82] Houghton AN. LIGHTing the way for tumor immunity. Nat Immunol 2004;5(2):123–4.

[83] Garbi N, Arnold B, Gordon S, et al. CpG motifs as proinflammatory factors render autochthonous tumors permissive for infiltration and destruction. J Immunol 2004;172(10): 5861–9.

[84] Yu P, Lee Y, Liu W, et al. Intra-tumor depletion of CD4 + cells unmasks tumor immunogenicity leading to the rejection of late-stage tumors. J Exp Med 2005;201(5): 779–91.

[85] Antony PA, Piccirillo CA, Akpinarli A, et al. CD8 + T cell immunity against a tumor/self-antigen is augmented by CD4 + T helper cells and hindered by naturally occurring T regulatory cells. J Immunol 2005;174(5):2591–601.

[86] Gattinoni L, Finkelstein SE, Klebanoff CA, et al. Removal of homeostatic cytokine sinks by lymphodepletion enhances the efficacy of adoptively transferred tumor-specific CD8 + T cells. J Exp Med 2005;202(7):907–12.

[87] Gattinoni L, Klebanoff CA, Palmer DC, et al. Acquisition of full effector function in vitro paradoxically impairs the in vivo antitumor efficacy of adoptively transferred CD8 + T cells. J Clin Invest 2005;115(6):1616–26.

[88] Klebanoff CA, Gattinoni L, Torabi-Parizi P, et al. Central memory self/tumor-reactive CD8 + T cells confer superior antitumor immunity compared with effector memory T cells. Proc Natl Acad Sci U S A 2005;102(27):9571–6.

[89] Danna EA, Sinha P, Gilbert M, et al. Surgical removal of primary tumor reverses tumor-induced immunosuppression despite the presence of metastatic disease. Cancer Res 2004;64(6):2205–11.

[90] Bursuker I, North RJ. Generation and decay of the immune response to a progressive fibrosarcoma. II. Failure to demonstrate postexcision immunity after the onset of T cell-mediated suppression of immunity. J Exp Med 1984;159(5):1312–21.

[91] Mullen CA, Rowley DA, Schreiber H. Highly immunogenic regressor tumor cells can prevent development of postsurgical tumor immunity. Cell Immunol 1989;119:101–13.

[92] Salvadori S, Martinelli G, Zier K. Resection of solid tumors reverses T cell defects and restores protective immunity. J Immunol 2000;164(4):2214–20.

[93] Golumbek PT, Lazenby AJ, Levitsky HI, et al. Treatment of established renal cancer by tumor cells engineered to secrete interleukin-4. Science 1991;254:713–6.

[94] van Mierlo GJ, den Boer AT, Medema JP, et al. CD40 stimulation leads to effective therapy of CD40(-) tumors through induction of strong systemic cytotoxic T lymphocyte immunity. Proc Natl Acad Sci U S A 2002;99:5561–6.

[95] Riethmüller G, Schneider-Gadicke E, Schlimok G, et al. Randomised trial of monoclonal antibody for adjuvant therapy of resected Dukes' C colorectal carcinoma. German Cancer Aid 17–1A Study Group. Lancet 1994;343:1177–83.

[96] Riethmuller G, Holz E, Schlimok G, et al. Monoclonal antibody therapy for resected Dukes' C colorectal cancer: seven-year outcome of a multicenter randomized trial. J Clin Oncol 1998;16:1788–94.

[97] Herlyn DM, Steplewski Z, Herlyn MF, et al. Inhibition of growth of colorectal carcinoma in nude mice by monoclonal antibody. Cancer Res 1980;40:717–21.

[98] Piccart-Gebhart MJ, Procter M, Leyland-Jones B, et al. Trastuzumab after adjuvant chemotherapy in HER2-positive breast cancer. N Engl J Med 2005;353(16):1659–72.

[99] Romond EH, Perez EA, Bryant J, et al. Trastuzumab plus adjuvant chemotherapy for operable HER2-positive breast cancer. N Engl J Med 2005;353(16):1673–84.

[100] Riethmuller G, Klein CA. Early cancer cell dissemination and late metastatic relapse: clinical reflections and biological approaches to the dormancy problem in patients. Semin Cancer Biol 2001;11:307–11.

[101] Klein CA, Blankenstein TJ, Schmidt-Kittler O, et al. Genetic heterogeneity of single disseminated tumour cells in minimal residual cancer. Lancet 2002;360(9334):683–9.

[102] Schmidt-Kittler O, Ragg T, Daskalakis A, et al. From latent disseminated cells to overt metastasis: genetic analysis of systemic breast cancer progression. Proc Natl Acad Sci U S A 2003;100(13):7737–42.

[103] Deichman GI, Kluchareva TE. Prevention of tumour induction in Sv 40-infected hamsters. Nature 1964;202:1126–8.

[104] Deichman GI, Kluchareva TE. Immunological determinants of oncogenesis in hamsters infected with Sv40 virus. Virology 1964;24:131–7.

[105] Deichman GI. Immunological aspects of carcinogenesis by deoxyribonucleic acid tumor viruses. Adv Cancer Res 1969;12:101–36.

[106] Willimsky G, Blankenstein T. Sporadic immunogenic tumours avoid destruction by inducing T-cell tolerance. Nature 2005;437(7055):141–6.

[107] Boggio K, Nicoletti G, Di Carlo E, et al. Interleukin 12-mediated prevention of spontaneous mammary adenocarcinomas in two lines of Her-2/neu transgenic mice. J Exp Med 1998;188:589–96.

[108] Guy CT, Webster MA, Schaller M, et al. Expression of the neu protooncogene in the mammary epithelium of transgenic mice induces metastatic disease. Proc Natl Acad Sci U S A 1992;89(22):10578–82.

[109] Greenberg NM, DeMayo F, Finegold MJ, et al. Prostate cancer in a transgenic mouse. Proc Natl Acad Sci U S A 1995;92(8):3439–43.

[110] Siegel CT, Schreiber K, Meredith SC, et al. Enhanced growth of primary tumors in cancer-prone mice after immunization against the mutation region of an inherited oncoprotein. J Exp Med 2000;191:1945–56.

[111] Lowndes CM. Vaccines for cervical cancer. Epidemiol Infect 2006;134(1):1–12.

[112] Dhodapkar MV, Krasovsky J, Osman K, et al. Vigorous premalignancy-specific effector T cell response in the bone marrow of patients with monoclonal gammopathy. J Exp Med 2003;198(11):1753–7.

[113] Dhodapkar MV. Harnessing host immune responses to preneoplasia: promise and challenges. Cancer Immunol Immunother 2005;54(5):409–13.

[114] Potter M. Neoplastic development in plasma cells. Immunol Rev 2003;194:177–95.

Hematol Oncol Clin N Am 20 (2006) 585–612

HEMATOLOGY/ONCOLOGY CLINICS
OF NORTH AMERICA

Antitumor Antibodies in the Treatment of Cancer: Fc Receptors Link Opsonic Antibody with Cellular Immunity

Raphael Clynes, MD, PhD

Departments of Medicine and Microbiology, Columbia University, College of Physicians and Surgeons, 630 West 168th Street, New York, NY 10032, USA

T his is an appropriate time to recognize the biologic importance of antibodies as opsonins. In 2 years, we will reach the 100th anniversary of the 1908 Nobel Prize in Medicine, which was shared by Paul Ehrlich and Ilya Metchnikov, in "recognition of their work on immunity" specifically, their respective studies on antibodies and phagocytosis, which demonstrated the physiologic importance of the cellular response to antibody opsonized targets [1]. Ehrlich developed the conceptual framework of "antibodies"; he envisioned them as substances that are released by immune cells which recognize microbial constituents in a lock and key fashion, and provide them with "magic bullet" capacities. His ground-breaking studies of antibodies against diphtheria toxin culminated in a clinical trial of passive immunotherapy (transfer of immune sera) that revolutionized the treatment of childhood diphtheria at the turn of the nineteenth century. Serotherapy, the transfer of immune sera containing polyclonal microbial-specific antibodies into patients, was used in the preantibiotic era for common infectious diseases (eg, pneumococcal pneumonia). Transferred sera were xenogeneic, and were derived from horses and other nonhuman species. These therapies were beset with complications, including serum sickness, that resulted from the generation of a host humoral antibody response to the highly immunogenic immunoglobulins. Decades later these same xenogeneic immune responses also undermined the clinical usefulness of early clinical antitumor antibodies using mouse immunoglobulins.

Ehrlich believed, based on in vitro observations with bacteria and serum components, that antibody eradicated microbes through the activation of other humoral microcidal substances, which he termed complement. But Ehrlich came to recognize the validity of Metchnikov's observations that the cytolytic capacity of antibodies was not due to serum components, but rather was mediated by phagocytic cells upon recognition of the antibody-opsonized targets. Or as Metchnikov stated, "the microbes, impregnated with [antibodies] and

E-mail address: rc645@columbia.edu

0889-8588/06/$ – see front matter
doi:10.1016/j.hoc.2006.02.010

the complement, fall an easy prey to the white corpuscles. The mixture of the two substances serves most of all to prepare the phagocytosis" [1]. Thus, the shared Nobel Prize of 1908 recognizes the importance in host immunity of the capacities of antibodies to provide protection to microbial pathogens through the induction of the cellular response.

This article discusses recent work suggesting that antibody therapeutics in cancer achieve tumor cell killing through engagement of the cellular Fcγ receptors (FγRs), the cellular receptors linking IgG-opsonins with immune effector cell ativation, as Metchikov proposed. Recent engineering efforts aimed at optimization of this link, have generated novel antibodies with improved binding characteristics for the Fc receptors for IgG (FcγR), which offer the hope that enhanced antibody-triggered effector responses may prove achievable.

THE EMERGENCE OF ANTIBODIES AS A THERAPEUTIC IN CANCER

The era of antibody therapy in cancer was ushered in with the advent of monoclonal hybridoma technology that was developed by Kohler and Milstein in 1975 [2]. With this technology, immortalized antibody-producing cells (B-cell hybridomas) that are derived from an immunized mouse can be selected for production of monoclonal antibodies that demonstrate high affinity and specific binding to target. Hybridoma technology using murine B cells continues to be a common method in the development of tumor-specific antibodies, because immortalization of human B cells that produce antibodies with defined antigen specificities has remained technically elusive.

The therapeutic potential of monoclonal antibodies raised against tumor antigens was realized quickly in rodent models and was the subject of clinical investigation in melanoma [3] and lymphoma as early as 1981 [4,5]. These clinical trials showed promising activity and transient responses; however, subsequent years of study failed to show durable clinical benefit. There were some notable exceptions, including patients who had B-cell lymphoma who were treated with anti-idiotype antibodies, some of whom remain alive today (Ron Levy, MD, personal communication, 2005). Nevertheless, the overall early record of antitumor antibodies was poor in solid tumors, and provoked the widely held view that IgG-mediated cellular effector responses were incapable of mediating meaningful tumor shrinkages. The clinical development of the first two antitumor antibodies that were approved by the U.S. Food and Drug Administration (FDA), Herceptin and Rituxan, was instead inspired by their potential ability to use other mechanistic pathways to limit tumor growth, specifically by inducing cellular apoptosis or growth arrest. Thus, recognition of critical growth regulatory membrane proteins, rather than induction of protective immune responses, was believed to be a requisite of effective antibody therapy.

However, recent data suggests that the potential mechanistic contributions of the immune effector response may prove to be highly relevant, because antibodies that lack the capacity to inhibit cell line growth in vitro [6] can induce meaningful clinical responses. Further, for Rituxan, there is ample evidence in mouse models and in the human that argue for important FcγR-mediated immune contributions. The more recent success of antibody therapeutics likely relates not merely to a poor choice of antigenic targets in earlier clinical work, but rather to the intrinsic immunogenicity of these early monoclonal antibodies, which were derived exclusively from mouse B-cell hybridomas. These highly immunogenic proteins induced human antimouse antibody responses (HAMA), which form immune complexes with the tumor antibodies that are cleared rapidly from the blood. Thus, unfavorable pharmacokinetics were manifested during repetitive administrations, which decreased the serologic half-life from 2 to 3 weeks to minutes. These obstacles were overcome by engineering the more recent clinically successful antibodies on a human IgG1 backbone.

Further development of mouse-derived antibodies has continued, however, by exploiting the general capacity of antibodies as targeting agents of "immunoconjugates" to deliver attached toxic payloads, including radioisotopes or chemical toxins. The two radioimmunoconjugates that are approved by the FDA, the CD20-specific Bexxar and Zevalin, are murine IgG1 antibodies that are conjugated to I^{131} and Y^{90}, respectively. These approaches are favored theoretically by efficient tumor site targeting combined with rapid serologic clearance, which would maximize tumor targeted killing while minimizing systemic toxicity [7]. Engineered antibodies with altered Fc domains with reduced affinities for the neonatal Fc receptor for IgG (FcRn) [8], the endothelial receptor that is responsible for maintaining antibody homeostasis, may be a useful future platform for immunoconjugates. The requirement of naked antibodies for repetitive dosing necessitated reduced immunogenicity, which has been accomplished by genetic engineering approaches that prompted the renaissance of antitumor antibodies in cancer.

ANTIBODY STRUCTURE AND FUNCTION

Targeting of protective antibodies is achieved by the remarkable specificity that is provided by the antigen-binding pocket, which is formed by the hypervariable domains of the immunoglobulin heavy and light chains contained within the Fab domains (fragment antibody-binding). The immunoglobulin heavy and light chain genes are each generated during B-cell differentiation by recombination of variable (V), diversity, and junctional gene segments. The diversity of the antibody repertoire is a consequence of the combinatorial effects of these gene rearrangements that occur during B-cell development, their precise nucleotide junctional sites, and the subsequent somatic mutational process that is triggered during the antigen-dependent germinal center response. These junctional sites and hypervariable portions of the V_H and V_L regions of the heavy and light chains regions provide the complementarity determining regions (CDRs 1–3), which together form the interacting sites with antigen, and provide a unique structural configuration for the antigen-binding region of each antibody. The protective capacity of the antigen-binding Fab region is limited to neutralization functions, cellular receptor engagement, or blockade. The capacity of antibodies to elicit a protective immune response is mediated by the Fc-domain, which is formed by the invariant or constant regions (C_{H2} and C_{H3}) of the dimeric IgG heavy chains. The Fc domains contribute the effector domains of the IgG molecule, which provide the binding sites for complement and Fc receptors that are critical for antibody homeostasis in vivo and linking antigen engagement with the immune effector response.

The critical requirement for Fc–FcγR interactions for antibody-mediated biologic function in vivo was demonstrated in models of infectious immunity, autoimmunity, and tumor immunity [9]. As a consequence of Fc–FcγR interactions and complement activation, antibody-opsonized microbes are cleared by phagocytic cells and local and systemic inflammatory responses are induced. The importance of complement and Fc receptors in host defense in infectious immunity is demonstrated by the enhanced susceptibility of FcγR-deficient and complement mice to viral and bacterial infections [10–15]. FcγR activation also is pivotal to autoantibody-triggered inflammation in acute [16] and chronic models of inflammation [17]. In tumor models, lack of Fc receptor engagement abrogates the protective capacity of passive antibody immunotherapy [18], a phenomenon that was first achieved in mice in 1980 [19–21]. Nevertheless, clinical success awaited the development of engineered antibodies with reduced immunogenicity.

ELIMINATION OF IMMUNOGENICITY BY ANTIBODY ENGINEERING

Reduced immunogenicity has been accomplished with three approaches. "Chimeric" antibodies [22–24] are generated from the mouse B-cell hybridoma parent antibody by a genetic swap of the constant regions of the murine heavy and light chains with the corresponding human IgG1 and κ chains. This resulted in proteins that contain 33% mouse sequences, and HAMA largely has been avoided. The first FDA-approved antitumor antibody, the anti-CD20 antibody Rituxan, was formed from its mouse parent IgG, 2B8, in this manner. Further refinements were accomplished in "humanized" antibodies by CDR sequence grafting. Because the contact sites within the antigen-binding cleft are formed by only a small portion of the variable domains, CDR grafting produces humanized antibodies with less than 10% mouse sequences, and thus, reduced immunogenicity. In this approach the CDR-containing sequences are introduced by site-directed mutagenesis into the framework regions of the genes that encode the human heavy and light chains [24–28]. Herceptin is a humanized antibody that contains only the CDR regions of its mouse parent, 4D5. Most recently, "fully humanized antibodies" have been developed as enabled by the genetic manipulation of the mouse. This allowed the introduction of large portions of the human chromosomes that encode the human immunoglobulin variable regions, diversity, joining sequences, and constant regions into the mouse genome. The endogenous murine IgH and kappa genes were disabled in these mice by insertional mutagenesis. Thus, immunization of these mice results in the generation of B cells that produce high-affinity antibodies that are encoded by human antibody genes. The humanized antibodies that are in clinical development were developed in mice whose transgenes contain many fewer variable gene segments than are naturally present in the human [29–31]. The resultant induced antibody repertoire is predicted to be constrained, which may limit the generation of antibodies with optimal affinity. This has not prevented the development of high-affinity humanized antibodies, including 33 that are in clinical development. Perhaps this is because the structural diversity of CDR2 and -3 seem to be attributable primarily to junctional diversity and somatic mutation, rather than to combinatorial diversity. Recent improvements of the antibody variable region repertoire has been accomplished by transfer of chromosomes or chromosome fragments, which contain the entire human heavy chain and light chain loci, into murine embryonic stem cells [32–35].

ANTIGENIC TARGET

In the absence of membrane permeabilization, antibodies traverse cell membranes poorly; this makes only extracellular and membrane-bound targets readily accessible to antitumor antibodies. Ideally, the target should be expressed preferentially by tumor cells to allow specific targeting in vivo. This would minimize untoward toxicities, eliminate the possibility of an antigenic "sink" that is provided by binding to nontumor cells, and diminish antibody delivery to tumor sites. Other potential factors that limit antibody therapy include antigenic modulation and generation of antigen loss variants. Antigenic modulation—the loss of cell surface expression that is due to receptor-mediated endocytosis—eliminates the antigen and the antibody from the cell surface. This is relevant to antibodies that are specific for cytokine receptors, including the epidermal growth factor (EGF) and insulin growth factor receptors (IGFR). Loss of surface antibodies unavailable to effectors, but is believed to underlie the tumor cell growth arrest/apoptosis that results from loss of persistent IGF and EGF family receptor signaling. The term "antigen loss variant" refers to the observation that antigen-negative cancer cells can be selected for during active cancer immunotherapy. Tumor cells are intrinsically genetically unstable, which allows for a high rate of generation of antigenic variants that have acquired or lost expression of individual proteins. Genetic instability may be central to the ability of tumors to overcome the selective pressure of immunosurveillance, which otherwise would eliminate immunogenic clones. Similarly, under the additional selective pressures of active or passive immunotherapy, antigen-expressing tumors are killed selectively, which allows for the potential emergence of antigen loss variants. This provides a rationale for the targeting of surface proteins that are critical to the transformed phenotype of the malignant cell. The emergence of HER-2–negative resistant variants has not been observed in patients who undergo Herceptin therapy, which argues for an essential contribution of HER-2 signaling in HER-2–positive breast cancer. Reports have noted that treatment of B-cell lymphoma with anti-CD20 antibodies can result in the loss of CD20 antigen expression [36–38].

Antigens that are expressed uniquely by tumors include the novel gene products derived from mutational mechanisms (eg, bcr/abl, ras) may be the most attractive targets for immunotherapy. Many of these novel proteins are intracellular and remain inaccessible to antibody; the B-cell receptor and T-cell receptor idiotype is a notable exception, and is expressed uniquely on cell surface of the malignant B- or T-cell clone. Other antigens that are merely preferentially expressed at tumor sites also have proven to be viable targets in preclinical and clinical studies. These include shared differentiation antigens (eg, tyrosinase-related proteins [TRPs] that are expressed by melanoma and normal melanocytes, CD20 that is expressed by B cells, and CD52 that is expressed by B- and T-lymphoid cells). Elimination is accompanied by depletion of the normal cellular counterparts. Thus, effective antimelanoma tumor immunity by anti–TRP-1 antibodies is accompanied by the development of depigmentation [39]. Similarly, anti-CD20 antibody treatment is accompanied by rapid and prolonged depletion of normal B cells. A humoral immunodeficiency is not clinically apparent in these patients, because of the persistence of CD20-negative antibody-producing plasma cells. Immunodeficiency has been a more serious clinical problem in patients who were treated with anti-CD52 antibodies as a consequence of rapid depletion of CD52-bearing normal T cells. Cancer testes genes are attractive candidates for active immunotherapy in cancer because of their restricted expression to cancer cells in the adult.

Targeting cell surface proteins whose signaling is crucial to intrinsic tumorigenicity provides advantages beyond induction of immune effector responses. The opportunity that is provided by targeted antibodies to bind to critical external faces of membrane receptors has enabled signaling blockade by competitive blockade with ligand or by inducing receptor internalization. Thus, the anti-EGF receptors (EGFR) antibody C225 blocks EGF signaling by blocking EGF binding and by inducing cell surface internalization and intracellular degradation of the receptor. The anti–HER-2/neu antibody Herceptin blocks ligand-induced signaling and promotes internalization, which prevent its interaction with other EGFR family members. The monoclonal antibody (mAb) 2C4, which is in late-stage clinical development, binds HER-2/neu but does not prevent ligand binding; instead, it prevents homedimeric and heterodimeric assembly of HER-2 with other EGFR family members. For tumors that are addicted to EGFR-mediated signaling for the maintenance of the transformed phenotype, antibody-mediated pharmacologic blockade of EGF-mediated signaling represents a clear therapeutic mechanism, and was the basis for their clinical development. Yet, the additional component of the Fc domain in the induction of host immunologic antitumor responses also may contribute to the ability of this class of antisignaling antibodies. It will be of interest to compare mechanistically the immunologic responses that are induced by panimutumab and Erbitux, both of which target EGFR, but differ in their Fc domains. Erbitux is a chimerized IgG1 antibody that is capable of interacting with FcγRs and comple-

Table 1
FDA-approved antitumor antibodies

Monoclonal antibody name	Trade name	Approved in	Used to treat	Construct	Isotype	Target
Rituximab[a]	Rituxan	1997	Non-Hodgkin's lymphoma	Chimeric	IgG1	CD20
Trastuzumab[a]	Herceptin	1998	Breast cancer	Humanized	IgG1	HER-2
Gemtuzumab ozogamicin[b]	Mylotarg	2000	Acute myelogenous leukemia	Humanized	IgG4	CD33
Alemtuzumab[a]	Campath	2001	Chronic lymphocytic leukemia	Humanized	IgG1	CD52
Ibritumomab tiuxetan[b]	Zevalin	2002	Non-Hodgkin's lymphoma	Mouse	IgG1	CD20
Tositumomab[b]	Bexxar	2003	Non-Hodgkin's lymphoma	Mouse	IgG2a	CD20
Cetuximab[a]	Erbitux	2004	Colorectal cancer	Chimeric	IgG1	EGFR
Bevacizumab[a]	Avastin	2004	Colorectal cancer	Humanized	IgG1	VEGF- A

Abbreviation: VEGF, vascular endothelial growth factor.

[a] The five "naked antibodies" are of the human IgG1 subclass and are expected to have FcγR-and complement-binding capacities.

[b] The three antibodies are immunoconjugates; Zevalin and Bexxar are radiolabled mAb's that deliver ^{90}Y (ibritumomomab tiuxetan) and ^{131}Y (tositumomab), respectively. The third mAb conjugate is a humanized IgG4 mAb that is conjugated to a cytotoxic calicheamicin derivative (gemtuzumab ozogamicin).

ment triggering antibody-dependent cellular cytotoxicity (ADCC) and complement-dependent toxicity (CDC) in vitro. Panitumab is a fully human IgG2 mAb that has poor affinity for FcγRs and complement; therefore, ADCC and CDC would not be expected to contribute to its biologic activity. Comparisons of the biologic activity of these two antibodies may prove revealing of important Fc-mediated contributions to tumor responses.

Eight mAb's are approved by the FDA for use in patients who have cancer (Table 1). Although the clinical experience is immature, the potency of this class of therapeutics as single agents seems to be greater for lymphoid malignancies than for solid tumors. Response rates for single-agent Rituxan as front-line therapy in low-grade lymphoma have ranged from 50% to 75% [40–43]. In contrast, single-agent Herceptin therapy of metastatic breast adenocarcinoma produced complete remissions in only 15% of patients [44]. Although combination therapies, including active cytotoxic agents and antitumor antibodies, have provided higher response rates [45–47] in lymphoma and in metastatic breast cancer [48], an understanding of the underlying mechanisms of action may allow for the development of more successful regimens. This article does not focus on the clinical evaluation of these antibodies nor of the many other antibodies that

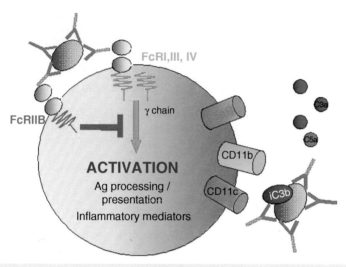

Fig. 1. Antibody-opsonized tumor targets can interact with cellular Fc and complement receptors.

are in clinical development, but discusses the mechanistic contributions of the Fc domains to tumor responses (Fig. 1).

HUMAN Fc RECEPTORS

Three different human Fc receptor subtypes for IgG trigger cellular activation when cross-linked by IgG: FcγRI, FcγRIIA, and FcγRIIIA. Activation is initiated by recruitment of src-family protein tyrosine kinases by way of immunoglobulin-tyrosine activation motifs (ITAMs) that are present in the cytoplasmic domain, in the case of FcγRIIA, or by an associated FcγR (for FcγRI and FcγRIIIA). FcγRIIIB is expressed on neutrophils but this GPI-linked receptor has no apparent intrinsic signaling capacity; however, it may contribute by enhancing antibody binding and recruitment to signaling membrane microdomains on neutrophils. FcγRIIB is expressed ubiquitously on hematopoietic cells, and contains an immunoglobulin tyrosine inhibitory motif (ITIM) that dominantly inhibits ITAM-containing receptors, including FcγRI, FcγIIA, and FcγIII, as well as surface immunoglobulin on B cells. Inhibition is mediated by recruitment of phosphotases, including the inositol phosphatase SHIP and the tyrosine phosphatase SHP-1 [49]. Thus, antibody-triggered responses are regulated reciprocally by the three activating Fc receptors and the inhibitory Fc receptor, which are coexpressed on hematopoietic cells (Tables 2 and 3). T helper cell (Th)1-type cytokines, including granulocyte/macrophage colony-stimulating factor (GM-CSF) and interferon (IFN)-γ, induce upregulation of activating FcγRs, whereas the Th2-type cytokines interleukin (IL)-4 and IL-13 induce FcγRIIB [50,51]. Transforming growth factor (TGF)-β, which induces alternatively activated macrophages, down-regulates activating FcγR expression [52], whereas IL-10 increases the expression of activating and inhibitory FcγRs

Table 2
Human Fc receptors and functional polymorphic alleles

	Isotype preference	Function	Polymorphisms	Functional consequences	Clinical autoimmunity/ infection	Clinical antitumor mAb efficacy
FcRI (CD64)	IgG1=3>4≫2	Myeloid cell activation	None described			
FcRIIA (CD32)	IgG1=3≫2≫4	Myeloid cell activation	His/Arg A.A. 131	H131 has higher affinity for IgG2	R131 allele associated with SLE, Guillain-Barré, MS	H/H higher RR for Rituximab
FcRIIB1	IgG1=3>4>2	B-cell inhibition	Ile/Thr A.A. 232 -343 G/C promoter	↓FcRIIB expression ?	Thr/Thr and C/C associated with SLE	?
FcRIIB2	IgG1=3>4>2	Myeloid cell inhibition	Ile/Thr A.A. 232 -343 G/C promoter	↓FcRIIB expression	Thr/Thr and C/C associated with SLE	
FcRIIIA (CD16)	IgG1=3≫2,4	Myeloid cell & NK activation	Val/Phe A.A. 158	Valine conveys higher affinity for IgG1	Phe/Phe conveys susceptibility to RA and SLE	V/V higher RR for Rituximab
FcRIIIB	IgG1=3≫2,4	Cooperate with other FcRs?	NA1/NA2	NA1 conveys enhanced IgG1 and IgG3 phagocytosis	NA2/NA2 associated with recurrent infection	?

Abbreviations: A.A., amino acid; Arg, arginine; G/C, guanine versus cytosine; His, histidine; Ile, isoleucine; MS, multiple sclerosis; NA, neutrophil antigen; RA, rheumatoid arthritis; SLE, systemic lupus erythematosus; Thr, threonine.

Table 3
Cellular expression of human Fc receptors

	MΦ	NK	PMN	Dendritic cell	B cell	Endocytosis/ phagocytosis	Regulation by cytokines
FcRI (CD64)	+	–	+	+	–	Yes/yes	↑ IFN-γ, GM-CSF G-CSF, ↓ TGF-β
FcRIIA (CD32)	+	–	+	+	–	Yes/yes	↓ IL-4
FcRIIB1	–	–	–	–	+	No/no	↓ IL-4
FcRIIB2	+	–	–	+	–	Yes/no	↑ IL-4, ↑ IL-13, ↓ IFN-γ
FcRIIIA (CD16)	+	+	+	+	–	Yes/yes	↑ IFN-γ, ↓ TGF-β
FcRIIIB	–	–	+	–	–	No/no	ND

Abbreviations: +, present; –, absent; MΦ, macrophage; ND, not determined; PMN, polymorphonuclear cell.

[50]. Thus, the magnitude of antibody-mediated effector responses is context-dependent and regulated in tissues by locally produced cytokines. The consequences of immune complex engagement depend on effector cell type, the nature of the immune complex, and the relative expression levels of activating/inhibitory FcγRs. Soluble immune complexes can induce inflammatory responses by activation of myeloid-derived cells, including production of cytokines, chemokines, reactive oxygen and nitrogen species, prostaglandins, and leukotrienes. Soluble immune complexes also can drive T-cell responses through enhancement of major histocompatibility complex (MHC) class II antigen presentation by macrophages, B cells, follicular dendritic cells (DCs) and MHC classes I and II antigen presentation by DCs. On macrophages and neutrophils, antibody-opsonized microorganisms are phagocytosed, whereas these same cells, as well as natural killer (NK) cells, can trigger ADCC of antibody-opsonized tumor cells.

The intracellular domains amongst individual activating and inhibitory FcγR family members are highly divergent, which is consistent with discordant signaling consequences; however, the extracellular domains have a high degree of sequence identity, and thus, comparable affinities for IgG-containing immune complexes. FcγRI contains a third extracellular domain that confers high-affinity binding for monomeric IgG (dissociation constant [Kd] 10^{-9}). Thus as is the case with the high-affinity IgE receptor, FcγRI likely is bound in vivo by monomeric IgG, which is present in mg/mL concentrations in the blood and in the interstitial fluid. Engagement of FcγRI by immune complexes or antibody-opsonized cells would require displacement of previously bound IgG; however, the avidity of FcγRI for multivalent ligand is at least 10-fold higher than for monomeric IgG. In the human, FcγRI is expressed on monocytes and granulocytes, and its expression is increased significantly with IFN-γ or granulocyte colony-stimulating factor (G-CSF).

The "so-called" low-affinity FcγRs—FcγRIIA, FcγRIIB, FcγRIIIA and FcγRIIIB—have lower affinity for monomeric IgG (Kd 10^{-6}); however, their affinity for complexed IgG is comparable to that of FcγRI. Thus, the various FcγRs should compete equally for immune complex binding. Although binding affinities of the various FcγRs are dependent on IgG subclass, this has not been established for the human system. IgG1 and IgG3 bind all FcγRs in the human, whereas IgG2 and IgG4 bind poorly. FcγRIIA and FcγRIIIA are expressed on monocyte and granulocyte cells. FcγRIIIA is the unique FcγR that is expressed on NK cells, and therefore, it must be entirely responsible for the antibody-mediated activation of these cells.

MURINE IgG RECEPTORS

Recent data in murine systems provided insights into the biologic mechanisms of antitumor antibodies; therefore, a description of the highly related FcγR family in the mouse is required. As in humans, the inhibitory FcγRIIB contains an ITIM motif in its intracellular domain, and is responsible for limiting activating FcγR-signaling through recruitment of SHIP. Three activating FcγRs for IgG have been described for the mouse—FcγRI, III, and IV—all of which are expressed as a heteromeric multisubunit complex. Each FcγRα-chain is dependent on the coexpressed γ chain for its cell surface expression and ITAM-mediated signaling capacity.

Fcγ Receptor I

Similar to the human, in which the low-affinity FcγRs contain two extracellular domains, mouse FcγRI contains three extracellular domains that are responsible for ligand binding, and is distinguished from the lower affinity FcγRs by its high affinity for monomeric IgG. FcγRI is not expressed on granulocytes in the mouse, but as in the human, it is inducibly expressed on monocyte lineage cells with cytokines. In the mouse, FcγRI has preferential affinity for mouse IgG2a. Accordingly, FcγRI$^{-/-}$ animals have reduced, but not abolished, IgG2a-mediated responses to cytotoxic antibodies in models of macrophage-mediated ADCC in vitro and hemolytic anemia in vivo [53]. FcγRI does not seem to play a role in the effector responses to other subclasses of murine IgG that are known to bind FcγRs (eg, IgG1 and IgG2b). A recent report suggests that FcγRI is the primary FcγR that is responsible for the in vivo activity of the antimelanoma IgG2a antibody TA99 [54].

Fcγ Receptor III

As in the human, murine FcγRIII is expressed on monocyte- and granulocyte-lineage cells, and is the sole FcγR on NK cells. It has a higher affinity for murine IgG1 and IgG2b than for IgG2a. Until the recent identification of FcγRIV, FcγRIII had been presumed to be responsible for IgG1- and IgG2b-mediated effector functions. FcγRIII$^{-/-}$ mice have reduced IgG1-mediated responses to cytotoxic antibodies by NK cells and macrophages in vitro and in vivo models of hemolytic anemia [55–59]; however, FcγRIV likely is responsible for the biologic activity of IgG2b in vivo.

Fcγ Receptor IV

The persistent effector function in FcγRI$^{-/-}$, FcγRIII$^{-/-}$ double knockout mice suggested the existence of a third IgG receptor [53]. The functional importance of the recently identified FcγR, FcγRIV, was established in recent reports using a specific FcγRIV-blocking antibody in vivo [60]. This receptor has intermediate affinities for IgG2a and IgG2b and fails to bind IgG1. Pathogenic clearance of platelets by antiplatelet antibodies of the IgG2a and IgG2b subclass were blocked completely by a blocking anti-FcγRIV antibody, whereas IgG1 antiplatelet antibodies required FcγRIII and were unaffected by anti-FcγRIV antibodies. As with other activating FcγRs, the expression of FcγRIV on monocytes is up-regulated by IFN-γ. Amongst the IgG receptors, murine FcγRIV has the greatest homology to human FcγRIII, and blocking antihuman FcγRIII antibodies were effective in an individual case report of immune thrombocytopenic purpura [61].

Fcγ RECEPTOR CONTRIBUTIONS TO TUMOR IMMUNITY ARE DEPENDENT ON ANTITUMOR ANTIBODY IgG SUBCLASS

The importance of Fc receptor engagement for antibody-mediated tumor immunity was demonstrated using tyrosinase related protein-1 (TRP-1/gp75) as model tumor antigen in the B16 melanoma lung metastases model. In both passive models of antibody-mediated protection using an IgG2a mAb, TA99, and in actively gp75-immunized mice, antitumor responses were abolished in FcγRγ$^{-/-}$ mice, which are deficient in all three activating FcγRs. Thus, even a polyclonal collection of antibodies, with diverse specificities and antibody subclasses, strictly required activating FcγRs for efficacy [18]. In nude mouse xenograft models the activity of Herceptin and Rituxan were reduced greatly in FcγRγ$^{-/-}$ mice. Further an engineered anti–HER-2 antibody which contained a single amino acid substitution in the Fc domain that abolished FcγR binding activity completely was ineffective in mediating tumor protection in vivo, despite its retained capacity to inhibit the growth of HER-2–expressing breast cancer cell lines in vitro. Thus, the presence of intact Fc domains and activating FcγRs were required for antitumor responses in vivo [62]. The presence of the inhibitory FcγR limits the therapeutic benefit of low-dose tumor antibodies, including TA99 and Herceptin (the mouse parent IgG1 4D5 and the humanized IgG1 trastuzumab). FcγRIIB$^{-/-}$ mice were protected fully at a 10-fold reduced dose of antibody. The prediction of this work was that antitumor responses could be improved by antibody engineering that might generate Fc domains that preferentially bind activating Fc receptors at the expense of binding the inhibitory FcγRIIB (high activating/inhibitory [A/I] index) [63].

Recent work by the Ravetch group, using switch variants of the mAb TA99 of the IgG1, IgG2a, and IgG2b subclasses, showed that the potency of each subclass reflects its affinities for specific FcγRs that are responsible for mediating tumor responses in vivo depend on IgG subclass [63]. IgG1-mediated protection required FcγRIII, but there was little role for FcγRI or FcγIV; this is consistent with the preferential affinity of IgG1 for FcγRIII. IgG1-mediated protection was enhanced dramatically in FcγRIIB$^{-/-}$ mice, presumably because of the competitive balance for binding in favor of FcγRIIB. IgG2a responses were completely independent of FcγRIII expression; they were impaired minimally in FcγRI-

Table 4
Relative affinities of murine IgG subclasses and Fc receptors

	FcRI	FcRIIB	FcRIII	FcRIV	A/I ratio
IgG1	–	++	+	–	0.1
IgG2a	+++	+/–	–	+++	69
IgG2b	–	+	–	+++	7

The relative affinities of monomeric IgG subclasses for murine FcγRs are shown. The A/I ratio is the ratio of the affinity of FcγRIII/FcγRIIB binding for IgG1, and FcγRIV/FcγRIIB binding for IgG2a and 2b. –, +/–, +, ++ and +++ denote relative binding affinities, increasing from left to right. *Data from* Nimmerjahn F, Ravetch JV. Divergent immunoglobulin G subclass activity through selective Fc receptor binding. Science 2005;310(5753):1510–2.

deficient animals, whereas more impressive inhibition was demonstrated with in vivo blockade of FcγRIV. At full doses of antibody there was no appreciable effect of FcγRII deficiency, because IgG2a has the lowest affinity for FcγRIIB. The IgG2a TA99 variant was the most potent antitumor antibody, which probably reflects its low affinity for FcγRIIB. Efficacy of the IgG2b antibody also was inhibited with FcγRIV blocking antibodies but as with IgG1, responses were limited by the presence of FcγRIIB. Thus, the protective capacities of IgG depend critically on subclass. Th1-mediated adjuvants preferentially induce IgG2a responses, and the protective capacity of this subclass has been recognized for years. This can be explained by its high A/I index, which is reflective of its high affinity for FcγRIV and low affinity for the inhibitory receptor FcγRIIB (Table 4). A similar distinction between the human IgGs (IgG1 versus IgG3) that bind FcγRs has not been demonstrated, but suggests that alterations of human Fc domains might accomplish preferential engagement of specific activating FcγRs.

ROLE OF COMPLEMENT IN ANTITUMOR RESPONSES
Human IgG1 and IgG3 bind C1q and initiate the classic complement activation pathway, which leads to the generation of C3b on the surface of antibody-opsonized cells. CDC can be demonstrated in vitro with CD20-expressing B-cell lines and in primary cultures of circulating tumor cells from patients [64]. In principle, the mechanism of cell death—in the absence of cellular effectors—could be mediated by formation of the C5–C9 membrane attack complex (MAC). Cytolysis that is due to MAC formation on the surface of cells is inhibited by a series of membrane proteins that efficiently prevent ultimate formation of the MAC. CD59 inhibits formation of MAC, whereas CD35 (complement receptor type I), CD46 (membrane cofactor protein), and CD55 (decay accelerating protein) inactivate the enzymatic activity of surface-bound C3b to form C3bi.

Much of the work on the potential mechanistic contributions of complement has been investigated in the CD20 system. Two tumor models suggested a contributory role for complement. Genetic evidence was provided using C1q-deficient mice which lacked protective rituximab responses against challenge with a human CD20–transfected T thymoma cell line [65]. In nude mouse xenograft studies, rituximab-mediated protection was reduced dramatically in mice that were depleted of complement with cobra venom factor [66]. Increased CD20 expression on cellular targets has correlated with rituximab-mediated CDC sensitivity [64,67]. Cragg and colleagues noted that the capacity of CD20 antibodies to induce cytolytic MAC correlates with their propensity to recruit CD20 into membrane lipid rat microdomains [68,69]. Blockade of the complement inhibitory proteins CD55 and CD59 enhanced rituximab-mediated CDC in vitro [70]. The notion that Rituxan resistance could be explained by levels of expression of complement inhibitory proteins on the surface of tumor cells gathered support from in vitro investigation of CD59 levels and rituximab sensitivity of cell lines [71]. No correlations were identified when samples were tested directly to examine whether clinical responses of patients who were treated with Rituxan were associated with in vitro CDC susceptibility or levels of membrane expression of the complement inhibitory proteins CD44, CD35, or CD59 [72]. The mechanistic importance of complement versus FcγR in vivo may depend on the target cell and the anatomic location. Although depletion of follicular B cells did not require complement in the mouse human CD20 transgenic system [73–75], anti-CD20 mAb clearance of marginal zone B cells was inefficient and dependent on an intact complement system [74].

The presence of multiple inhibitory proteins prevent MAC formation and direct complement-mediated cytolysis; other complement functional pathways remain intact. Although the C3 fragment C3bi is enzymatically inactive, it remains on the cell surface and functions as an opsonin for uptake by cellular effectors that bear receptors for C3 fragments, including CD11b (Mac-1), CD11c, and CR1 (CD35). The presence of opsonic C3 fragments promotes a synergistic interaction between Mac-1 and FcγR-mediated signaling, which enhances FcγR-mediated phagocytosis, cellular migration, and ADCC [76,77]. CD11b-deficient mice showed impaired protection by mAb TA99 in the lung metastases [78]. This could be due to impaired effector recruitment to tumor sites or reduced ADCC activity upon FcγR engagement. Recent work suggests another potential positive interaction between the complement system and FcγR-mediated activation of the effector response. The generation of C5a during acute immune complex–mediated inflammatory responses induces up-regulation of activating FcγRs and reduced surface expression of inhibitory FcγRs on macrophages [79]. Thus, C5a would be predicted to increase effector cell responsiveness to FcγR engagement.

CLINICAL RELEVANCE OF HUMAN Fc RECEPTOR POLYMORPHISMS

Complete genetic loss of FcγR is rare, and has been described for FcγRI and FcγRIIIB in only a few individuals without significant clinical consequence. Several polymorphic alleles have been described, some fairly common, which may be associated with increased risk of autoimmune states (see Table 2) (reviewed in [16]). Negative studies have been reported as well, which showed no link between systemic lupus erythematosus and polymorphic alleles. Some of these polymorphisms lead to altered affinities for IgG. Recent data from four clinical studies–two in follicular lymphoma and one each in Waldenström's macroglobulinemia and chronic lymphocytic leukemia (CLL)–revealed potential impact on antitumor antibody clinical responses in patients who were treated with Rituxan. Cartron and colleagues [80] reported the first genetic study that assessed responses to Rituximab in patients who had follicular lymphoma and harbored one of two different polymorphic FcγRIIIA alleles. These alleles differ in a single amino acid substitution at position 158. The presence of valine (val; V), rather than phenylalanine (phe; F), at position 158 conveys a higher affinity for human IgG1. If Fc receptor engagement was pivotal to the biologic activity one would predict that response rates would be higher in patients who have the homozygous val/val haplotype. In this small study, objective responses (OR) 1 year after treatment were significantly higher ($P=.03$) in patients who had the val/val haplotype (90% OR in 10 patients) than in those who harbored val/phe or phe/phe (51% OR in 40 patients). These data were confirmed and extended in a larger study assessing the contributions of both FcγRIIIA-158 and FcγRIIA-131 polymorphic alleles to response rates in patients who had follicular lymphoma and were treated with Rituxan in a second-line setting [81]. In patients who expressed FcγRIIIA-158V/V, 9 of 12 patients (75%) had durable objective responses at 12 months, whereas just 16 of 62 patients (26%) responded if they were FcγRIII F/V or -F/F carriers. In the same study, the presence of the homozygous FcγRIIA-131H/H haplotype was associated with favorable responses rates (55% versus 26%, $P=.027$). The FcγRIIA-H131–containing variant has a higher affinity for human IgG2 than does the FcγRIIA-R131 polymorph [81]. Differential affinities for human IgG1 have not been reported. In an analysis of patients who had follicular lymphoma and were immunized actively with idiotype-based (Id) vaccines, the Levy group noted that progression-free survival was associated with induction of an anti-Id humoral response as well as FcγR haplotype. Patients with a FcRIIIa-158V/V genotype had a longer progression-free survival than did those with V/F or F/F genotypes (V/V, 8.21 years versus V/F, 3.38 years; $P=.004$; versus F/F, 4.47 years; $P=.035$). In a study of 58 patients who had Waldenström's macroglobulinemia and were treated with Rituxan [82], a higher response rate was seen in patients who harbored the homozygous FcγRIIIA-158V/V haplotype (-V/V [40%] and -V/F [35%] versus -F/F [9%]; $P=.03$). These latter three trials all concurred that the FcγRIIIA-V/V haplotype was protective, and that there was no evidence for a gene dosage effect; the FcγRIIIA-158F/V and -F/F carriers had similarly reduced response rates. Thus three studies in follicular lymphoma have implicated FcγRIIIA as a determinant of response rates (FcγRIIIA-158V/V haplotype conferring protection), and one study has implicated FcγRIIA (FcγRIIA 131H/H haplotype conferring protection). A small study in patients who had CLL suggested that FcγγR allelic status did not contribute to clinical outcome after treatment with Alemtuzumab [83] or Rituximab [84], which may reflect other non-FcγR–related mechanistic contributions in this disease. In light of the potential derivation of these transformed CLL cells from normal B-1 cell populations, complement, and not FcγR-engagement, was important in the clearance of marginal zone B cells in the human CD20 transgenic mouse [74].

The available genetic data from patients and mice imply that preferential engagement of activating Fc receptors modulates antitumor responses in vivo. The mechanistic importance of FcγR-mediated ADCC and overall tumor response rates are likely to vary considerably according to the nature of the primary tumor and the sites of disease.

CELLULAR MECHANISMS OF Fcγ RECEPTOR–MEDIATED TUMOR IMMUNITY

Induction of antibody-opsonized tumor cell killing by cellular effectors (ADCC) can be accomplished in vitro with several hematopoietic lineage cells, including granulocytes, monocytes, and NK cells. A variety of molecular mediators of cellular toxicity is elaborated after FcγR engagement on cellular effectors, depending on cell type. NK cells produce FasL and perforin/granzyme. Activated macrophages express tumor necrosis factor (TNF) family members, including TNF and TRAIL, as well as reactive oxygen species, NO, and proinflammatory cytokines. FcγR-triggered granulocyte and mast cell degranulation results in the elaboration of several proteases, reactive oxygen species, and small molecular mediators of inflammation that can contribute to cytotoxicity. Thus, many FcγR-bearing hematopoietic cell types might contribute in vivo—separately or in an organized manner—to induce tumor shrinkages (Fig. 2). Clinical data are lacking in this area, and mouse models have provided only limited insight.

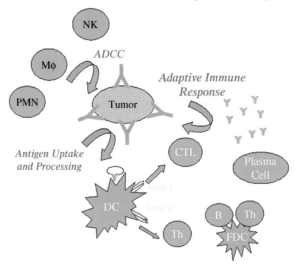

Fig. 2. Fc receptor–mediated activation of cellular effectors and antigen-presenting cells. Fc receptor engagement on NK cells, macrophages, and neutrophils can trigger ADCC or direct tumor cell killing, whereas uptake of antibody-opsonized antigen can lead to DC-mediated induction of tumor antigen-specific CD4 and CD8 responses.
Abbreviations: MΦ, macrophage; NK, natural killer cell; PMN, polymorphonuclear cell.

Macrophages are required for clearance of opsonized red blood cells and platelets, which occurs by way of phagocytosis in the spleen or liver. Similarly macrophages have been implicated in the Rituxan-mediated clearance of normal B cells from the blood. Liposomal clodronate treatment, which is toxic for splenic and hepatic macrophages, greatly reduced anti-CD20–mediated B-cell clearance [73,74]. Splenectomy had little effect on clearance, which implicated the liver as the site of clearance [74]. Enhancing macrophage-mediated phago-cytosis or ADCC might be accomplished with cytokines, including IFN-γ [85] and GM-CSF, which activate monocyte/macrophage cells and preferentially up-regulate activating FcγR expression.

Some murine studies implicated neutrophils as potential mediators of tumor responses in vivo [77,78,86,87], and their numbers and activity can be increased potently by G-CSF. A single-arm clinical investigation of combined treatment with Rituxan and G-CSF showed acceptable toxicity profiles [86,88,89]. FcγRI, FcγRIIA, and FcγRIIIA can mediate ADCC by neutrophils, and FcγRI-mediated ADCC was enhanced significantly in neutrophils that were obtained from individuals who were treated with G-CSF [90,91] and upon treatment with GM-CSF [92]. IgG and IgA can induce neutrophil-mediated ADCC because of their expression of the FcγRs and the IgA Fc receptor FcαRI [86,93–95]. Bispecific antibodies targeted by dual Fab specificities for tumor antigen and FcγRI (or to FcαRI) can arm neutrophils for specific lysis of antigen-bearing cells [96].

IL-2–activated NK cells efficiently induce ADCC in vitro, and mice depleted of NK cells were not protected from melanoma metastases with the mAb TA99 [97]. FcγRIII is the sole FcγR on NK cells; therefore, the enhanced tumor responses in FcγRIIB$^{-/-}$ mice after treatment with Herceptin or TA99 argues against a singular contribution of NK cells. Although NK cells lack expression of the inhibitory FcγRIIB, enhancing the contributions of NK cell–mediated ADCC in vivo may be possible by blocking other inhibitory receptors on these cells. Anti-CD20–mediated B-cell clearance in mice was not impaired in perforin-deficient mice nor in beige mice (which exhibit dysfunctional vesicular exocytosis), which suggested that the NK perforin/granzyme system was not involved [73]. Thus, animal data do not support a direct cytopathic role for NK cells; however, they may contribute indirectly in their roles as producers of large quantities of cytokines (including, for example, IFN-γ and TNFα). As a result, NK activation could spur secondary activation of other TNF- and IFN-γ–responsive effectors, including monocyte lineage cells. Several cytokines (IL-2, -12, -15, -21) can activate NK cells, which leads to improved ADCC function and increased IFN-γ production. Combined treatment of IL-2 with antitumor antibodies was more effective than antibody alone in ADCC assays in vitro and in tumor animal models that used several tumor targets, including anti-CD20 [98,99] and HER-2 [100]. Toxicities of systemic IL-2 and IL-12 are a significant obstacle to their clinical use [99,101–110], but at least one trial reported increased response rates that correlated with NK cell expansion [104]. In an effort to improve the therapeutic index of cytokine therapy, antitumor antibody-cytokine fusions have been developed to deliver cytokine to tumor sites selectively, which enables local, but not systemic, activation of cellular effectors [111].

Much of what we know about antibody-mediated effector responses are derived from acute inflammatory models and in vitro ADCC assay models, the immediate tumor cell killing of peripheral blood effectors. Both models seem inappropriate given the chronic administration of antitumor antibodies and the timing of the clinical responses. An alternative view is that antitumor antibodies could alter chronic inflammatory responses in tumor stroma, which may alter the local tolerogenic environment and enhance T-cell–mediated antitumor cellular immunity. Thus, the potential importance of FcγRs as antigen uptake receptors on antigen-presenting cells, especially DCs, has been a recent area of investigation. Specific antitumor CD8 responses can be induced after antitumor antibody treatment, presumably as the result of FcγR-mediated uptake by antigen-presenting cells [112]. Selective targeting of antigens through activating FcγRs on DCs accomplishes the two tasks of an effective vaccine (ie, delivery of antigen to DCs coupled with a DC activation signal, or adjuvant). Antitumor antibodies would be expected to enhance the uptake of tumor antigen by DCs quantitatively, either by endocytosis of soluble immune complexes or by phagocytosis of opsonized cells or cellular debris. Uptake by activating FcγRs on DCs rapidly accesses the antigen-processing machinery, which allows for presentation on MHC classes I and II, and is coupled with an ITAM-mediated DC activation signal [113]. In vitro work demonstrated that FcγR-mediated phagocytosis of opsonized myeloma cells could enhance the presentation of multiple tumor antigens to patient-derived T cells [114]. In animal model systems, immunization with DCs that acquired tumor antigens by way of endocytosis [115,116] or phagocytosis [117] induced CD4- and CD8-mediated tumor immunity. Ongoing studies in the author's laboratory and elsewhere (unpublished data of Ron Levy, Stanford University and Lou Wiener, Fox Chase Cancer Center) are investigating whether treatment with antitumor antibodies modulate the antitumor B- or T-cell response in patients. Because antibody-opsonized apoptotic cells can be phagocytosed by DCs with the resultant induction of T-cell responses, this pathway might be exploited by the combined use of antitumor antibodies with an inducer of tumor cell apoptosis, including chemotherapy, radiation, or using more defined blockers of signals that are essential for tumor cell viability (eg, growth receptor blockade, kinase inhibitors, antiangiogenics). Uptake of apoptotic cells by DCs ordinarily delivers a tolerogenic signal to T cells; however, the uptake of antibody-opsonized apoptotic cells may result in DC activation in vivo, and tilt the balance of tolerance toward the induction of a tumor-specific effector T-cell response. Thus, passive antibody immunotherapy would be expected to enhance the uptake of tumor antigen into DCs, which provides the opportunity for a vaccinelike effect with induction of tumor-specific B and T cells.

Fc ENGINEERING

Several engineering approaches are being pursued to capitalize on the ability of antibodies to target tumor beds and allow selective delivery of toxic payloads or localized enzymatic activation of cytotoxic drugs [7]. This article focuses on the engineering efforts that are aimed at optimizing immune effector responses of naked antibodies.

Interaction of antibodies with activating Fc receptors induce effector cell activation, whereas interactions with inhibitory FcγRs are likely to limit these responses. Thus, the primary goal of Fc engineering is the generation of Fc domain–containing antibodies with favorable binding avidities for FcγRs. It is not clear to which of the activating FcγRs that the antibodies should be tailored for targeting, but reduced binding to FcγRIIB while maintaining or enhancing binding to FcγRs should improve efficacy. Largely, the focus on optimizing Fc domain function for potential antitumor applications has focused on human IgG1. The binding sites on human IgG1 for human FcγRs, complement, and FcRn have been mapped by alanine scanning mutagenesis across the entire C_H1 and C_H2 domain [118]. This comprehensive and elegant study identified several residues at contact sites that were required to maintain FcγR-binding capability. All were within the C_H2 domain and clustered near the hinge region. These included previously described residues at the hinge region (residues 216–238) and sites of N-linked glycosylation (Asp297) that are known to interact directly with FcγR surfaces [119]. Substitution of alanine at these sites disrupted binding to all FcγRs. A few residues were identified, which when altered to alanine, had potentially favorable characteristics—either improved binding to activating FcγR or reduced binding to inhibitory FcγRIIB. Although several combinatorial variants can be imagined, the best binding IgG1 variant reported combined alanine scanning mutations at Ser-298, Glu-333, and Lys-334. This triple mutant bound to FcγRIIIA with a 1.5-fold greater affinity, and exhibited a greater improvement in binding to the low-affinity variant FcγRIIIA (Phe-158) polymorph. Furthermore, this IgG1 variant demonstrated improved ADCC function with comparable cytotoxicity achieved at 10-fold reduced concentrations of antibody when using resting NK cells from peripheral blood as effectors. Because NK cells express FcγRIIIA uniquely and lack expression of other FcγRs, the functional ADCC assay confirmed the ability of this IgG1 variant to engage FcγRIII, but did not address whether the antibody has an improved profile for other FcγR-bearing cellular effectors, including monocytes or granulocytes. Nevertheless, the reduced binding to FcγRIIB in vitro predicts that this variant, and others that bear amino acid substitutions that result in favorable FcγR-binding profiles, will induce enhanced ADCC activity in vivo. Preclinical development of this Fc variant is ongoing; amino acid substitutions that use amino acids other than alanine seem likely to provide further improved FcγR-binding characteristics.

Another fruitful direction in antibody engineering has been glycoengineering–modifications of the carbohydrate side chains that are attached posttranslationally. Human IgG1 contains several asparagines with sites for N-linked glycosylation. Aglycosylated antibodies are impaired for FcγR binding and have abolished ADCC activity [120,121]. In particular, the N-linked carbohydrate at Asparagine 297 in C_H2 contributes directly to FcγR binding, and amino acid substitutions at this site cripple FcγR binding. Manipulation of these essential carbohydrate moieties resulted in glycoengineered IgG1 Fc domains with improved FcγR-binding characteristics and enhanced ADCC activity in vivo [63,122]. All of the approaches accomplish the inclusion of low fucose–containing carbohydrates in the branched-chain oligosaccharides. Recombinant antibodies (humanized and chimeric) are produced most commonly by Chinese hamster ovary (CHO) cell transfectants. The generation of CHO producer cell variants [123] with altered glycosylation enzymatic capacities enabled production of antibodies with novel low-fucose oligosaccharide moieties and improved FcγR binding characteristics. Umana and colleagues overexpressed beta 1, 4-N Acetylglucosaminyl transferase III (GnT-III) in antibody-producing CHO cells; this led to increased levels of bisected, nonfucosylated oligosaccharides that exhibited improved ADCC function in vitro and reduced CDC activity [124,125]. GnT-III transferase in the produced cell line led to the addition of a bisecting N-acetylglucosamine (GlcNAc) residue that has an important influence on multiple subsequent enzymatic glycosylation reactions in the Golgi complex of the cell, especially the inhibition of Golgi α-mannosidase II, α1,6 fucosyltransferase, or galactosyl-transferases. Yamane-Ohnuki and colleagues [126] achieved a reduction of core fucosylation by recombinant antibody expression in CHO cells that lacked core-fucosyl transferase activity, whereas Mori and colleagues [127] maximized effector functions of expressed antibodies using fucosyl transferase–specific short interfering RNA. Both strategies resulted in an increased ADCC. Carbohydrate motifs on FcγRIIIA contribute to the selective improvement of the dissociation rates [128] of low-fucosylated antibodies [129]. Low fucose–containing antibodies of all four IgG subclasses enhanced ADCC, and can mediate ADCC at reduced epitope density and preferentially in FcγRIIIA F/F polymorphs [130]. The defucosylated variant of murine IgG2b, which had a threefold enhanced relative affinity, was equally effective in FcγRIIB$^{-/-}$ mice because it was reduced greatly for FcγRIIB binding [63].

By combining both engineering approaches, amino acid substitutions and altered fucosylation would be predicted to generate antibodies with even more favorable binding characteristics. Although intrinsic tumor resistance may be difficult to overcome, it is hoped that these engineered antibodies will improve overall response rates, particularly in patients with unfavorable FcγR polymorphisms or in tumor-types that express the tumor antigen only weakly. Finally, designer antibodies are being engineered with heightened CDC activity that is due to improved C1q binding [131,132] or improved serologic half-lives that are due to increased FcRn binding [133]. Most of these engineering approaches have focused on IgG1, but it is possible that modifications of other IgG subclasses will prove superior in the coupling of antibodies and the induction of antitumor cellular immune responses (Box 1). The real hope of these improvements is that the high response rates that are seen for Rituxan in lymphoma can be extended to solid tumor types that have not enjoyed comparable success.

BOX 1: STRATEGIES TO ENHANCE ANTITUMOR ANTIBODY EFFICACY

Tumor Site

Optimization of antibody delivery, antigenic target density, and overcoming "antiapoptotic" program

Antibody

Alter Fc glycosylation and primary amino acid sequence to optimize engagement of activating Fc receptors and C1q

Effector Cell

Increase number and ADCC activity
Natural killer cell (IL-2, IFN-γ, IL-12), macrophage (GM-CSF, IFN-γ), polymorphonuclear cell (G-CSF)

Antigen-Presenting cell/T cell

"Th1 promoting adjuvants" type I and II IFNs, IL-12, Toll-like receptor-antagonist-agonists; induction of tumor cell apoptosis for driving antibody-mediated cross-presentation

Preclinical evaluation of antibodies with improved Fc domains is difficult because the ideal animal model should express human FcγRs. Clinical testing of these Fc domain variants to identify an optimal Fc domain will be complicated by their use in various antigenic-targeting platforms, which prevents a direct head-to-head comparison. In this pursuit, however, clinical evaluation may reveal a theoretic concern, that an affinity "wall" will be broached with these approaches; if engineered antibodies (monomeric/dimeric or small aggregates) trigger widespread FcγR engagement on monocytes, granulocytes, or platelets, this likely would have deleterious consequences. This might give pause to the effort of affinity maximization, and require instead a compromised approach reminiscent of nature's own evolutionary solution to the problem of optimizing FcγR function of the opposing low-affinity FcγR receptors to balance maximally protective antimicrobial responses without induction of untoward inflammation [134].

SUMMARY

The promise of antigen-specific targeting of tumors—initially spurred by hybridoma technology that was developed by Kohler and Milstein in the 1970s—was not fulfilled clinically for 20 years, coincident with the use of "humanized" or "chimerized" antibodies which eliminated mouse protein immunogenicity. In the past decade, the use of these engineered mAb's has provided patients with clinical responses, and added significantly to the therapeutic arsenal in cancer. Several recent important advances in the understanding of Fc-FcγR interactions in vivo provide the framework for the discussion of potential approaches that are designed to improve their clinical usefulness.

The heavy chain is used most often for "naked antibody" constructs is human IgG1. This IgG subclass has favorable pharmacokinetics with a serum half-life of 7 to 14 days. IgG1 also has high affinity for human Fc receptors and for the first component of complement, C1q. Thus, mAb's that are developed with the human IgG1 "backbone" predictably lead to activation of immune effector functions that are mediated by complement and Fc receptors. Recent data from murine models demonstrate that interactions with Fc receptors are required for antitumor efficacy in vivo. This prompted efforts to re-engineer novel antibody-Fc domains with optimized interactions with Fc receptors. The promise of these next generations of antitumor antibodies is that stronger immune effector responses will lead to improved efficacy.

References

[1] Metchnikov I. On the present state of immunity in infectious diseases. Nobel Lecture December 11, 1908. Available at: http://nobelprize.org/medicine/laureates/1908/. Accessed April 24, 2006.

[2] Kohler G, Milstein C. Continuous cultures of fused cells secreting antibody of predefined specificity. Nature 1975;256(5517):495–7.

[3] Houghton AN, Mintzer D, Cordon-Cardo C, et al. Mouse monoclonal IgG3 antibody detecting GD3 ganglioside: a phase I trial in patients with malignant melanoma. Proc Natl Acad Sci U S A 1985;82(4):1242–6.

[4] Miller RA, Levy R. Response of cutaneous T cell lymphoma to therapy with hybridoma monoclonal antibody. Lancet 1981;2(8240):226–30.

[5] Miller RA, Maloney DG, Warnke R, et al. Treatment of B-cell lymphoma with monoclonal anti-idiotype antibody. N Engl J Med 1982;306(9):517–22.

[6] Rowan WC, Hale G, Tite JP, et al. Cross-linking of the CAMPATH-1 antigen (CD52) triggers activation of normal human T lymphocytes. Int Immunol 1995;7(1):69–77.

[7] Wu AM, Senter PD. Arming antibodies: prospects and challenges for immunoconjugates. Nat Biotechnol 2005;23(9):1137–46.

[8] Vaccaro C, Zhou J, Ober RJ, et al. Engineering the Fc region of immunoglobulin G to modulate in vivo antibody levels. Nat Biotechnol 2005;23(10):1283–8.

[9] Ravetch JV, Bolland S. IgG Fc receptors. Annu Rev Immunol 2001;19:275–90.

[10] Suresh M, Molina H, Salvato MS, et al. Complement component 3 is required for optimal expansion of CD8 T cells during a systemic viral infection. J Immunol 2003;170(2): 788–94.

[11] Kopf M, Abel B, Gallimore A, et al. Complement component C3 promotes T-cell priming and lung migration to control acute influenza virus infection. Nat Med 2002;8(4):373–8.

[12] Wessels MR, Butko P, Ma M, et al. Studies of group B streptococcal infection in mice deficient in complement component C3 or C4 demonstrate an essential role for complement in both innate and acquired immunity. Proc Natl Acad Sci U S A 1995;92(25): 11490–4.

[13] Huber VC, Lynch JM, Bucher DJ, et al. Fc receptor-mediated phagocytosis makes a significant contribution to clearance of influenza virus infections. J Immunol 2001;166(12): 7381–8.

[14] Saeland E, Vidarsson G, Leusen JH, et al. Central role of complement in passive protection by human IgG1 and IgG2 anti-pneumococcal antibodies in mice. J Immunol 2003;170(12):6158–64.

[15] Prodeus AP, Zhou X, Maurer M, et al. Impaired mast cell-dependent natural immunity in complement C3-deficient mice. Nature 1997;390(6656):172–5.

[16] Takai T, Li M, Sylvestre D, et al. FcR gamma chain deletion results in pleiotrophic effector cell defects. Cell 1994;76(3):519–29.

[17] Clynes R, Dumitru C, Ravetch JV. Uncoupling of immune complex formation and kidney damage in autoimmune glomerulonephritis. Science 1998;279(5353):1052–4.
[18] Clynes R, Takechi Y, Moroi Y, et al. Fc receptors are required in passive and active immunity to melanoma. Proc Natl Acad Sci U S A 1998;95(2):652–6.
[19] Herlyn DM, Steplewski Z, Herlyn MF, et al. Inhibition of growth of colorectal carcinoma in nude mice by monoclonal antibody. Cancer Res 1980;40(3):717–21.
[20] Moshakis V, McIlhinney RA, Raghavan D, et al. Localization of human tumour xenografts after i.v. administration of radiolabeled monoclonal antibodies. Br J Cancer 1981;44(1): 91–9.
[21] Trowbridge IS, Domingo DL. Anti-transferrin receptor monoclonal antibody and toxin-antibody conjugates affect growth of human tumour cells. Nature 1981;294(5837): 171–3.
[22] Boulianne GL, Hozumi N, Shulman MJ. Production of functional chimaeric mouse/human antibody. Nature 1984;312(5995):643–6.
[23] Morrison SL, Johnson MJ, Herzenberg LA, et al. Chimeric human antibody molecules: mouse antigen-binding domains with human constant region domains. Proc Natl Acad Sci U S A 1984;81(21):6851–5.
[24] Neuberger MS, Williams GT, Mitchell EB, et al. A hapten-specific chimaeric IgE antibody with human physiological effector function. Nature 1985;314(6008):268–70.
[25] Jones PT, Dear PH, Foote J, et al. Replacing the complementarity-determining regions in a human antibody with those from a mouse. Nature 1986;321(6069):522–5.
[26] Verhoeyen M, Milstein C, Winter G. Reshaping human antibodies: grafting an anti-lysozyme activity. Science 1988;239(4847):1534–6.
[27] Riechmann L, Clark M, Waldmann H, et al. Reshaping human antibodies for therapy. Nature 1988;332(6162):323–7.
[28] Hale G, Dyer MJ, Clark MR, et al. Remission induction in non-Hodgkin lymphoma with reshaped human monoclonal antibody CAMPATH-1H. Lancet 1988;2(8625): 1394–9.
[29] Fishwild DM, O'Donnell SL, Bengoechea T, et al. High-avidity human IgG kappa monoclonal antibodies from a novel strain of minilocus transgenic mice. Nat Biotechnol 1996; 14(7):845–51.
[30] Lonberg N, Taylor LD, Harding FA, et al. Antigen-specific human antibodies from mice comprising four distinct genetic modifications. Nature 1994;368(6474):856–9.
[31] Green LL, Hardy MC, Maynard-Currie CE, et al. Antigen-specific human monoclonal antibodies from mice engineered with human Ig heavy and light chain YACs. Nat Genet 1994;7(1):13–21.
[32] Tomizuka K, Yoshida H, Uejima H, et al. Functional expression and germline transmission of a human chromosome fragment in chimaeric mice. Nat Genet 1997;16(2): 133–43.
[33] Tomizuka K, Shinohara T, Yoshida H, et al. Double trans-chromosomic mice: maintenance of two individual human chromosome fragments containing Ig heavy and kappa loci and expression of fully human antibodies. Proc Natl Acad Sci U S A 2000;97(2):722–7.
[34] Kuroiwa Y, Tomizuka K, Shinohara T, et al. Manipulation of human minichromosomes to carry greater than megabase-sized chromosome inserts. Nat Biotechnol 2000;18(10): 1086–90.
[35] Nicholson IC, Zou X, Popov AV, et al. Antibody repertoires of four- and five-feature translocus mice carrying human immunoglobulin heavy chain and kappa and lambda light chain yeast artificial chromosomes. J Immunol 1999;163(12):6898–906.
[36] Davis TA, Czerwinski DK, Levy R. Therapy of B-cell lymphoma with anti-CD20 antibodies can result in the loss of CD20 antigen expression. Clin Cancer Res 1999; 5(3):611–5.
[37] Massengale WT, McBurney E, Gurtler J. CD20-negative relapse of cutaneous B-cell lymphoma after anti-CD20 monoclonal antibody therapy. J Am Acad Dermatol 2002;46(3): 441–3.

[38] Kinoshita T, Nagai H, Murate T, et al. CD20-negative relapse in B-cell lymphoma after treatment with Rituximab. J Clin Oncol 1998;16(12):3916.

[39] Trcka J, Moroi Y, Clynes RA, et al. Redundant and alternative roles for activating Fc receptors and complement in an antibody-dependent model of autoimmune vitiligo. Immunity 2002;16(6):861–8.

[40] Berinstein NL, Grillo-Lopez AJ, White CA, et al. Association of serum Rituximab (IDEC-C2B8) concentration and anti-tumor response in the treatment of recurrent low-grade or follicular non- Hodgkin's lymphoma. Ann Oncol 1998;9(9):995–1001.

[41] Colombat P, Salles G, Brousse N, et al. Rituximab (anti-CD20 monoclonal antibody) as single first-line therapy for patients with follicular lymphoma with a low tumor burden: clinical and molecular evaluation. Blood 2001;97(1):101–6.

[42] Hainsworth JD. Rituximab as first-line systemic therapy for patients with low-grade lymphoma. Semin Oncol 2000;27(6, Suppl 12):25–9.

[43] Hainsworth JD. Rituximab as first-line and maintenance therapy for patients with indolent non-Hodgkin's lymphoma: interim follow-up of a multicenter phase II trial. Semin Oncol 2002;29(1 Suppl 2):25–9.

[44] Cobleigh MA, Vogel CL, Tripathy D, et al. Multinational study of the efficacy and safety of humanized anti-HER2 monoclonal antibody in women who have HER2-overexpressing metastatic breast cancer that has progressed after chemotherapy for metastatic disease. J Clin Oncol 1999;17(9):2639–48.

[45] Vose JM, Link BK, Grossbard ML, et al. Phase II study of rituximab in combination with chop chemotherapy in patients with previously untreated, aggressive non-Hodgkin's lymphoma. J Clin Oncol 2001;19(2):389–97.

[46] Czuczman MS. CHOP plus rituximab chemoimmunotherapy of indolent B-cell lymphoma. Semin Oncol 1999;26(5 Suppl 14):88–96.

[47] Coiffier B. Rituximab in the treatment of diffuse large B-cell lymphomas. Semin Oncol 2002;29(1 Suppl 2):30–5.

[48] Carson WE, Parihar R, Lindemann MJ, et al. Interleukin-2 enhances the natural killer cell response to Herceptin- coated Her2/neu-positive breast cancer cells. Eur J Immunol 2001;31(10):3016–25.

[49] Ravetch JV, Lanier LL. Immune inhibitory receptors. Science 2000;290(5489):84–9.

[50] Liu Y, Masuda E, Blank MC, et al. Cytokine-mediated regulation of activating and inhibitory Fc gamma receptors in human monocytes. J Leukoc Biol 2005;77(5): 767–76.

[51] Pricop L, Redecha P, Teillaud JL, et al. Differential modulation of stimulatory and inhibitory Fc gamma receptors on human monocytes by Th1 and Th2 cytokines. J Immunol 2001; 166(1):531–7.

[52] Tridandapani S, Wardrop R, Baran CP, et al. TGF-beta 1 suppresses [correction of supresses] myeloid Fc gamma receptor function by regulating the expression and function of the common gamma-subunit. J Immunol 2003;170(9):4572–7.

[53] Ioan-Facsinay A, de Kimpe SJ, Hellwig SM, et al. FcgammaRI (CD64) contributes substantially to severity of arthritis, hypersensitivity responses, and protection from bacterial infection. Immunity 2002;16(3):391–402.

[54] Bevaart L, Jansen MJ, van Vugt MJ, et al. The high-affinity IgG receptor, Fc{gamma}RI, plays a central role in antibody therapy of experimental melanoma. Cancer Res 2006; 66(3):1261–4.

[55] Fossati-Jimack L, Ioan-Facsinay A, Reininger L, et al. Markedly different pathogenicity of four immunoglobulin G isotype-switch variants of an antierythrocyte autoantibody is based on their capacity to interact in vivo with the low-affinity Fcgamma receptor III. J Exp Med 2000;191(8):1293–302.

[56] Hazenbos WL, Gessner JE, Hofhuis FM, et al. Impaired IgG-dependent anaphylaxis and Arthus reaction in Fc gamma RIII (CD16) deficient mice. Immunity 1996;5(2):181–8.

[57] Hazenbos WL, Heijnen IA, Meyer D, et al. Murine IgG1 complexes trigger immune effector functions predominantly via Fc gamma RIII (CD16). J Immunol 1998;161(6):3026–32.

[58] Meyer D, Schiller C, Westermann J, et al. FcgammaRIII (CD16)-deficient mice show IgG isotype-dependent protection to experimental autoimmune hemolytic anemia. Blood 1998;92(11):3997–4002.
[59] Verbeek JS, Hazenbos WL, Capel PJ, et al. The role of FcR in immunity: lessons from gene targeting in mice. Res Immunol 1997;148(7):466–74.
[60] Nimmerjahn F, Bruhns P, Horiuchi K, et al. FcgammaRIV: a novel FcR with distinct IgG subclass specificity. Immunity 2005;23(1):41–51.
[61] Soubrane C, Tourani JM, Andrieu JM, et al. Biologic response to anti-CD16 monoclonal antibody therapy in a human immunodeficiency virus-related immune thrombocytopenic purpura patient. Blood 1993;81(1):15–9.
[62] Clynes RA, Towers TL, Presta LG, et al. Inhibitory Fc receptors modulate in vivo cytoxicity against tumor targets. Nat Med 2000;6(4):443–6.
[63] Nimmerjahn F, Ravetch JV. Divergent immunoglobulin G subclass activity through selective Fc receptor binding. Science 2005;310(5753):1510–2.
[64] Golay J, Lazzari M, Facchinetti V, et al. CD20 levels determine the in vitro susceptibility to rituximab and complement of B-cell chronic lymphocytic leukemia: further regulation by CD55 and CD59. Blood 2001;98(12):3383–9.
[65] Di Gaetano N, Cittera E, Nota R, et al. Complement activation determines the therapeutic activity of rituximab in vivo. J Immunol 2003;171(3):1581–7.
[66] Cragg MS, Glennie MJ. Antibody specificity controls in vivo effector mechanisms of anti-CD20 reagents. Blood 2004;103(7):2738–43.
[67] Bellosillo B, Villamor N, Lopez-Guillermo A, et al. Complement-mediated cell death induced by rituximab in B-cell lymphoproliferative disorders is mediated in vitro by a caspase- independent mechanism involving the generation of reactive oxygen species. Blood 2001;98(9):2771–7.
[68] Cragg MS, Morgan SM, Chan HT, et al. Complement-mediated lysis by anti-CD20 mAb correlates with segregation into lipid rafts. Blood 2003;101(3):1045–52.
[69] Teeling JL, French RR, Cragg MS, et al. Characterization of new human CD20 monoclonal antibodies with potent cytolytic activity against non-Hodgkin lymphomas. Blood 2004;104(6):1793–800.
[70] Golay J, Zaffaroni L, Vaccari T, et al. Biologic response of B lymphoma cells to anti-CD20 monoclonal antibody rituximab in vitro: CD55 and CD59 regulate complement-mediated cell lysis. Blood 2000;95(12):3900–8.
[71] Treon SP, Mitsiades C, Mitsiades N, et al. Tumor cell expression of cd59 is associated with resistance to CD20 serotherapy in patients with B-cell malignancies. J Immunother 2001;24(3):263–71.
[72] Weng WK, Levy R. Expression of complement inhibitors CD46, CD55, and CD59 on tumor cells does not predict clinical outcome after rituximab treatment in follicular non-Hodgkin lymphoma. Blood 2001;98(5):1352–7.
[73] Uchida J, Hamaguchi Y, Oliver JA, et al. The innate mononuclear phagocyte network depletes B lymphocytes through Fc receptor-dependent mechanisms during anti-CD20 antibody immunotherapy. J Exp Med 2004;199(12):1659–69.
[74] Gong Q, Ou Q, Ye S, et al. Importance of cellular microenvironment and circulatory dynamics in B cell immunotherapy. J Immunol 2005;174(2):817–26.
[75] Hamaguchi Y, Uchida J, Cain DW, et al. The peritoneal cavity provides a protective niche for B1 and conventional B lymphocytes during anti-CD20 immunotherapy in mice. J Immunol 2005;174(7):4389–99.
[76] Ottonello L, Epstein AL, Dapino P, et al. Monoclonal Lym-1 antibody-dependent cytolysis by neutrophils exposed to granulocyte-macrophage colony-stimulating factor: intervention of FcgammaRII (CD32), CD11b-CD18 integrins, and CD66b glycoproteins. Blood 1999;93(10):3505–11.
[77] van Spriel AB, Leusen JH, van Egmond M, et al. Mac-1 (CD11b/CD18) is essential for Fc receptor-mediated neutrophil cytotoxicity and immunologic synapse formation. Blood 2001;97(8):2478–86.

[78] van Spriel AB, van Ojik HH, Bakker A, et al. Mac-1 (CD11b/CD18) is crucial for effective Fc receptor-mediated immunity to melanoma. Blood 2003;101(1):253–8.

[79] Schmidt RE, Gessner JE. Fc receptors and their interaction with complement in autoimmunity. Immunol Lett 2005;100(1):56–67.

[80] Cartron G, Dacheux L, Salles G, et al. Therapeutic activity of humanized anti-CD20 monoclonal antibody and polymorphism in IgG Fc receptor FcgammaRIIIa gene. Blood 2002;99(3):754–8.

[81] Weng WK, Levy R. Two immunoglobulin G fragment C receptor polymorphisms independently predict response to rituximab in patients with follicular lymphoma. J Clin Oncol 2003;21(21):3940–7.

[82] Treon SP, Hansen M, Branagan AR, et al. Polymorphisms in FcgammaRIIIA (CD16) receptor expression are associated with clinical response to rituximab in Waldenstrom's macroglobulinemia. J Clin Oncol 2005;23(3):474–81.

[83] Farag SS, Flinn IW, Modali R, et al. Fc gamma RIIIa and Fc gamma RIIa polymorphisms do not predict response to rituximab in B-cell chronic lymphocytic leukemia. Blood 2004;103(4):1472–4.

[84] Lin TS, Flinn IW, Modali R, et al. FCGR3A and FCGR2A polymorphisms may not correlate with response to alemtuzumab in chronic lymphocytic leukemia. Blood 2005;105(1): 289–91.

[85] Schiff DE, Rae J, Martin TR, et al. Increased phagocyte Fc gammaRI expression and improved Fc gamma-receptor-mediated phagocytosis after in vivo recombinant human interferon-gamma treatment of normal human subjects. Blood 1997;90(8):3187–94.

[86] Otten MA, Rudolph E, Dechant M, et al. Immature neutrophils mediate tumor cell killing via IgA but not IgG Fc receptors. J Immunol 2005;174(9):5472–80.

[87] Hernandez-Ilizaliturri FJ, Jupudy V, Ostberg J, et al. Neutrophils contribute to the biological antitumor activity of rituximab in a non-Hodgkin's lymphoma severe combined immunodeficiency mouse model. Clin Cancer Res 2003;9(16 Pt 1):5866–73.

[88] Niitsu N, Hayama M, Okamoto M, et al. Phase I study of Rituximab-CHOP regimen in combination with granulocyte colony-stimulating factor in patients with follicular lymphoma. Clin Cancer Res 2004;10(12 Pt 1):4077–82.

[89] van der Kolk LE, Grillo-Lopez AJ, Baars JW, et al. Treatment of relapsed B-cell non-Hodgkin's lymphoma with a combination of chimeric anti-CD20 monoclonal antibodies (rituximab) and G-CSF: final report on safety and efficacy. Leukemia 2003;17(8): 1658–64.

[90] Valerius T, Elsasser D, Repp R, et al. HLA class II antibodies recruit G-CSF activated neutrophils for treatment of B cell malignancies. Leuk Lymphoma 1997;26(3–4):261–9.

[91] Stockmeyer B, Valerius T, Repp R, et al. Preclinical studies with Fc(gamma)R bispecific antibodies and granulocyte colony-stimulating factor-primed neutrophils as effector cells against HER-2/neu overexpressing breast cancer. Cancer Res 1997;57(4):696–701.

[92] Ottonello L, Epstein AL, Mancini M, et al. Chimaeric Lym-1 monoclonal antibody-mediated cytolysis by neutrophils from G-CSF-treated patients: stimulation by GM-CSF and role of Fc gamma -receptors. Br J Cancer 2001;85(3):463–9.

[93] Valerius T, Stockmeyer B, van Spriel AB, et al. FcalphaRI (CD89) as a novel trigger molecule for bispecific antibody therapy. Blood 1997;90(11):4485–92.

[94] Stockmeyer B, Dechant M, van Egmond M, et al. Triggering Fc alpha-receptor I (CD89) recruits neutrophils as effector cells for CD20-directed antibody therapy. J Immunol 2000;165(10):5954–61.

[95] Dechant M, Valerius T. IgA antibodies for cancer therapy. Crit Rev Oncol Hematol 2001; 39(1–2):69–77.

[96] Heijnen IA, Rijks LJ, Schiel A, et al. Generation of HER-2/neu-specific cytotoxic neutrophils in vivo: efficient arming of neutrophils by combined administration of granulocyte colony-stimulating factor and Fcgamma receptor I bispecific antibodies. J Immunol 1997; 159(11):5629–39.

[97] Hara I, Takechi Y, Houghton AN. Implicating a role for immune recognition of self in

tumor rejection: passive immunization against the brown locus protein. J Exp Med 1995;
182(5):1609–14.

[98] Hooijberg E, Sein JJ, van den Berk PC, et al. Eradication of large human B cell tumors in
nude mice with unconjugated CD20 monoclonal antibodies and interleukin 2. Cancer
Res 1995;55(12):2627–34.

[99] Eisenbeis CF, Grainger A, Fischer B, et al. Combination immunotherapy of B-cell non-
Hodgkin's lymphoma with rituximab and interleukin-2: a preclinical and phase I study.
Clin Cancer Res 2004;10(18 Pt 1):6101–10.

[100] Carson WE, Parihar R, Lindemann MJ, et al. Interleukin-2 enhances the natural killer cell
response to Herceptin-coated Her2/neu-positive breast cancer cells. Eur J Immunol 2001;
31(10):3016–25.

[101] Soiffer RJ, Chapman PB, Murray C, et al. Administration of R24 monoclonal antibody and low-dose interleukin 2 for malignant melanoma. Clin Cancer Res 1997;3(1):
17–24.

[102] Fleming GF, Meropol NJ, Rosner GL, et al. A phase I trial of escalating doses of
trastuzumab combined with daily subcutaneous interleukin 2: report of cancer and
leukemia group B 9661. Clin Cancer Res 2002;8(12):3718–27.

[103] Repka T, Chiorean EG, Gay J, et al. Trastuzumab and interleukin-2 in HER2-positive
metastatic breast cancer: a pilot study. Clin Cancer Res 2003;9(7):2440–6.

[104] Gluck WL, Hurst D, Yuen A, et al. Phase I studies of interleukin (IL)-2 and rituximab in
B-cell non-Hodgkin's lymphoma: IL-2 mediated natural killer cell expansion correlations
with clinical response. Clin Cancer Res 2004;10(7):2253–64.

[105] Golay J, Manganini M, Facchinetti V, et al. Rituximab-mediated antibody-dependent
cellular cytotoxicity against neoplastic B cells is stimulated strongly by interleukin-2.
Haematologica 2003;88(9):1002–12.

[106] Friedberg JW, Neuberg D, Gribben JG, et al. Combination immunotherapy with rituximab and interleukin 2 in patients with relapsed or refractory follicular non-Hodgkin's
lymphoma. Br J Haematol 2002;117(4):828–34.

[107] Keilholz U, Szelenyi H, Siehl J, et al. Rapid regression of chemotherapy refractory
lymphocyte predominant Hodgkin's disease after administration of rituximab (anti CD 20
mono-clonal antibody) and interleukin-2. Leuk Lymphoma 1999;35(5–6):641–2.

[108] Kossman SE, Scheinberg DA, Jurcic JG, et al. A phase I trial of humanized monoclonal
antibody HuM195 (anti-CD33) with low-dose interleukin 2 in acute myelogenous leukemia. Clin Cancer Res 1999;5(10):2748–55.

[109] Ansell SM. Adding cytokines to monoclonal antibody therapy: does the concurrent
administration of interleukin-12 add to the efficacy of rituximab in B-cell non-Hodgkin
lymphoma? Leuk Lymphoma 2003;44(8):1309–15.

[110] Ansell SM, Witzig TE, Kurtin PJ, et al. Phase 1 study of interleukin-12 in combination with
rituximab in patients with B-cell non-Hodgkin lymphoma. Blood 2002;99(1):67–74.

[111] Dela Cruz JS, Huang TH, Penichet ML, et al. Antibody-cytokine fusion proteins: innovative
weapons in the war against cancer. Clin Exp Med 2004;4(2):57–64.

[112] Vasovic LV, Dyall R, Clynes RA, et al. Synergy between an antibody and CD8+ cells in
eliminating an established tumor. Eur J Immunol 1997;27(2):374–82.

[113] Regnault A, Lankar D, Lacabanne V, et al. Fcgamma receptor-mediated induction of
dendritic cell maturation and major histocompatibility complex class I-restricted antigen
presentation after immune complex internalization. J Exp Med 1999;189(2):371–80.

[114] Dhodapkar KM, Krasovsky J, Williamson B, et al. Antitumor monoclonal antibodies
enhance cross-presentation ofcellular antigens and the generation of myeloma-specific
killer T cells by dendritic cells. J Exp Med 2002;195(1):125–33.

[115] Rafiq K, Bergtold A, Clynes R. Immune complex-mediated antigen presentation induces
tumor immunity. J Clin Invest 2002;110(1):71–9.

[116] Kalergis AM, Ravetch JV. Inducing tumor immunity through the selective engagement of
activating Fcgamma receptors on dendritic cells. J Exp Med 2002;195(12):1653–9.

[117] Akiyama K, Ebihara S, Yada A, et al. Targeting apoptotic tumor cells to Fc gamma R

provides efficient and versatile vaccination against tumors by dendritic cells. J Immunol 2003;170(4):1641–8.

[118] Shields RL, Namenuk AK, Hong K, et al. High resolution mapping of the binding site on human IgG1 for Fc gamma RI, Fc gamma RII, Fc gamma RIII, and FcRn and design of IgG1 variants with improved binding to the Fc gamma R. J Biol Chem 2001;276(9): 6591–604.

[119] Presta LG, Shields RL, Namenuk AK, et al. Engineering therapeutic antibodies for improved function. Biochem Soc Trans 2002;30(4):487–90.

[120] Lund J, Takahashi N, Pound JD, et al. Multiple interactions of IgG with its core oligosaccharide can modulate recognition by complement and human Fc gamma receptor I and influence the synthesis of its oligosaccharide chains. J Immunol 1996;157(11): 4963–9.

[121] Radaev S, Sun PD. Recognition of IgG by Fcgamma receptor. The role of Fc glycosylation and the binding of peptide inhibitors. J Biol Chem 2001;276(19):16478–83.

[122] Niwa R, Shoji-Hosaka E, Sakurada M, et al. Defucosylated chimeric anti-CC chemokine receptor 4 IgG1 with enhanced antibody-dependent cellular cytotoxicity shows potent therapeutic activity to T-cell leukemia and lymphoma. Cancer Res 2004;64(6):2127–33.

[123] Shields RL, Lai J, Keck R, et al. Lack of fucose on human IgG1 n-linked oligosaccharide improves binding to human Fcgamma RIII and antibody-dependent cellular toxicity. J Biol Chem 2002;277(30):26733–40.

[124] Umana P, Jean-Mairet J, Moudry R, et al. Engineered glycoforms of an antineuroblastoma IgG1 with optimized antibody-dependent cellular cytotoxic activity. Nat Biotechnol 1999;17(2):176–80.

[125] Schuster M, Umana P, Ferrara C, et al. Improved effector functions of a therapeutic monoclonal Lewis Y-specific antibody by glycoform engineering. Cancer Res 2005; 65(17):7934–41.

[126] Yamane-Ohnuki N, Kinoshita S, Inoue-Urakubo M, et al. Establishment of FUT8 knockout Chinese hamster ovary cells: an ideal host cell line for producing completely defucosylated antibodies with enhanced antibody-dependent cellular cytotoxicity. Biotechnol Bioeng 2004;87(5):614–22.

[127] Mori K, Kuni-Kamochi R, Yamane-Ohnuki N, et al. Engineering Chinese hamster ovary cells to maximize effector function of produced antibodies using FUT8 siRNA. Biotechnol Bioeng 2004;88(7):901–8.

[128] Okazaki A, Shoji-Hosaka E, Nakamura K, et al. Fucose depletion from human IgG1 oligosaccharide enhances binding enthalpy and association rate between IgG1 and FcgammaRIIIa. J Mol Biol 2004;336(5):1239–49.

[129] Ferrara C, Stuart F, Sondermann P, et al. The carbohydrate at Fcgamma RIIIa ASN162: an element required for high affinity binding to non-fucosylated IgG glycoforms. J Biol Chem 2006;281(8):5032–6.

[130] Niwa R, Hatanaka S, Shoji-Hosaka E, et al. Enhancement of the antibody-dependent cellular cytotoxicity of low-fucose IgG1 Is independent of FcgammaRIIIa functional polymorphism. Clin Cancer Res 2004;10(18 Pt 1):6248–55.

[131] Idusogie EE, Wong PY, Presta LG, et al. Engineered antibodies with increased activity to recruit complement. J Immunol 2001;166(4):2571–5.

[132] Idusogie EE, Presta LG, Gazzano-Santoro H, et al. Mapping of the C1q binding site on rituxan, a chimeric antibody with a human IgG1 Fc. J Immunol 2000;164(8):4178–84.

[133] Ghetie V, Popov S, Borvak J, et al. Increasing the serum persistence of an IgG fragment by random mutagenesis. Nat Biotechnol 1997;15(7):637–40.

[134] Clatworthy MR, Smith KG. FcgammaRIIb balances efficient pathogen clearance and the cytokine-mediated consequences of sepsis. J Exp Med 2004;199(5):717–23.

Hematol Oncol Clin N Am 20 (2006) 613–636

HEMATOLOGY/ONCOLOGY CLINICS
OF NORTH AMERICA

ELSEVIER
SAUNDERS

DNA Vaccines Against Cancer

Rodica Stan, PhD[a], Jedd D. Wolchok, MD, PhD[a,b],
Adam D. Cohen, MD[a,b,*]

[a]Department of Medicine, Memorial Sloan-Kettering Cancer Center, New York, NY, USA
[b]Weill Medical College of Cornell University, New York, NY, USA

T he origins of cancer immunotherapy are routinely traced to Dr. William Coley [1], who in 1893 published his initial observations on the use of bacterial toxins to treat patients who had cancer. Since then, investigators have focused on harnessing the power of the immune system and channeling it into the quest for better treatments for cancer. The field of cancer immunotherapy emerged and developed based on preclinical and clinical studies demonstrating that:

1. The immune system is able to recognize and eliminate tumors of various histologic types in animal models
2. The incidence of tumor formation is higher in immunodeficient mice
3. Treatment of melanoma and renal cell carcinoma with cytokines such as interleukin (IL)-2 and interferon (IFN)-alpha results in modest but reproducible response rates
4. Antibodies and tumor-infiltrating lymphocytes recognizing a host of tumor antigens can be isolated from patients who have cancer

Furthermore, success in cancer immunotherapy was reported with passive immunotherapies, such as donor leukocyte infusion after allogeneic stem cell transplantation, and monoclonal antibodies, such as rituximab, in patients who had hematologic malignancies. Despite the variety of immunization strategies designed to induce antitumor immunity, active immunotherapy has shown only anecdotal success in clinical studies [2]. This article reviews a more recent approach to the active immunotherapy of cancer, DNA vaccination.

DNA vaccines are bacterially derived plasmids that encode one or more antigens of interest. Numerous studies showed that plasmid-based DNA immunization can elicit immune responses in animals. Studies of DNA vaccines encoding human growth hormone or human α1-antitrypsin [3] and pathogen-derived antigens from influenza [4,5], malaria [6–9], tuberculosis [10], Ebola virus [11], rabies [12], lymphocytic choriomeningitis virus [13,14], herpes simplex virus [15],

* Corresponding author. Memorial Sloan-Kettering Cancer Center, 1275 York Avenue, New York, NY 10021. E-mail address: cohena@mskcc.org (A.D. Cohen).

0889-8588/06/$ – see front matter
doi:10.1016/j.hoc.2006.02.004

HIV-1 [16], and hepatitis B [17] demonstrated that this approach could generate antibody as well as CD4+ and CD8+ T-cell responses. Furthermore, DNA immunization was efficient in protecting from pathogenic microbial challenge, and its efficiency led to its application in various models of infectious disease. The safety and immunogenicity of DNA vaccines against HIV, malaria, and hepatitis B virus have been demonstrated in nonhuman primates as well as in human clinical trials [18–20].

DNA vaccination strategies also have been developed for cancer immunotherapy. This area of investigation has benefited from recent research identifying

Table 1
Tumor antigens targeted by DNA vaccines

Antigen	Therapeutic application	References
Tyrosinase	Melanoma	[21,22]
gp75/TRP-1	Melanoma	[23,24]
DCT/TRP-2	Melanoma	[25,26]
gp100	Melanoma	[27–31]
MelanA/MART-1	Melanoma	[32]
CEA	Epithelial cancers (colorectal, lung, breast, head and neck, pancreas, gastric)	[33–36]
PSA	Prostate carcinoma	[37,38]
PSMA	Prostate, renal cell carcinoma	[39,40]
Her2/neu (erbB2)	Epithelial cancers (breast, ovarian, pancreas, lung)	[41–46]
MUC1	Epithelial cancers (breast, colorectal, ovarian, pancreas)	[47,48]
Ig idiotype	B-cell NHL, myeloma	[49–51]
TCR idiotype	T cell NHL	[52]
CD20	B-cell NHL	[53]
PML/RARα	APL	[54]
bcr-abl	CML, Ph + ALL	[55]
HPV E6, E7	Cervical carcinoma	[56–58]
MAGE-1, Mage-b	Melanoma; myeloma; renal cell, lung, breast, colon, bladder, ovarian cancer	[59,60]
AFP	Hepatocellular carcinoma, germ cell tumors, cholangiocarcinoma, ovarian	[61,62]
WT1	Acute leukemias	[63]
Survivin	Most carcinomas; melanoma; neuroblastoma; CLL; NHL	[64]
p53	Multiple carcinomas (gastric, colorectal, pancreas, esophageal, cholangiocarcinoma)	[65,66]
Mutant ras	Melanoma, pancreas, colorectal, thyroid, lung, cholangiocarcinoma	[67,68]

Abbreviations: AFP, alpha fetoprotein; APL, acute promyelocytic leukemia; CEA, carcinoembryonic antigen; CLL, chronic lymphocytic leukemia; CML, chronic myelogenous leukemia; DCT, dopachrome tautomerase; HPV, human papillomavirus; Ig, immunoglobulin; MAGE, melanoma antigen; MART-1, melanoma antigen recognized by T cells 1; MUC1, mucin 1; NHL, non-Hodgkin's lymphoma; Ph + ALL, Philadelphia chromosome-positive acute lymphoblastic leukemia; PSA, prostate-specific antigen; PSMA, prostate-specific membrane antigen; TCR, T-cell receptor; TRP-1, tyrosinase-related protein 1; TRP-2, tyrosinase-related protein 2; WT1, Wilms' tumor 1.

tumor antigens and a better understanding of the mechanisms that prevent immune responses to malignancies. DNA vaccines targeting numerous tumor antigens have been extensively investigated in disease models such as melanoma, epithelial cancers (eg, breast, colon, and lung cancers), and hematologic cancers (Table 1).

MECHANISM OF ACTION OF DNA VACCINES

In most cases, DNA vaccines consist of plasmid DNA encoding the genes of interest under the control of a constitutively active promoter. In one commonly used technique, the DNA is coated onto gold microprojectiles and is injected into mouse skin using particle-mediated delivery or a "gene gun." Although originally developed as a method to introduce DNA into plant cells, particle-mediated delivery rapidly became a convenient method for efficient gene transfer into the epidermis and superficial dermis of mammalian skin. Most clinical studies to date have used intramuscular immunization; however, with the development of a "gene gun" device for human clinical use, more frequent trials of particle-mediated delivery are expected. Regardless of the route of administration, once the DNA enters the skin or muscle professional antigen-presenting cells (APCs), particularly dendritic cells (DCs), are able to present the transcribed and translated antigen in the proper context of major histocompatibility complex (MHC) and costimulatory molecules. The bacterial and plasmid DNA itself contains immunostimulatory sequences that may act as a potent immunologic adjuvant in the immune response [69].

The mechanism by which DNA vaccines induce immune responses is not fully understood, but it is clear that an initial step in the induction of immunity is the activation of the innate immune response caused by the presence of the "CpG motifs," hypomethylated cytosine-guanine (CpG) dinucleotides flanked by particular surrounding motifs. They bind to Toll-like receptor (TLR) 9 on B cells and DCs, ultimately leading to the production of interferons and interleukins. Studies in mouse models emphasize the role of bone marrow–derived APCs in the priming of immune responses by DNA vaccines. One such mechanism is based on cross-priming, whereby the gene product encoded by the DNA vaccine is secreted from transfected myocytes or keratinocytes and then is taken up by APCs such as DCs. DCs process the antigen and migrate to regional lymph nodes, where they can prime naive T cells [70,71]. In addition, APCs residing at the site of immunization can be transfected directly by plasmid, leading to endogenous transcription, translation, and antigenic processing of the encoded protein [72,73].

DNA vaccines are usually administered intramuscularly or intradermally by gene gun or needle. Some authors have suggested that intradermal and intramuscular injections induce a predominantly T-helper cell 1 (Th1) response and cellular immunity, whereas gene-gun mediated and intradermal DNA immunization triggers mainly T-helper cell 2 (Th2)-type response and humoral immunity [74–77]. This difference may result from the amount of plasmid DNA used for vaccination and the associated CpG motifs, the site of administration, the immunologic "bias" of the particular mouse strain used, or the nature of the antigen, rather than the route of administration [76,78–81].

DNA VACCINES AGAINST CANCER: THE PROBLEM OF "SELF"

Tumor antigens identified in recent years as potential targets for active immunization include viral antigens (eg, human papillomavirus 16 E6) [56], mutated oncogenes (eg, CDK4, β-catenin) [82,83], products of gene translocations (eg, bcr-abl) [84], and cancer-testes antigens (eg, melanoma antigen-A1, NY-ESO-1) (see Table 1) [85,86] These tumor antigens represent attractive targets for immune therapy with DNA vaccines because they contain novel epitopes or epitopes previously sequestered in immune-privileged sites. Nevertheless, the most prevalent tumor antigens are true "self" antigens, widely expressed molecules that are overexpressed on cancer cells (eg, carcinoembryonic antigen [CEA], mucin 1, her2/neu), or differentiation antigens gp 100, tyrosinase, prostate-specific membrane antigen [PSMA]) expressed only on specific tumors and their normal cell counterparts. Most high-avidity T and B lymphocytes specific for these tumor antigens have already been deleted from the immune repertoire through central tolerance during development. Therefore, these tumor antigens are indistinguishable from "self." Most self-reactive lymphocytes managing to escape central tolerance normally have low avidity and are maintained in the repertoire in an anergic state. This state of peripheral tolerance is possible because of the absence of proper costimulation in the presence of regulatory T cells [87]. Overcoming this type of tolerance is one of the most significant challenges for active immunization against cancer.

DNA VACCINES AGAINST MELANOMA ANTIGENS

Melanoma differentiation antigens are among the most extensively studied tumor antigens. They include tyrosinase, tyrosinase-related protein 1 (TRP-1)/gp75, TRP-2/dopachrome tautomerase (DCT), gp100, and melanA/melanoma antigen recognized by T cells 1 (MART-1). These antigens are expressed only in melanomas and normal melanocytes, with higher levels in melanoma cell lines and in samples from patients who have primary melanoma. Melanoma differentiation antigens are recognized by T cells or antibodies derived from melanoma patients [88–92], making them attractive targets for cancer vaccination strategies. In an early study of immunization against melanoma tumor antigens, active immunization of mice against TRP-1/gp75 with an unaltered syngeneic (ie, mouse) form of the antigen did not induce immune responses. When mice were immunized with xenogeneic (ie, human) TRP-1/gp75 protein (87% homology with the mouse protein), however, they developed antibodies that recognized both human and mouse TRP-1/gp75 [92]. These immunized mice were also protected from an otherwise lethal tumor challenge with the poorly immunogenic syngeneic B16 melanoma cell line [93]. In addition, mice immunized with human TRP-1/gp75, but not with the mouse counterpart, developed autoimmunity (visible as coat depigmentation), confirming that tolerance to this melanosomal self-protein had been broken.

Following this initial study, these authors [23,25,27] and others [26,28,29] demonstrated that DNA vaccines encoding xenogeneic orthologues of these melanoma differentiation antigens were an effective way to break tolerance and induce protective tumor immunity. Immunization of mice with a DNA plasmid encoding human TRP-1/gp75 led to production of antigen-specific autoantibodies and a significant decrease in the number of B16 lung metastases compared with unimmunized mice or mice immunized with a mouse TRP-1/gp75 DNA vaccine [23]. Similar protective immunity was reported with DNA vaccines encoding human TRP-2 or gp100, although with these antigens tumor immunity was mediated primarily by CD8+ T cells. Of note, immunization with the human TRP-2 plasmid led to a significant decrease in B16 lung metastases even when started 4 or 10 days after tumor challenge, when metastases were already established [25,27]. Xenogeneic melanoma DNA vaccines have also been studied preclinically in an outbred dog population with spontaneously arising melanoma. Tumor regressions and prolonged survival compared with historical controls were reported [21]. All these studies showed that xenogeneic DNA immunization can generate both antibody and T-cell responses to melanosomal self-antigens leading to protective tumor immunity and autoimmunity.

One mechanism by which xenogeneic immunization may break tolerance to self is through key amino acid differences in MHC class I or class II epitopes that lead to higher affinity for native MHC molecules than the syngeneic peptide. These so-called "heteroclitic epitopes" represent another strategy by which poorly recognized self-antigens can be altered to become immunogenic. For example, the human form of the MHC class I– restricted $gp100_{25-33}$ epitope, **KVP**RNQDWL, binds more strongly to the mouse D^b MHC class I molecule than the native mouse peptide, **EGS**RNQDWL. A DNA vaccine encoding a site-specific mutant of human gp100, in which amino acids KVP were changed to EGS, present at the same position in mouse gp100, lost its ability to induce tumor protection. Similarly, a "minigene" construct encoding only the human $gp100_{25-33}$ epitope was sufficient to induce cytotoxic T-lymphocyte (CTL) responses and protect from tumor challenge, whereas the mouse $gp100_{25-33}$ minigene had no effect [30]. In this system, a single heteroclitic epitope therefore is both necessary and sufficient to break tolerance and induce tumor immunity. These results suggest that using site-specific mutagenesis to alter known and potential MHC class I epitopes to enhance binding may be a promising strategy to optimize DNA vaccines against cancer antigens.

DNA VACCINES AGAINST OTHER TUMOR ANTIGENS

CEA is expressed in normal fetal and adult gastrointestinal tissue and is over-expressed in numerous epithelial malignancies, including colorectal, pancreas, gastric, breast, non–small cell lung, and head and neck carcinomas [94]. DNA vaccination against human CEA was shown to elicit humoral and T-cell responses as well as protective immunity against a human CEA–transduced mouse colon cancer cell line [33]. In a more relevant CEA-transgenic mouse model, widespread expression of human CEA led to a state of peripheral tolerance similar to that induced by a self-antigen. In this model, a CEA-encoding DNA vaccine could break tolerance and lead to protective immunity against CEA-expressing MC38 colon or Lewis lung carcinomas when the plasmid was administered orally through a bacterial carrier system (attenuated *Salmonella typhimurium*) [34,35]. Similar to the plasmid backbone of DNA vaccines, the bacterial carrier probably provides natural "danger" signals, such as lipopoly-saccharide and CpG motifs, which stimulate innate immunity and provide the inflammatory signals necessary to overcome tolerance.

Another well-studied antigen used for DNA vaccination is the product of the oncogene her-2/neu (erbB-2), which is overexpressed in a number of epithelial cancers, including breast, ovarian, lung, and pancreatic cancer. This oncogene is recognized by naturally arising antibodies and T cells in patients who have cancer [95,96]. Targeting this antigen for immunotherapy is supported by the success of trastuzumab, a humanized monoclonal antibody specific for the her-2/neu protein, both alone and together with chemotherapy, in improving response rates and survival of women who have breast carcinoma that overexpresses her-2/neu [97,98]. DNA vaccines encoding human or rat her-2/neu successfully generate immunity against her-2/neu in mice, leading to protection from sub-sequent challenge with a her-2/neu–expressing tumor [41–43]. In addition, vaccination with her-2/neu DNA slowed or even reversed the growth of spon-taneously arising mammary carcinomas in rat-neu transgenic mouse models [44–46]. Protective immunity was mediated by antibodies and T cells and was induced by plasmids encoding truncated her-2/neu proteins lacking the cyto-plasmic tyrosine kinase domain, which diminishes the concerns about transfect-ing host cells with a potential oncogene. Therefore, active immunotherapy targeting her-2/neu in patients who have cancers overexpressing her-2/neu is of significant importance, and initial clinical trials of this approach have already begun at the University of Washington Fred Hutchinson Cancer Center (M.L. Disis, MD, personal communication, 2005).

DNA immunization is also being used to target hematologic malignancies. Among the DNA vaccines most frequently explored in this setting are those encoding a unique portion of light- and heavy-chain variable-region sequences derived from the clone-specific immunoglobulin expressed in immunoglobulin-producing malignancies (ie, B-cell lymphomas and multiple myeloma). This unique immunoglobulin fragment, called "idiotype" (Id), is expressed only by the clonally rearranged neoplastic cell and represents a true tumor- and patient-specific antigen, because the neoplastic cells of each patient who has lymphoma or myeloma express a unique Id. Syrengelas and colleagues [49] were the first to demonstrate that a DNA vaccine encoding a murine B-cell lymphoma Id could induce anti-Id antibodies and protection from tumor challenge. Later studies reported strong anti-Id antibodies and tumor rejection in other murine lym-phoma and myeloma models with plasmids encoding single-chain variable-region fragments fused to fragment C of tetanus toxin [50,51]. A DNA vaccine encoding the clonotypic T-cell receptor Vα and Vβ sequences from a murine T-cell lymphoma fused to fragment C of tetanus toxin also induced antibody-mediated immunity from in vivo tumor challenge [52]. Another study showed that immunization of mice with DNA plasmids encoding CD20 (full-length or minigene) generated CD20-specific cytotoxic CD8+ T cells and modest tumor protection in the A20 murine B-cell lymphoma model [53]. CD20 is a surface molecule expressed by many B-cell lymphomas and has been successfully targeted with the monoclonal antibody rituximab for therapy.

CLINICAL STUDIES OF DNA VACCINES AGAINST CANCER

Despite the abundance of preclinical studies with DNA vaccines, only a limited number of reports have been published about DNA vaccine trials in cancer [22,31,32,36,37,39,99–101]. A phase I study of DNA immunization in patients who had metastatic melanoma evaluated a plasmid encoding mutated human gp100 [31]. Two mutations were introduced in the *gp100* gene (at positions 210 and 288) to produce heteroclitic epitopes with increased binding affinity for the HLA-A*0201 class I molecule. The study enrolled 22 HLA-A*0201–positive patients who received the DNA vaccine monthly for 4 months intramuscularly ($n = 10$) or intradermally ($n = 12$). Of the five patients who finished treatment, three were evaluable, but none showed gp100-specific CD8+ T-cell responses to the immunodominant $gp100_{209-217}$ or $gp100_{280-288}$ peptides, as measured by an in vitro restimulation assay. The safety and immunogenicity of a DNA vaccine encoding two human tyrosinase peptides was evaluated in another phase I trial that enrolled 26 patients who had stage IV melanoma [22]. The vaccine was administered as a continuous 4-day infusion into an inguinal lymph node, repeated every 2 weeks for four treatments, and was well tolerated. Of the total 24 evaluable patients, 11 (46%) had increased peptide-specific T-cell responses, as measured by tetramer assay. No objective tumor responses were observed. Another phase I DNA vaccine trial evaluated escalating doses of a MART-1 plasmid vaccine (100, 300, and 1000 µg) in 12 patients who had resected high-risk melanoma [32]. The DNA vaccine, which was administered intramuscularly every 6 weeks for four immunizations, was well tolerated. Nevertheless, no significant T-cell or antibody responses were noted to MART-1 or to a control hepatitis B surface antigen (HBsAg) DNA vaccine that was administered concurrently.

In a phase I/II study in patients who had advanced prostate cancer, immunization with DNA constructs encoding the extracellular domain of human PSMA or PSMA plus the costimulatory molecule CD86 induced delayed-type hypersensitivity responses, but the plasmids were less effective than a replication-deficient adenovirus vector expressing PSMA [39]. Another phase I clinical trial evaluated DNA vaccines encoding the prostate-specific antigen (PSA) administered together with the cytokines granulocyte-macrophage colony-stimulating factor (GM-CSF) and IL-2 as vaccine adjuvants in patients who had hormone-refractory prostate cancer. The vaccine was administered monthly for five immunizations, and the vaccines and adjuvants were given concomitantly. Three of the eight evaluable patients showed PSA-specific cellular immune responses measured by IFN-γ production by activated T cells. Two other patients treated in the highest dose group (900 μg DNA) experienced a rise in anti-PSA IgG, one of whom had a decline in serum PSA levels. No clinical responses were described [37,99].

A DNA vaccine encoding a chimeric Id protein, the variable heavy and light chains from each patient's tumor linked to a mouse heavy- and light-chain constant region, was evaluated in a phase I clinical trial that enrolled 12 patients who had B-cell lymphoma [100]. Nine of these patients (75%) developed anti-mouse immunoglobulin responses, and six (50%) developed modest anti-Id humoral or T-cell responses which usually were not solely specific for the patients' own Id. DNA vaccination was well tolerated, with mild-to-moderate injection-site reactions being the only adverse effect.

In a phase I study in patients who had metastatic colon cancer, a dual-expression plasmid encoding CEA and HbsAg induced T-cell proliferative responses to CEA in 4 of 17 patients (24%), but no anti-CEA antibodies or objective clinical responses were reported [36].

Several clinical trials of xenogeneic DNA vaccines are under way at Memorial Sloan-Kettering Cancer Center. Accrual and treatment have already been completed for two studies in patients who have melanoma and who received DNA vaccines encoding the melanosomal differentiation antigens tyrosinase or TRP-1/gp75. Both vaccines were well tolerated and proved safe to use. Analysis of immune responses is under way. Two additional studies with DNA vaccines in patients who have melanoma are ongoing: one evaluates the safety and immunogenicity of gp100 DNA, and the other one evaluates immunization with GM-CSF DNA in combination with MHC class I–restricted peptides from tyrosinase and gp100. In addition, a phase I clinical trial with PSMA DNA for patients who have prostate cancer and one with PSMA DNA for patients who have renal cell cancer are being performed at this center. Results from these studies will provide extensive knowledge about the xenogeneic DNA vaccine approach in humans.

So far, these initial clinical trials with DNA vaccines have shown they are safe and well tolerated in patients who have cancer, but immune and clinical responses are rare. It is possible that the DNA vaccines have been tested in a less optimal patient population (ie, in patients who had advanced metastatic disease or who had been extensively pretreated with chemotherapy or immunotherapy). On the other hand, delayed-type hypersensitivity responses and lymphoproliferation assays commonly used to evaluate immune responses in these initial trials may lack the sensitivity required to detect vaccine-induced immune responses. For more refined detection and measurement of changes in antigen-specific T-cell frequency, techniques such as ELISPOT, intracellular cytokine assays, or tetramer assays may be better suited. Other important factors for DNA vaccines that need to be considered and that require more extensive studies are the optimal administration schedule, administration site (intramuscular, intradermal, or subcutaneous), and delivery method (needle and syringe, particle bombardment, or needle-free jet injection). Furthermore, although the dose in which the vaccines are administered may be the most influential factor of immunogenicity, thus far the doses used (100–1800 µg) have been approximately one to two orders of magnitude lower (on a per-weight basis) than those commonly used in mice. To overcome this limitation, trials are being planned delivering the DNA vaccines to patients using electroporation or particle-mediated transfer. Both methods have been described in detail, and it is clear that they dramatically amplify immune responses to DNA vaccines in the preclinical setting [102–104].

The first-generation DNA vaccines have demonstrated efficacy in murine tumor models, but they may simply lack the potency necessary to treat a growing tumor with its complement of predominantly self-antigens effectively. This limited success may result, at least in part, from the absence of strong elicited immune responses and, in some cases, from the undesired polarized immune response (antibodies versus T cells instead of a combination of the two). The presence of numerous immunosuppressive and immune-escape mechanisms used by tumors in vivo [105] and the differential expression on mouse and human DC subsets of TLR9, the receptor for immunostimulatory CpG motifs present on plasmid vectors [106,107], may also hinder the potency of DNA vaccines in patients. Optimizing the structure of DNA vaccines and the use of DNA vaccines together with adjuvants are probably the most important steps in the generation of effective antitumor immunity in patients who have cancer.

MODULATING IMMUNITY TO DNA VACCINES

Although tumor antigens are weakly immunogenic, and the immune repertoire in patients may be tolerized, DNA vaccines offer the opportunity to add genes encoding molecules aimed at overcoming these constraints. One of the inherent advantages of plasmid DNA as a vaccine vector is its malleability. Thus, immunization with DNA vaccines can be manipulated to enhance the magnitude of the induced immune response and to change its type (cellular versus humoral immunity; Th1- versus Th2-type response). The ability to modulate DNA vaccine–induced immunity has been demonstrated using a number of different approaches (Table 2):

1. Coimmunization with plasmids encoding the antigen and cytokine or costimulatory molecules
2. Fusion of antigens to bacterial or viral products that provide Th epitopes, alter antigen trafficking, or stimulate innate immunity
3. Use of monoclonal antibodies to block inhibitory T-cell signaling, among others

Some of these approaches are described briefly here.

Cytokines, Chemokines, and Costimulatory Molecules

Adjuvants have always been required for vaccines using purified proteins. For DNA vaccines, although there is a natural stimulus of innate pathways from the CpG motifs, additional adjuvant activity has been extensively explored. Cytokine- and chemokine-expressing plasmids have been studied as "genetic" or "molecular" adjuvants designed to augment DNA vaccine–induced immunity

Table 2
Modulating immunity to DNA vaccines

Approach	Rationale / comment	References
Cytokine/chemokine genetic adjuvants		
IL-2	T-cell activation and proliferation	[108–114]
IL-4	Th2 bias; B-cell activation	[111,114]
IL-12	Th1 bias; enhances NK cell and CTL activity	[109,111,113, 115–117]
IL-15	Stimulates effector and memory CD8+ T cells	[109,113,118]
IL-18	CD4+ T-cell proliferation and IFN-γ production	[109,116,117, 119,120]
GM-CSF	Monocyte and DC recruitment & activation	[111,113,121,122]
IFN-γ	Macrophage activation; upregulation of MHC complexes	[111,116]
Flt3L	Expands and matures DCs	[57,113,123–126]
MIP-1α	Recruits monocytes and DCs; synergistic with Flt3L plasmid	[125,127–129]
RANTES	Recruits monocytes, T cells	[127,130,131]
MCP-1	Recruits monocytes	[127,129,130]
SLC/CCL21	CCR7 ligand; recruits and activates DCs	[64,109,129,132]
Costimulatory/adhesion molecule		
B7.1/B7.2 (CD80/CD86)	Costimulates T-cell activation	[133–135]
CD40 ligand	Activates/matures APCs	[136–138]
ICAM-1 or LFA-3	Facilitate T cell–APC interactions	[139]
Bacterial/viral products	(All enhance innate immunity)	
Tetanus toxoid FrC	Additional T-helper epitopes	[50–52]
HSV VP22	Intercellular spread of antigen	[58]
Pseudomonas exotoxin	Alters endosomal trafficking to enhance cross-presentation of antigen	[140,141]
Alphaviral replicase	Augments antigen expression; creates dsRNA (TLR3 agonist)	[24]
Klebsiella OmpA	Induces DC maturation and IL-12 production	[142]
Attenuated Salmonella typhimurium	Oral delivery vehicle; mucosal and systemic immunity	[34,35,143,144]
Mycobacterial HSP70	Enhances MHC class I presentation of antigen	[145]
Block negative T-cell signaling		
Anti-CTLA4 mAb	Blocks B7-CTLA4 interaction; enhances expansion of activated T cells	[169]
Anti-GITR mAb	Inhibits Tregs; costimulates activated effector T cells	[148a,177]
Other strategies		
Imiquimod/resiquimod	TLR7 agonist DC maturation	[148–150]
Flagellin	TLR5 agonist	[151]

(continued on next page)

Table 2 (continued)		
Approach	Rationale / comment	References
VEGFR2-, Fra-1-, or PDGF-B-expressing plasmids	Target endothelial cells; anti-angiogenesis	[152–154]
BCL-xL plasmid	Inhibits apoptosis and prolongs DC survival	[155]
Electroporation	Enhances plasmid delivery/ expression	[45,156]
Low-dose cyclophosphamide	Inhibits Tregs or boosts T-cell homeostatic proliferation	[154,157]

Abbreviations: APC, antigen-presenting cell; BCL-xL, Bcl-2 related gene (long alternatively spliced variant of Bcl-x gene); CCL21, chemokine (C-C motif) ligand 21; CTL, cytotoxic T lymphocyte; CTLA4, cytotoxic T lymphocyte antigen 4; DC, dendritic cell; dsRNA, double-stranded RNA; Flt3L, fms-like tyrosine kinase 3 ligand; Fra-1, fos-related antigen 1; FrC, fragment C; GITR, glucocorticoid-induced tumor necrosis factor receptor; GM-CSF, granulocyte/monocyte-colony stimulating factor; HSP70, heat shock protein 70; HSV, herpes simplex virus; ICAM-1, intracellular adhesion molecule 1; IFN, interferon; LFA-3, lymphocyte function associated 3; mAb, monoclonal antibody; MCP-1, monocyte chemoattractant protein 1; MHC, major histocompatibility complex; MIP, macrophage inflammatory protein; NK, natural killer; OmpA, outer membrane protein A; PDGF-B, platelet-derived growth factor B; RANTES, regulated upon activation, normal T-cell expressed, and presumably secreted; SLC, secondary lymphoid tissue cytokine; TLR, toll-like receptor; Tregs, CD4+/CD25+ regulatory T cells; VEGFR2, vascular endothelial growth factor receptor 2.

(see Table 2) [74,108,158,159]. They are normally administered simultaneously with or shortly after DNA immunization, either as separate plasmids or in bicistronic vectors with the DNA vaccine. Delivery of the cytokine from a DNA construct, rather than as recombinant protein, may allow lower manufacturing costs and the ability to generate high concentrations of cytokine at the immunization site and draining lymph nodes (where the immune response is being primed). These local, rather than systemic, effects can be enhanced further by using DNA vectors that fuse the cytokine to the Fc portion of an IgG immunoglobulin, thus theoretically increasing the stability of the protein and extending its in vivo half-life [109,110,133a,148a].

Some of the best-studied molecular adjuvants in the setting of DNA vaccines are IL-2, IL-12, and GM-CSF DNA. A wide range of effects is seen with these adjuvants. When given in combination with DNA vaccines, they enhance protection from infectious pathogens and rejection of tumors in both rodent and nonhuman primate models [38,75,108–155,158,159]; they currently are being tested as vaccine adjuvants in clinical trials.

Although IL-2 constructs can enhance humoral and cellular immunity, IL-12 plasmids contribute mainly to the increase in cytotoxic T-cell responses and the generation of memory T cells. When administered before the first vaccination to recruit DCs and other APCs to the immunization site [122,160], GM-CSF constructs led to an augmentation in priming for antibody and T-cell responses. Cytokines, such as IL-15, IL-18, and fms-like tyrosine kinase 3 (flt3) ligand, have produced encouraging results in studies of DNA vaccines in animal models. IL-15 plays an important role in enhancing both effector and memory CD8+ T-cell responses [113,118]. Several studies have demonstrated that IL-18 augments antigen-specific lymphoproliferative responses and production of the Th1 cytokines IL-2 and IFN-γ [38,116,119,120]. Coadministration of a PSA DNA vaccine with another plasmid expressing IL-18 in a mouse tumor model showed tumor protection mediated by both CD4+ and CD8+ T cells in all treated mice [161]. The flt3 ligand expands and matures DCs recruited to the site of immunization, thus leading to increased priming of humoral and T-cell responses [113,120,123–125].

Chemokines are chemoattractant molecules that regulate the trafficking of leukocytes, including monocytes, lymphocytes, DCs, eosinophils, and neutrophils. They play a significant role in the induction of nonspecific inflammatory responses and in adaptive immunity [162]. Plasmids encoding the chemokine receptor (CCR)1/CCR5 agonists macrophage inflammatory protein (MIP)-1α, MIP-1β, and regulated upon activation, normal T-cell expressed, and presumably secreted (RANTES), the CCR2 agonist monocyte chemoattractant protein-1, and the CCR7 agonist secondary lymphoid tissue cytokine/chemokine (C-C motif) ligand 21, among others, demonstrated potent adjuvant activity in preclinical studies when coinjected with DNA vaccines. This effect may be explained by the enhanced recruitment of APCs to the immunization site and increased production of inflammatory cytokines, such as IFN-γ [64,125,127–131,163]. Intramuscular injection of an HIV-1 envelope DNA vaccine without adjuvants recruited few DCs to the injection site and elicited low-frequency, envelope-specific immune responses in mice [125]. Coadministration of plasmids encoding the chemokine MIP-1α and the DC-specific growth factor flt3L with the DNA vaccine resulted in the recruitment, expansion, and activation of large numbers of DCs at the site of inoculation. Consistent with these findings, coadministration of these plasmid cytokine and chemokine acted synergistically to augment markedly the cellular and humoral immune responses elicited by the DNA vaccine and to increase protection against challenge with recombinant vaccinia virus. This study demonstrated that combining chemokine and cytokine genetic adjuvants can further enhance the effect of the DNA vaccines.

Codelivery of CD80 or CD86 genes together with DNA immunization can also boost antigen-specific cellular immune responses by improving the antigen-presenting potential of transfected host cells [133,134,138]. Costimulatory molecules such as CD80 (B7.1) and CD86 (B7.2) are expressed by activated APCs and are critical for the activation of naive T lymphocytes through secondary signaling through CD28. CD40 is another costimulatory molecule that is expressed on APCs, such as B cells, macrophages, and DCs. CD40 ligand (CD40L)/CD154 is expressed by helper CD4+ T cells. Ligation of CD40 sends an activation and maturation stimulus to the APC, enabling it to activate naive CD8+ T cells more effectively in a process termed "licensing" [164–166]. Therefore, studies evaluating DNA immunization with CD40L, either as a separate plasmid or as part of a bi-cistronic plasmid expressing the antigen also, demonstrated increased antibody and cytotoxic T-lymphocyte responses and improved protection from viral or tumor challenge [136–138,166].

Bacterial and Viral Products

Immunogenicity of DNA vaccines may be enhanced by combining the antigen of interest with a component from an infectious organism. This strategy has the advantage of providing both universal Th epitopes and inherent "danger" signals engendered by a microbial product. As mentioned previously, fusion of immunoglobulin Id genes to fragment C of tetanus toxin, which contains a "promiscuous" MHC class II–binding epitope, induced protective immunity in mouse models of lymphoma and myeloma and is currently being evaluated in clinical trials [50,51]. Herpesvirus VP22 tegument protein and the translocation domain of *Pseudomonas* exotoxin A also have been fused to tumor antigens and studied in animal models. They alter inter- or intracellular antigen trafficking, respectively, and enhance MHC class I presentation. As a consequence, the fusion vaccines significantly enhanced antigen-specific CD8+ T-cell responses and improved protection from tumor challenge [58,133a,140,141]. In contrast to the lack of induced immunity with a DNA vaccine encoding syngeneic mouse gp75/TYRP1 (mgp75), the DNA vaccine expressing mgp75 under control of an alphaviral replicase enzyme was able to break tolerance, induced autoantibodies, and protected mice from challenge with B16 melanoma [24]. This effect was not the result of an anticipated enhanced antigen expression but probably resulted from the production of double-stranded RNA, which is a byproduct of replicase-mediated gene expression as well as a TLR3 agonist and a potent stimulator of innate immunity [167]. Oral delivery of DNA vaccines using an attenuated *Salmonella typhimurium* strain as a carrier also has led to the generation of strong T-cell responses against viral and tumor antigens and potentially may be used to induce specific mucosal immunity [34,35,143,144].

Targeting Negative Regulatory Mechanisms

Blocking inhibitory responses that lead to the suppression of anti-tumor immunity is another strategy that has been studied in relation to the modulation of DNA vaccination against cancer. In recent years, two such approaches that use monoclonal antibodies to target cytotoxic T-lymphocyte antigen 4 (CTLA-4) and glucocorticoid-induced tumor necrosis factor receptor family–related gene (GITR) have been studied in combination with DNA vaccination. CTLA-4 is a homologue of CD28 that binds to CD80 and CD86, and its expression is increased on CD4+ and CD8+ T cells after T-cell receptor (TCR)-mediated activation. CTLA-4 is also expressed constitutively on CD4+/CD25+ regulatory T cells (Tregs), although its exact function on these cells remains unclear. Ligation of CTLA-4 results in the inhibition of T-cell activation and is a checkpoint in controlling antigen-specific T-cell proliferation and effector activity [168]. It has been shown that combining anti-CTLA-4 antibody and xenogeneic DNA vaccines encoding melanoma or prostate differentiation antigens enhanced antigen-specific CD8+ T cell responses and tumor rejection [169].

This effect was observed only when the anti-CTLA-4 antibody was administered during the second or third of three weekly vaccinations and not when given before the initial DNA immunization. Thus, T cells may need to be activated in advance for this approach to become effective. Nevertheless, based on preclinical studies showing that antagonist anti-CTLA-4 antibodies enhance T-cell responses to whole-cell tumor vaccines in murine models [170], these antibodies are being evaluated alone or in combination with peptide vaccination in patients who have cancer. Results from these initial clinical trials are encouraging and demonstrate tumor immunity (significant clinical responses) and autoimmunity [171–173].

GITR belongs to the family of tumor necrosis factor receptors and has significant homology to the costimulatory molecules OX40, 4-1BB, and CD27. Similar to CTLA-4, GITR is expressed at low levels on resting CD4+ and CD8+ T cells, but its expression is increased after T-cell activation. It is also expressed constitutively at high levels on Tregs [174]. Ligation of GITR on activated T cells enhances costimulation and proliferation [175,176]. It is expected that use of an agonist anti-GITR antibody may enhance the effect of tumor immunotherapy by costimulating tumor-specific effector T cells and by inhibiting the immunosuppressive effects of Tregs. Sakaguchi and colleagues [177] have demonstrated that an agonist anti-GITR antibody can induce regression of early-stage, modestly immunogenic murine tumors. Moreover, this effect was enhanced by combining anti-GITR and anti-CTLA-4 treatments, supporting the hypothesis that the two antibodies may target distinct cell populations.

Studies from the authors' laboratory showed that when anti-GITR antibody was administered in combination with xenogeneic DNA vaccines encoding the melanoma differentiation antigens gp100 or TRP-2, primary and recall CD8+ T-cell responses were enhanced, and rejection of the poorly immunogenic B16 melanoma cell line was improved (Cohen AD, Diab A, Perales MA, et al, unpublished manuscript, 2006). Similar to CTLA-4 blockade, GITR ligation was not effective before the initial vaccination, re-emphasizing the requirement for prior activation of T cells. Nevertheless, these preclinical results strongly support the use of anti-GITR and anti-CTLA-4 antibodies in combination with DNA vaccines against cancer.

SUMMARY

DNA vaccines can be pictured as simple vehicles for in vivo transfection and antigen production. DNA vaccines present several advantages over other vaccination strategies against cancer. They are relatively inexpensive to prepare in large quantities and have better stability than protein or peptide vaccines. Because they encode the entire sequence of a tumor antigen, DNA vaccines also provide multiple potential epitopes for binding to MHC class I and class II molecules as well as to antibodies. DNA vaccines do not target an HLA-restricted patient population as peptide vaccines do, and unlike autologous tumor or DC vaccines, they do not require extensive ex vivo preparation of patient samples.

DNA vaccination avoids the need for in vitro growth of virulent microorganisms and purification and modification of protein/peptide preparations and also circumvents the impact on vaccine efficacy of pre-existing immunity to the carrier organism. Unlike live, modified viral vaccines, DNA vaccines do not induce potentially neutralizing immunity against immunodominant viral antigens and produce no concerns about virulence in immunosuppressed patients.

An additional advantage with DNA vaccines is that their bacterial plasmid backbone contains immunostimulatory sequences known as "CpG motifs." By binding mainly to TLR9 on B cells and DCs, the CpG motifs promote B-cell activation and lead to natural-killer cell and T-cell activation by DCs, which in turn produce interferons and interleukins [146,147,178]. Finally, by providing a natural, inflammatory "danger signal" that connects innate and acquired immunity, DNA vaccines containing immunostimulatory sequences in the form of CpG motifs attenuate the need for adjuvants [179].

DNA immunization has already proved to be an essential approach to cancer immunotherapy in preclinical models because it can deliver tumor antigens to specific processing pathways. Numerous strategies designed to optimize and augment the immunogenicity of these vaccines have been identified. A vast amount of laboratory data demonstrates that DNA vaccines have significant potency in stimulating innate and adaptive immunity against a wide variety of tumor antigens. Although this stimulation remains to be achieved in patients, early clinical trials in cancer have demonstrated the safety of DNA vaccination. Further studies must focus on testing the next generation of vaccines and adjuvant strategies in humans, with particular attention to determining the optimal dose, timing, and method of administration, because these parameters may differ significantly from those seen in animal models. Ultimately, combining DNA vaccination with other immunotherapeutic approaches, such as adoptive cellular therapy, other vaccines (eg, "prime-boost"), immunomodulatory chemotherapy, activation of innate immunity using TLRs, or anti-Treg strategies may be the most effective way to develop a comprehensive immune-based treatment regimen for cancer.

References

[1] Coley WB. For treatment of malignant tumors by repeated inoculations of erysipelas with a report of ten original cases. Am J Med Sci 1893;105:487–511.

[2] Rosenberg SA, Yang JC, Restifo NP. Cancer immunotherapy: moving beyond current vaccines. Nat Med 2004;10(9):909–15.

[3] Tang DC, DeVit M, Johnston SA. Genetic immunization is a simple method for eliciting an immune response. Nature 1992;356(6365):152–4.

[4] Ulmer JB, Donnelly JJ, Parker SE, et al. Heterologous protection against influenza by injection of DNA encoding a viral protein. Science 1993;259(5102):1745–9.

[5] Fynan EF, Webster RG, Fuller DH, et al. DNA vaccines: protective immunizations by parenteral, mucosal, and gene-gun immunizations. Proc Natl Acad Sci U S A 1993;90: 11478–82.

[6] Becker SI, Wang R, Hedstrom RC, et al. Protection of mice against *Plasmodium yoelii* sporozoite challenge with *P. yoelii* merozoite surface protein 1 DNA vaccines. Infect Immun 1998;66(7):3457–61.

[7] Doolan DL, Sedegah M, Hedstrom RC, et al. Circumventing genetic restriction of protection against malaria with multigene DNA immunization: CD8 + cell-, interferon gamma-, and nitric oxide-dependent immunity. J Exp Med 1996;183(4):1739–46.

[8] Gardner MJ, Doolan DL, Hedstrom RC, et al. DNA vaccines against malaria: immunogenicity and protection in a rodent model. J Pharm Sci 1996;85(12):1294–300.

[9] Sedegah M, Hedstrom R, Hobart P, et al. Protection against malaria by immunization with plasmid DNA encoding circumsporozoite protein. Proc Natl Acad Sci U S A 1994; 91(21):9866–70.

[10] Tascon RE, Colston MJ, Ragno S, et al. Vaccination against tuberculosis by DNA injection. Nat Med 1996;2(8):888–92.

[11] Xu L, Sanchez A, Yang Z, et al. Immunization for Ebola virus infection. Nat Med 1998; 4(1):37–42.

[12] Lodmell DL, Ray NB, Parnell MJ, et al. DNA immunization protects nonhuman primates against rabies virus. Nat Med 1998;4(8):949–52.

[13] Martins LP, Lau LL, Asano MS, et al. DNA vaccination against persistent viral infection. J Virol 1995;69(4):2574–82.

[14] Yokoyama M, Zhang J, Whitton JL. DNA immunization confers protection against lethal lymphocytic choriomeningitis virus infection. J Virol 1995;69(4):2684–8.

[15] Manickan E, Yu Z, Rouse RJ, et al. Induction of protective immunity against herpes simplex virus with DNA encoding the immediate early protein ICP 27. Viral Immunol 1995; 8(2):53–61.

[16] Wang B, Ugen KE, Srikantan V, et al. Gene inoculation generates immune responses against human immunodeficiency virus type 1. Proc Natl Acad Sci U S A 1993;90(9): 4156–60.

[17] Davis HL, Michel ML, Mancini M, et al. Direct gene transfer in skeletal muscle: plasmid DNA-based immunization against the hepatitis B virus surface antigen. Vaccine 1994; 12(16):1503–9.

[18] Wang R, Doolan DL, Le TP, et al. Induction of antigen-specific cytotoxic T lymphocytes in humans by a malaria DNA vaccine. Science 1998;282(5388):476–80.

[19] MacGregor RR, Boyer JD, Ugen KE, et al. First human trial of a DNA-based vaccine for treatment of human immunodeficiency virus type 1 infection: safety and host response. J Infect Dis 1998;178(1):92–100.

[20] Rottinghaus ST, Poland GA, Jacobson RM, et al. Hepatitis B DNA vaccine induces protective antibody responses in human non-responders to conventional vaccination. Vaccine 2003;21(31):4604–8.

[21] Bergman PJ, McKnight J, Novosad A, et al. Long-term survival of dogs with advanced malignant melanoma after DNA vaccination with xenogeneic human tyrosinase: a phase I trial. Clin Cancer Res 2003;9(4):1284–90.

[22] Tagawa ST, Lee P, Snively J, et al. Phase I study of intranodal delivery of a plasmid DNA vaccine for patients with stage IV melanoma. Cancer 2003;98(1):144–54.

[23] Weber LW, Bowne WB, Wolchok JD, et al. Tumor immunity and autoimmunity induced by immunization with homologous DNA. J Clin Invest 1998;102:1258–64.

[24] Leitner WW, Hwang LN, DeVeer MJ, et al. Alphavirus-based DNA vaccine breaks immunological tolerance by activating innate antiviral pathways. Nat Med 2003;9(1): 33–9.

[25] Bowne WB, Srinivasan R, Wolchok JD, et al. Coupling and uncoupling of tumor immunity and autoimmunity. J Exp Med 1999;190(11):1717–22.

[26] Steitz J, Bruck J, Steinbrink K, et al. Genetic immunization of mice with human tyrosinase-related protein 2: implications for the immunotherapy of melanoma. Int J Cancer 2000; 86(1):89–94.

[27] Hawkins WG, Gold JS, Dyall R, et al. Immunization with DNA coding for gp100 results in CD4 T-cell independent antitumor immunity. Surgery 2000;128(2):273–80.

[28] Rakhmilevich AL, Imboden M, Hao Z, et al. Effective particle-mediated vaccination against mouse melanoma by coadministration of plasmid DNA encoding Gp100

and granulocyte-macrophage colony-stimulating factor. Clin Cancer Res 2001;7(4): 952–61.

[29] Schreurs MW, de Boer AJ, Figdor CG, et al. Genetic vaccination against the melanocyte lineage-specific antigen gp100 induces cytotoxic T lymphocyte-mediated tumor protection. Cancer Res 1998;58(12):2509–14.

[30] Gold JS, Ferrone CR, Guevara-Patino JA, et al. A single heteroclitic epitope determines cancer immunity after xenogeneic DNA immunization against a tumor differentiation antigen. J Immunol 2003;170(10):5188–94.

[31] Rosenberg SA, Yang JC, Sherry RM, et al. Inability to immunize patients with metastatic melanoma using plasmid DNA encoding the gp100 melanoma-melanocyte antigen. Hum Gene Ther 2003;14(8):709–14.

[32] Triozzi PL, Aldrich W, Allen KO, et al. Phase I study of a plasmid DNA vaccine encoding MART-1 in patients with resected melanoma at risk for relapse. J Immunother 2005; 28(4):382–8.

[33] Conry RM, LoBuglio AF, Loechel F, et al. A carcinoembryonic antigen polynucleotide vaccine has in vivo antitumor activity. Gene Ther 1995;2(1):59–65.

[34] Niethammer AG, Primus FJ, Xiang R, et al. An oral DNA vaccine against human carcinoembryonic antigen (CEA) prevents growth and dissemination of Lewis lung carcinoma in CEA transgenic mice. Vaccine 2001;20(3–4):421–9.

[35] Zhou H, Luo Y, Mizutani M, et al. A novel transgenic mouse model for immunological evaluation of carcinoembryonic antigen-based DNA minigene vaccines. J Clin Invest 2004;113(12):1792–8.

[36] Conry RM, Curiel DT, Strong TV, et al. Safety and immunogenicity of a DNA vaccine encoding carcinoembryonic antigen and hepatitis B surface antigen in colorectal carcinoma patients. Clin Cancer Res 2002;8(9):2782–7.

[37] Pavlenko M, Roos AK, Lundqvist A, et al. A phase I trial of DNA vaccination with a plasmid expressing prostate-specific antigen in patients with hormone-refractory prostate cancer. Br J Cancer 2004;91(4):688–94.

[38] Kim JJ, Yang JS, Dang K, et al. Engineering enhancement of immune responses to DNA-based vaccines in a prostate cancer model in rhesus macaques through the use of cytokine gene adjuvants. Clin Cancer Res 2001;7(3 Suppl):882s–9s.

[39] Mincheff M, Tchakarov S, Zoubak S, et al. Naked DNA and adenoviral immunizations for immunotherapy of prostate cancer: a phase I/II clinical trial. Eur Urol 2000;38(2): 208–17.

[40] Gregor PD, Wolchok JD, Turaga V, et al. Induction of autoantibodies to syngeneic prostate-specific membrane antigen by xenogeneic vaccination. Int J Cancer 2005; 116(3):415–21.

[41] Chen Y, Hu D, Eling DJ, et al. DNA vaccines encoding full-length or truncated Neu induce protective immunity against Neu-expressing mammary tumors. Cancer Res 1998;58(9): 1965–71.

[42] Piechocki MP, Pilon SA, Wei WZ. Complementary antitumor immunity induced by plasmid DNA encoding secreted and cytoplasmic human ErbB-2. J Immunol 2001; 167(6):3367–74.

[43] Foy TM, Bannink J, Sutherland RA, et al. Vaccination with Her-2/neu DNA or protein subunits protects against growth of a Her-2/neu-expressing murine tumor. Vaccine 2001; 19(17–19):2598–606.

[44] Amici A, Venanzi FM, Concetti A. Genetic immunization against neu/erbB2 transgenic breast cancer. Cancer Immunol Immunother 1998;47(4):183–90.

[45] Quaglino E, Iezzi M, Mastini C, et al. Electroporated DNA vaccine clears away multi-focal mammary carcinomas in her-2/neu transgenic mice. Cancer Res 2004;64(8): 2858–64.

[46] Spadaro M, Ambrosino E, Iezzi M, et al. Cure of mammary carcinomas in Her-2 trans-genic mice through sequential stimulation of innate (neoadjuvant Interleukin-12) and adaptive (DNA vaccine electroporation) immunity. Clin Cancer Res 2005;11(5):1941–52.

[47] Johnen H, Kulbe H, Pecher G. Long-term tumor growth suppression in mice immunized with naked DNA of the human tumor antigen mucin (MUC1). Cancer Immunol Immunother 2001;50(7):356–60.

[48] Kontani K, Taguchi O, Ozaki Y, et al. Novel vaccination protocol consisting of injecting MUC1 DNA and nonprimed dendritic cells at the same region greatly enhanced MUC1-specific antitumor immunity in a murine model. Cancer Gene Ther 2002;9(4):330–7.

[49] Syrengelas AD, Chen TT, Levy R. DNA immunization induces protective immunity against B-cell lymphoma. Nat Med 1996;2(9):1038–41.

[50] King CA, Spellerberg MB, Zhu D, et al. DNA vaccines with single-chain Fv fused to fragment C of tetanus toxin induce protective immunity against lymphoma and myeloma. Nat Med 1998;4(11):1281–6.

[51] Stevenson FK, Ottensmeier CH, Johnson P, et al. DNA vaccines to attack cancer. Proc Natl Acad Sci U S A 2004;101(Suppl2):14646–52.

[52] Thirdborough SM, Radcliffe JN, Friedmann PS, et al. Vaccination with DNA encoding a single-chain TCR fusion protein induces anticlonotypic immunity and protects against T-cell lymphoma. Cancer Res 2002;62(6):1757–60.

[53] Palomba ML, Roberts WK, Dao T, et al. CD8 + T-cell-dependent immunity following xenogeneic DNA immunization against CD20 in a tumor challenge model of B-cell lymphoma. Clin Cancer Res 2005;11(1):370–9.

[54] Padua RA, Larghero J, Robin M, et al. PML-RARA-targeted DNA vaccine induces protective immunity in a mouse model of leukemia. Nat Med 2003;9(11):1413–7.

[55] Sun J-Y, Krouse RS, Forman SJ, et al. Immunogenicity of a p210BCR-ABL fusion domain candidate DNA vaccine targeted to dendritic cells by a recombinant adeno-associated virus vector in vitro. Cancer Res 2002;62(11):3175–83.

[56] Wlazlo AP, Deng H, Giles-Davis W, et al. DNA vaccines against the human papillomavirus type 16 E6 or E7 oncoproteins. Cancer Gene Ther 2004;11(6):457–64.

[57] Hung CF, Hsu KF, Cheng WF, et al. Enhancement of DNA vaccine potency by linkage of antigen gene to a gene encoding the extracellular domain of Fms-like tyrosine kinase 3-ligand. Cancer Res 2001;61(3):1080–8.

[58] Hung CF, Cheng WF, Chai CY, et al. Improving vaccine potency through intercellular spreading and enhanced MHC class I presentation of antigen. J Immunol 2001;166(9):5733–40.

[59] Park JH, Kim CJ, Lee JH, et al. Effective immunotherapy of cancer by DNA vaccination. Mol Cells 1999;9(4):384–91.

[60] Sypniewska RK, Hoflack L, Tarango M, et al. Prevention of metastases with a Mage-b DNA vaccine in a mouse breast tumor model: potential for breast cancer therapy. Breast Cancer Res Treat 2005;91(1):19–28.

[61] Hanke P, Serwe M, Dombrowski F, et al. DNA vaccination with AFP-encoding plasmid DNA prevents growth of subcutaneous AFP-expressing tumors and does not interfere with liver regeneration in mice. Cancer Gene Ther 2002;9(4):346–55.

[62] Meng WS, Butterfield LH, Ribas A, et al. Alpha-fetoprotein-specific tumor immunity induced by plasmid prime-adenovirus boost genetic vaccination. Cancer Res 2001; 61(24):8782–6.

[63] Tsuboi A, Oka Y, Ogawa H, et al. Cytotoxic T-lymphocyte responses elicited to Wilms' tumor gene WT1 product by DNA vaccination. J Clin Immunol 2000;20(3):195–202.

[64] Xiang R, Mizutani N, Luo Y, et al. A DNA vaccine targeting survivin combines apoptosis with suppression of angiogenesis in lung tumor eradication. Cancer Res 2005;65(2): 553–61.

[65] Deng H, Kowalczyk D, O I, et al. A modified DNA vaccine to p53 induces protective immunity to challenge with a chemically induced sarcoma cell line. Cell Immunol 2002; 215(1):20–31.

[66] Tuting T, Gambotto A, Robbins PD, et al. Co-delivery of T helper 1-biasing cytokine genes enhances the efficacy of gene gun immunization of mice: studies with the model tumor antigen beta-galactosidase and the BALB/c Meth A p53 tumor-specific antigen. Gene Ther 1999;6(4):629–36.

[67] Lindinger P, Mostbock S, Hammerl P, et al. Induction of murine ras oncogene peptide-specific T cell responses by immunization with plasmid DNA-based minigene vectors. Vaccine 2003;21(27–30):4285–96.

[68] Bristol JA, Orsini C, Lindinger P, et al. Identification of a ras oncogene peptide that contains both CD4(+) and CD8(+) T cell epitopes in a nested configuration and elicits both T cell subset responses by peptide or DNA immunization. Cell Immunol 2000; 205(2):73–83.

[69] Wloch MK, Pasquini S, Ertl HC, et al. The influence of DNA sequence on the immuno-stimulatory properties of plasmid DNA vectors. Hum Gene Ther 1998;9(10):1439–47.

[70] Casares S, Inaba K, Brumeanu TD, et al. Antigen presentation by dendritic cells after immunization with DNA encoding a major histocompatibility complex class II-restricted viral epitope. J Exp Med 1997;186(9):1481–6.

[71] Corr M, von Damm A, Lee DJ, et al. In vivo priming by DNA injection occurs pre-dominantly by antigen transfer. J Immunol 1999;163(9):4721–7.

[72] Porgador A, Irvine KR, Iwasaki A, et al. Predominant role for directly transfected dendritic cells in antigen presentation to CD8(+) T cells after gene gun immunization. J Exp Med 1998;188(6):1075–82.

[73] Akbari O, Panjwani N, Garcia S, et al. DNA vaccination: transfection and activation of dendritic cells as key events for immunity. J Exp Med 1999;189(1):169–78.

[74] Barry MA, Johnston SA. Biological features of genetic immunization. Vaccine 1997; 15(8):788–91.

[75] Cohen AD, Boyer JD, Weiner DB. Modulating the immune response to genetic immuni-zation. FASEB J 1998;12(15):1611–26.

[76] Feltquate DM, Heaney S, Webster RG, et al. Different T helper cell types and antibody isotypes generated by saline and gene gun DNA immunization. J Immunol 1997;158(5): 2278–84.

[77] Schirmbeck R, Reimann J. Modulation of gene-gun-mediated Th2 immunity to hepatitis B surface antigen by bacterial CpG motifs or IL-12. Intervirology 2001;44(2–3):115–23.

[78] Aberle JH, Aberle SW, Allison SL, et al. A DNA immunization model study with constructs expressing the tick-borne encephalitis virus envelope protein E in different physical forms. J Immunol 1999;163(12):6756–61.

[79] Haddad D, Liljeqvist S, Stahl S, et al. Differential induction of immunoglobulin G subclasses by immunization with DNA vectors containing or lacking a signal sequence. Immunol Lett 1998;61(2–3):201–4.

[80] Pertmer TM, Roberts TR, Haynes JR. Influenza virus nucleoprotein-specific immunoglobulin G subclass and cytokine responses elicited by DNA vaccination are dependent on the route of vector DNA delivery. J Virol 1996;70(9):6119–25.

[81] Zhou X, Zheng L, Liu L, et al. T helper 2 immunity to hepatitis B surface antigen primed by gene-gun-mediated DNA vaccination can be shifted towards T helper 1 immunity by codelivery of CpG motif-containing oligodeoxynucleotides. Scand J Immunol 2003; 58(3):350–7.

[82] Wolfel T, Hauer M, Schneider J, et al. A p16INK4a-insensitive CDK4 mutant targeted by cytolytic T lymphocytes in a human melanoma. Science 1995;269(5228):1281–4.

[83] Robbins PF, El-Gamil M, Li YF, et al. A mutated beta-catenin gene encodes a melanoma-specific antigen recognized by tumor infiltrating lymphocytes. J Exp Med 1996;183: 1185–92.

[84] Pinilla-Ibarz J, Cathcart K, Korontsvit T, et al. Vaccination of patients with chronic mye-logenous leukemia with bcr-abl oncogene breakpoint fusion peptides generates specific immune responses. Blood 2000;95(5):1781–7.

[85] Scanlan MJ, Gure AO, Jungbluth AA, et al. Cancer/testis antigens: an expanding family of targets for cancer immunotherapy. Immunol Rev 2002;188:22–32.

[86] Segal NH, Blachere NE, Guevara-Patino JA, et al. Identification of cancer-testis genes expressed by melanoma and soft tissue sarcoma using bioinformatics. Cancer Immun 2005;5:2.

[87] O'Garra A, Vieira P. Regulatory T cells and mechanisms of immune system control. Nat Med 2004;10(8):801–5.

[88] Brichard V, Van Pel A, Wolfel T, et al. The tyrosinase gene codes for an antigen recognized by autologous cytolytic T lymphocytes on HLA-A2 melanomas. J Exp Med 1993;178(2):489–95.

[89] Wang RF, Appella E, Kawakami Y, et al. Identification of TRP-2 as a human tumor antigen recognized by cytotoxic T lymphocytes. J Exp Med 1996;184(6):2207–16.

[90] Bakker AB, Schreurs MW, de Boer AJ, et al. Melanocyte lineage-specific antigen gp100 is recognized by melanoma-derived tumor-infiltrating lymphocytes. J Exp Med 1994; 179(3):1005–9.

[91] Kawakami Y, Eliyahu S, Delgado CH, et al. Cloning of the gene coding for a shared human melanoma antigen recognized by autologous T cells infiltrating into tumor. Proc Natl Acad Sci U S A 1994;91(9):3515–9.

[92] Vijayasaradhi S, Bouchard B, Houghton AN. The melanoma antigen gp75 is the human homologue of the mouse b (brown) locus gene product. J Exp Med 1990;171(4):1375–80.

[93] Naftzger C, Takechi Y, Kohda H, et al. Immune response to a differentiation antigen induced by altered antigen: a study of tumor rejection and autoimmunity. Proc Natl Acad Sci U S A 1996;93(25):14809–14.

[94] Marshall J. Carcinoembryonic antigen-based vaccines. Semin Oncol 2003;30(3Suppl 8): 30–6.

[95] Disis ML, Calenoff E, McLaughlin G, et al. Existent T-cell and antibody immunity to HER-2/neu protein in patients with breast cancer. Cancer Res 1994;54(1):16–20.

[96] Peoples GE, Goedegebuure PS, Smith R, et al. Breast and ovarian cancer-specific cytotoxic T lymphocytes recognize the same HER2/neu-derived peptide. Proc Natl Acad Sci U S A 1995;92(2):432–6.

[97] Slamon DJ, Leyland-Jones B, Shak S, et al. Use of chemotherapy plus a monoclonal antibody against HER2 for metastatic breast cancer that overexpresses HER2. N Engl J Med 2001;344(11):783–92.

[98] Vogel CL, Cobleigh MA, Tripathy D, et al. Efficacy and safety of trastuzumab as a single agent in first-line treatment of HER2-overexpressing metastatic breast cancer. J Clin Oncol 2002;20(3):719–26.

[99] Miller AM, Ozenci V, Kiessling R, et al. Immune monitoring in a phase 1 trial of a PSA DNA vaccine in patients with hormone-refractory prostate cancer. J Immunother 2005;28(4):389–95.

[100] Timmerman JM, Singh G, Hermanson G, et al. Immunogenicity of a plasmid DNA vaccine encoding chimeric idiotype in patients with B-cell lymphoma. Cancer Res 2002; 62(20):5845–52.

[101] Smith CL, Dunbar PR, Mirza F, et al. Recombinant modified vaccinia Ankara primes functionally activated CTL specific for a melanoma tumor antigen epitope in melanoma patients with a high risk of disease recurrence. Int J Cancer 2005;113(2):259–66.

[102] Dupuis M, Denis-Mize K, Woo C, et al. Distribution of DNA vaccines determines their immunogenicity after intramuscular injection in mice. J Immunol 2000;165(5):2850–8.

[103] Mathiesen I. Electropermeabilization of skeletal muscle enhances gene transfer in vivo. Gene Ther 1999;6(4):508–14.

[104] O'Hagan D, Singh M, Ugozzoli M, et al. Induction of potent immune responses by cationic microparticles with adsorbed human immunodeficiency virus DNA vaccines. J Virol 2001;75(19):9037–43.

[105] Zou W. Immunosuppressive networks in the tumour environment and their therapeutic relevance. Nat Rev Cancer 2005;5(4):263–74.

[106] Kadowaki N, Ho S, Antonenko S, et al. Subsets of human dendritic cell precursors express different Toll-like receptors and respond to different microbial antigens. J Exp Med 2001;194(6):863–70.

[107] Hochrein H, O'Keeffe M, Wagner H. Human and mouse plasmacytoid dendritic cells. Hum Immunol 2002;63(12):1103–10.

[108] Prud'homme GJ. DNA vaccination against tumors. J Gene Med 2005;7(1):3–17.

[109] Barouch DH, Santra S, Schmitz JE, et al. Control of viremia and prevention of clinical AIDS in rhesus monkeys by cytokine-augmented DNA vaccination. Science 2000;290: 486–92.

[110] Barouch DH, Truitt DM, Letvin NL. Expression kinetics of the interleukin-2/immunoglobulin (IL-2/Ig) plasmid cytokine adjuvant. Vaccine 2004;22(23–24):3092–7.

[111] Chow YH, Chiang BL, Lee YL, et al. Development of Th1 and Th2 populations and the nature of immune responses to hepatitis B virus DNA vaccines can be modulated by codelivery of various cytokine genes. J Immunol 1998;160(3):1320–9.

[112] Bertley FM, Kozlowski PA, Wang SW, et al. Control of simian/human immunodeficiency virus viremia and disease progression after IL-2-augmented DNA-modified vaccinia virus Ankara nasal vaccination in nonhuman primates. J Immunol 2004;172(6):3745–57.

[113] Moore AC, Kong WP, Chakrabarti BK, et al. Effects of antigen and genetic adjuvants on immune responses to human immunodeficiency virus DNA vaccines in mice. J Virol 2002; 76(1):243–50.

[114] Geissler M, Gesien A, Tokushige K, et al. Enhancement of cellular and humoral immune responses to hepatitis C virus core protein using DNA-based vaccines augmented with cytokine-expressing plasmids. J Immunol 1997;158(3):1231–7.

[115] Sin JI, Kim JJ, Arnold RL, et al. IL-12 gene as a DNA vaccine adjuvant in a herpes mouse model: IL-12 enhances Th1-type CD4 + T cell-mediated protective immunity against herpes simplex virus-2 challenge. J Immunol 1999;162(5):2912–21.

[116] Kim JJ, Nottingham LK, Tsai A, et al. Antigen-specific humoral and cellular immune responses can be modulated in rhesus macaques through the use of IFN-gamma, IL-12, or IL-18 gene adjuvants. J Med Primatol 1999;28(4–5):214–23.

[117] Kim JJ, Yang JS, Manson KH, et al. Modulation of antigen-specific cellular immune responses to DNA vaccination in rhesus macaques through the use of IL-2, IFN-gamma, or IL-4 gene adjuvants. Vaccine 2001;19(17–19):2496–505.

[118] Kutzler MA, Robinson TM, Chattergoon MA, et al. Coimmunization with an optimized IL-15 plasmid results in enhanced function and longevity of CD8 T cells that are partially independent of CD4 T cell help. J Immunol 2005;175(1):112–23.

[119] Billaut-Mulot O, Idziorek T, Loyens M, et al. Modulation of cellular and humoral immune responses to a multiepitopic HIV-1 DNA vaccine by interleukin-18 DNA immunization/ viral protein boost. Vaccine 2001;19(20–22):2803–11.

[120] Zhu M, Xu X, Liu H, et al. Enhancement of DNA vaccine potency against herpes simplex virus 1 by co-administration of an interleukin-18 expression plasmid as a genetic adjuvant. J Med Microbiol 2003;52(Pt 3):223–8.

[121] Weiss WR, Ishii KJ, Hedstrom RC, et al. A plasmid encoding murine granulocyte-macrophage colony-stimulating factor increases protection conferred by a malaria DNA vaccine. J Immunol 1998;161(5):2325–32.

[122] Perales MA, Fantuzzi G, Goldberg SM, et al. GM-CSF DNA induces specific patterns of cytokines and chemokines in the skin: implications for DNA vaccines. Cytokines Cell Mol Ther 2003;7(3):125–33.

[123] Sailaja G, Husain S, Nayak BP, et al. Long-term maintenance of gp120-specific immune responses by genetic vaccination with the HIV-1 envelope genes linked to the gene encoding Flt-3 ligand. J Immunol 2003;170(5):2496–507.

[124] Sang H, Pisarev VM, Munger C, et al. Regional, but not systemic recruitment/expansion of dendritic cells by a pluronic-formulated Flt3-ligand plasmid with vaccine adjuvant activity. Vaccine 2003;21(21–22):3019–29.

[125] Sumida SM, McKay PF, Truitt DM, et al. Recruitment and expansion of dendritic cells in vivo potentiate the immunogenicity of plasmid DNA vaccines. J Clin Invest 2004;114(9): 1334–42.

[126] Fong CL, Mok CL, Hui KM. Intramuscular immunization with plasmid coexpressing tumour antigen and Flt-3L results in potent tumour regression. Gene Ther 2006;13(3): 245–56.

[127] Kim JJ, Nottingham LK, Sin JI, et al. CD8 positive T cells influence antigen-specific immune responses through the expression of chemokines. J Clin Invest 1998;102(6): 1112–24.

[128] Lu Y, Xin KQ, Hamajima K, et al. Macrophage inflammatory protein-1alpha (MIP-1alpha) expression plasmid enhances DNA vaccine-induced immune response against HIV-1. Clin Exp Immunol 1999;115(2):335–41.

[129] Eo SK, Lee S, Chun S, et al. Modulation of immunity against herpes simplex virus infection via mucosal genetic transfer of plasmid DNA encoding chemokines. J Virol 2001;75(2): 569–78.

[130] Pinto AR, Reyes-Sandoval A, Ertl HC. Chemokines and TRANCE as genetic adjuvants for a DNA vaccine to rabies virus. Cell Immunol 2003;224(2):106–13.

[131] Sin J, Kim JJ, Pachuk C, et al. DNA vaccines encoding interleukin-8 and RANTES enhance antigen-specific Th1-type CD4(+) T-cell-mediated protective immunity against herpes simplex virus type 2 in vivo. J Virol 2000;74(23):11173–80.

[132] Yamano T, Kaneda Y, Huang S, et al. Enhancement of immunity by a DNA melanoma vaccine against TRP2 with CCL21 as an adjuvant. Mol Ther 2006;13(1):194–202 [Epub 2005 Aug 22].

[133] Conry RM, Widera G, LoBuglio AF, et al. Selected strategies to augment polynucleotide immunization. Gene Ther 1996;3(1):67–74.

[133a] Guevara-Patiño JA, Engelhorn ME, Turk MJ, et al. Optimization of a self antigen for presentation of multiple epitopes in cancer immunity. J Clin Invest 2006 [in press].

[134] Kim JJ, Bagarazzi ML, Trivedi N, et al. Engineering of in vivo immune responses to DNA immunization via codelivery of costimulatory molecule genes. Nat Biotechnol 1997; 15(7):641–6.

[135] Iwasaki A, Stiernholm BJN, Chan AK, et al. Enhanced CTL responses mediated by plasmid DNA immunogens encoding costimulatory molecules and cytokines. J Immunol 1997;158:4591–601.

[136] Mendoza RB, Cantwell MJ, Kipps TJ. Immunostimulatory effects of a plasmid expressing CD40 ligand (CD154) on gene immunization. J Immunol 1997;159(12): 5777–81.

[137] Xiang R, Primus FJ, Ruehlmann JM, et al. A dual-function DNA vaccine encoding carcinoembryonic antigen and CD40 ligand trimer induces T cell-mediated protective immunity against colon cancer in carcinoembryonic antigen-transgenic mice. J Immunol 2001;167(8):4560–5.

[138] Sin JI, Kim JJ, Zhang D, et al. Modulation of cellular responses by plasmid CD40L: CD40L plasmid vectors enhance antigen-specific helper T cell type 1 CD4 + T cell-mediated protective immunity against herpes simplex virus type 2 in vivo. Hum Gene Ther 2001; 12(9):1091–102.

[139] Kim JJ, Tsai A, Nottingham LK, et al. Intracellular adhesion molecule-1 modulates beta-chemokines and directly costimulates T cells in vivo. J Clin Invest 1999;103(6):869–77.

[140] Hung CF, Cheng WF, Hsu KF, et al. Cancer immunotherapy using a DNA vaccine encoding the translocation domain of a bacterial toxin linked to a tumor antigen. Cancer Res 2001;61(9):3698–703.

[141] Rohrbach F, Weth R, Kursar M, et al. Targeted delivery of the ErbB2/HER2 tumor antigen to professional APCs results in effective antitumor immunity. J Immunol 2005;174(9): 5481–9.

[142] Jeannin P, Renno T, Goetsch L, et al. OmpA targets dendritic cells, induces their maturation and delivers antigen into the MHC class I presentation pathway. Nat Immunol 2000;1(6):502–9.

[143] Xiang R, Lode HN, Chao TH, et al. An autologous oral DNA vaccine protects against murine melanoma. Proc Natl Acad Sci U S A 2000;97(10):5492–7.

[144] Woo PC, Wong LP, Zheng BJ, et al. Unique immunogenicity of hepatitis B virus DNA vaccine presented by live-attenuated Salmonella typhimurium. Vaccine 2001;19(20–22): 2945–54.

[145] Chen CH, Wang TL, Hung CF, et al. Enhancement of DNA vaccine potency by linkage of antigen gene to an HSP70 gene. Cancer Res 2000;60(4):1035–42.

[146] Krieg AM, Yi A-K, Matson S, et al. CpG motifs in bacterial DNA trigger direct B-cell activation. Nature 1995;374:546–9.

[147] Sato Y, Roman M, Tighe H, et al. Immunostimulatory DNA sequences necessary for effective intradermal gene immunization. Science 1996;273(5273):352–4.

[148] Otero M, Calarota SA, Felber B, et al. Resiquimod is a modest adjuvant for HIV-1 gag-based genetic immunization in a mouse model. Vaccine 2004;22(13–14):1782–90.

[148a] Cohen AD, Diab A, Perales M-A, et al. Agonist anti-GITR antibody enhances vaccine-induced CD8+ T cell responses and tumor immunity. Cancer Res 2006 [in press].

[149] Zuber AK, Brave A, Engstrom G, et al. Topical delivery of imiquimod to a mouse model as a novel adjuvant for human immunodeficiency virus (HIV) DNA. Vaccine 2004; 22(13–14):1791–8.

[150] Thomsen LL, Topley P, Daly MG, et al. Imiquimod and resiquimod in a mouse model: adjuvants for DNA vaccination by particle-mediated immunotherapeutic delivery. Vaccine 2004;22(13–14):1799–809.

[151] Applequist SE, Rollman E, Wareing MD, et al. Activation of innate immunity, inflammation, and potentiation of DNA vaccination through mammalian expression of the TLR5 agonist flagellin. J Immunol 2005;175(6):3882–91.

[152] Niethammer AG, Xiang R, Becker JC, et al. A DNA vaccine against VEGF receptor 2 prevents effective angiogenesis and inhibits tumor growth. Nat Med 2002;8(12): 1369–75.

[153] Luo Y, Zhou H, Mizutani M, et al. Transcription factor Fos-related antigen 1 is an effective target for a breast cancer vaccine. Proc Natl Acad Sci U S A 2003;100(15): 8850–5.

[154] Loeffler M, Kruger JA, Reisfeld RA. Immunostimulatory effects of low-dose cyclophosphamide are controlled by inducible nitric oxide synthase. Cancer Res 2005;65(12): 5027–30.

[155] Kim TW, Hung C-F, Boyd D, et al. Enhancing DNA vaccine potency by combining a strategy to prolong dendritic cell life with intracellular targeting strategies. J Immunol 2003;171(6):2970–6.

[156] Widera G, Austin M, Rabussay D, et al. Increased DNA vaccine delivery and immunogenicity by electroporation in vivo. J Immunol 2000;164(9):4635–40.

[157] Hermans IF, Chong TW, Palmowski MJ, et al. Synergistic effect of metronomic dosing of cyclophosphamide combined with specific antitumor immunotherapy in a murine melanoma model. Cancer Res 2003;63(23):8408–13.

[158] Toka FN, Pack CD, Rouse BT. Molecular adjuvants for mucosal immunity. Immunol Rev 2004;199:100–12.

[159] Calarota SA, Weiner DB. Enhancement of human immunodeficiency virus type 1-DNA vaccine potency through incorporation of T-helper 1 molecular adjuvants. Immunol Rev 2004;199:84–99.

[160] Bowne WB, Wolchok JD, Hawkins WG, et al. Injection of DNA encoding granulocyte-macrophage colony-stimulating factor recruits dendritic cells for immune adjuvant effects. Cytokines Cell Mol Ther 1999;5:217–25.

[161] Marshall DJ, Rudnick KA, McCarthy SG, et al. Interleukin-18 enhances Th1 immunity and tumor protection of a DNA vaccine. Vaccine 2006;24(3):244–53 [Epub 2005 Aug 15].

[162] Zlotnik A, Yoshie O. Chemokines: a new classification system and their role in immunity. Immunity 2000;12(2):121–7.

[163] Eo SK, Lee S, Kumaraguru U, et al. Immunopotentiation of DNA vaccine against herpes simplex virus via co-delivery of plasmid DNA expressing CCR7 ligands. Vaccine 2001; 19(32):4685–93.

[164] Schoenberger SP, Toes REM, van der Voort EIH, et al. T-cell help for cytotoxic T lymphocytes is mediated by CD40–CD40L interactions. Nature 1998;393:480–3.

[165] Bennett SRM, Carbone FR, Karamalis F, et al. Help for cytotoxic-T-cell responses is mediated by CD40 signaling. Nature 1998;393:478–80.

[166] Ridge JP, Di Rosa F, Matzinger P. A conditioned dendritic cell can be a temporal bridge between a CD4 + T helper and a T-killer cell. Nature 1998;393:474–8.

[167] Alexopoulou L, Holt AC, Medzhitov R, et al. Recognition of double-stranded RNA and activation of NF-[kappa]B by Toll-like receptor 3. Nature 2001;413:732.

[168] Egen JG, Kuhns MS, Allison JP. CTLA-4: new insights into its biological function and use in tumor immunotherapy. Nat Immunol 2002;3(7):611–8.

[169] Gregor PD, Wolchok JD, Ferrone CR, et al. CTLA-4 blockade in combination with xeno-geneic DNA vaccines enhances T-cell responses, tumor immunity and autoimmunity to self antigens in animal and cellular model systems. Vaccine 2004;22(13–14):1700–8.

[170] van Elsas A, Hurwitz AA, Allison JP. Combination immunotherapy of B16 melanoma using anti-cytotoxic T lymphocyte-associated antigen 4 (CTLA-4) and granulocyte/macro-phage colony-stimulating factor (GM-CSF)-producing vaccines induces rejection of sub-cutaneous and metastatic tumors accompanied by autoimmune depigmentation. J Exp Med 1999;190(3):355–66.

[171] Phan GQ, Yang JC, Sherry RM, et al. Cancer regression and autoimmunity induced by cytotoxic T lymphocyte-associated antigen 4 blockade in patients with metastatic mela-noma. Proc Natl Acad Sci U S A 2003;100(14):8372–7.

[172] Hodi FS, Mihm MC, Soiffer RJ, et al. Biologic activity of cytotoxic T lymphocyte-associated antigen 4 antibody blockade in previously vaccinated metastatic melanoma and ovarian carcinoma patients. Proc Natl Acad Sci U S A 2003;100(8):4712–7.

[173] Attia P, Phan GQ, Maker AV, et al. Autoimmunity correlates with tumor regression in patients with metastatic melanoma treated with anti-cytotoxic T-lymphocyte antigen-4. J Clin Oncol 2005;23(25):6043–53.

[174] Nocentini G, Riccardi C. GITR: a multifaceted regulator of immunity belonging to the tumor necrosis factor receptor superfamily. Eur J Immunol 2005;35(4):1016–22.

[175] Shimizu J, Yamazaki S, Takahashi T, et al. Stimulation of CD25(+)CD4(+) regulatory T cells through GITR breaks immunological self-tolerance. Nat Immunol 2002;3(2):135–42.

[176] McHugh RS, Whitters MJ, Piccirillo CA, et al. CD4(+)CD25(+) immunoregulatory T cells: gene expression analysis reveals a functional role for the glucocorticoid-induced TNF receptor. Immunity 2002;16(2):311–23.

[177] Ko K, Yamazaki S, Nakamura K, et al. Treatment of advanced tumors with agonistic anti-GITR mAb and its effects on tumor-infiltrating Foxp3 + CD25 + CD4 + regulatory T cells. J Exp Med 2005;202(7):885–91.

[178] Hemmi H, Takeuchi O, Kawai T, et al. A Toll-like receptor recognizes bacterial DNA. Nature 2000;408:740–5.

[179] Liu L, Zhou X, Liu H, et al. CpG motif acts as a 'danger signal' and provides a T helper type 1-biased microenvironment for DNA vaccination. Immunology 2005;115(2):223–30.

Hematol Oncol Clin N Am 20 (2006) 637–659

HEMATOLOGY/ONCOLOGY CLINICS
OF NORTH AMERICA

Heat Shock Protein–Based Cancer Vaccines

Kelvin P. Lee, MD[a,b,*], Luis E. Raez, MD[b], Eckhard R. Podack, MD, PhD[a]

[a]*Department of Microbiology and Immunology, University of Miami Miller School of Medicine, Miami, FL, USA*
[b]*Division of Hematology and Oncology, Department of Medicine, University of Miami Miller School of Medicine, Miami, FL, USA*

The ability to duplicate the remarkable success of infectious disease vaccines in cancer, with durably robust and highly specific antitumor immune responses, has been long held as one of the keys in developing true "magic bullet" cancer therapies. This article attempts to explain why cancer vaccines have failed (so far), delineates the increasingly complex barriers that prevent the eliciting of effective antitumor immunity, and examines the ability of heat shock protein (HSP)–based vaccines to overcome these barriers. This article is not a definitive compendium of the huge body of relevant literature, but rather focuses on the major concepts underlying active specific immunotherapy in general and HSP vaccines in particular.

THE FAILURE OF CANCER VACCINES
"Although every field has suffered, cancer has had the greatest chasm between hope and reality" [1]. Vaccines against a constellation of infectious diseases have shown remarkable efficacy. The morbidity from measles has declined from 503,282 cases in the preimmunization era (baseline twentieth century annual morbidity) to 89 cases postimmunization (1998) [2]. This ability to elicit highly effective and durable immune responses has long been the compelling rationale to test vaccine approaches in other diseases, in particular, cancer. Despite the myriad of vaccine-based strategies that have shown potent ability to eradicate tumors in preclinical animal models (including established and metastatic disease), however, in humans there has been little meaningful efficacy against non–virally mediated cancers in more than 35 years of clinical testing. Although there are important caveats regarding the study populations (typically late-stage patients with compromised immune systems) and immunotherapy clinical trial design [3], responses have been limited primarily to tumors known to be immunologically sensitive (melanoma, renal cell carcinoma). Even in these cancers,

* Corresponding author. 1550 NW 10th Avenue, Papanicolaou Building, Room 211 (M710), Miami, FL 33136. *E-mail address:* klee@med.miami.edu (K.P. Lee).

0889-8588/06/$ – see front matter
doi:10.1016/j.hoc.2006.02.007

clinically significant reduction in tumor burden (not to mention improvement in patient survival) has been the exception more than the rule. This lack of therapeutic efficacy is not due to the general inability of the human immune system to kill cancer cells; allogeneic bone marrow transplantation shows that antitumor responses can control or eradicate disease effectively and result in significantly improved clinical outcomes in hematologic malignancies and solid tumors [4,5]. Rather, the generation of robust endogenous antitumor responses (possibly at the cost of significant autoimmune toxicity, as suggested by the strong correlation between graft-versus-host disease and leukemia control in allogeneic bone marrow transplantation) faces different and perhaps more intractable obstacles.

Development of all vaccines faces two basic hurdles—identification and delivery of the appropriate antigen and prodding the immune system to respond effectively to the immunization. In contrast to infectious disease vaccines, in which the pathogen antigens are readily recognized as "foreign" by the immune system, these hurdles are significantly higher in the setting of autologous "self" tumors, in which most (if not all) cellular proteins are normal and weakly immunogenic to nonimmunogenic. For cancer vaccines (and in contrast to measles vaccines), identifying useful tumor antigens is thoroughly entangled with getting an immune response against them from a therapeutic and a toxicity (ie, autoimmunity) standpoint. It was the early hope that if tumor-specific/associated antigens could be identified and T cell tolerance/passive unresponsiveness could be broken, cancer vaccines would be as effective as their infectious disease counterparts.

Tumor Antigens and Vaccine Formulation

The first generation of cancer vaccines comprised predominately of defined specific protein or synthetic peptide formulations intended to elicit $CD8^+$ cytotoxic T lymphocyte (CTL) antitumor immune responses. Of particular focus were antigens derived from unique tumor proteins (eg, antibody idiotypic regions in myeloma and lymphoma [6,7]) or oncofetal (eg, carcinoembryonic antigen [8]) and cancer/testis antigens (eg, MAGE-3 [9], NY-ESO-1 [10]), with the rationale that they would be largely specific for the cancer cells (less toxicity), and that tolerance to them may be more readily broken compared with more ubiquitous proteins (more efficacy). Using anti-idiotype vaccination in multiple myeloma as an illustrative example, evidence for anti-idiotype T cell responses and a reduction in circulating clonotypic B cells [11] could be detected in most immunized patients [7,11–13]. Changes in serum paraprotein as a measure of overall myeloma cell burden were not affected [11], however, and an improvement in other clinical parameters (eg, time to relapse, disease-free survival) in either the minimal residual disease or relapsed setting have not yet been reported. Although antitumor immune responses can be generated, several aspects of the vaccine formulation itself may have blunted the clinical response.

These first vaccines were typically monovalent to better deliver higher concentrations of the relevant antigen better, a limitation for polyvalent vaccines such as whole cell lysates. The tradeoff is that the immune response is narrowly targeted to a single antigen. This targeting may allow subclones to escape this response by downregulating expression/effective presentation of the antigen [14,15], especially if the target antigens are not essential for cell survival. Second, synthetic MHC I restricted peptides do not elicit significant CD4$^+$ T cell responses, and it is becoming increasingly clear that CD4$^+$ T cell help plays an important role in initiating and maintaining CD8$^+$ antitumor responses [16]. Similarly, these vaccines do not target activation of the innate immune system (in particular natural killer [NK cells], but also macrophages), whereas increasing evidence suggests there are crucial and synergistic interactions between innate and adaptive responses in endogenous antitumor immunity (ie, immunosurveillance [17,18]) and vaccine-elicited responses [19,20]. Finally, adjuvants are an essential component of protein/peptide vaccines, and the adjuvants available for human use (eg, incomplete Freund's, alum, granulocyte-macrophage colony-stimulating factor [GM-CSF]) [21] are not as potent as those available in animal models (ie, complete Freund's). Understanding of the critical importance of professional antigen presenting cell (APC) activation through pathogen-associated molecular pattern (PAMP) receptors, such as the Toll-like receptors (TLR), for generating immune responses [22–24] has yielded new mechanistic insight into how adjuvants are working. This insight has led to the next generation of vaccine approaches that more directly activate the APC (in particular dendritic cells [DC]) or incorporate molecular components of activated APC (eg, costimulatory ligands and cytokines) into the vaccine itself.

The Antigen Presenting Cell Gateway

The initial focus of active specific immunotherapy was activation of CD8$^+$ CTL. Antigen presentation by APC, although a complex molecular process, generally was regarded as a constant and not a variable. With the identification of DC as the primary professional APC for naive T cell activation [25], it is now clear that DC play an active and possible decisive role in determining antigen-specific T cell activation (including Th1/Th2 skewing) versus tolerance or deletion, as well as activating innate NK responses [26–28]. Major efforts to use antigen-pulsed, ex vivo–derived DC as cellular vaccines are under way and are described elsewhere in this issue. For molecular vaccines, DC (and other professional APC) are the gateway by which the vaccines gain access to the immune system, and how a vaccine modulates DC function would have a significant impact on its efficacy. In this regard, the two most important aspects of DC biology (among the multitude of relevant ones) are DC activation and antigen presentation/cross-presentation.

Among the various DC subsets, the CD11c$^+$ "myeloid" DC are likely to be most involved in eliciting vaccine responses. These DC can be differentiated from numerous hematopoietic precursors (as least in vitro [29]) into unactivated (also called immature) tissue-resident DC that are highly efficient in antigen uptake but are nonimmunogenic to tolerogenic [22,30]. Simply delivering antigens to unactivated DC may not be a neutral event, but an immunoinhibitory one. To become immunogenic (which includes trafficking from peripheral sites to the T cell areas within lymph nodes), DC need to be activated (or matured) by a "danger signal" [31], of which activation of TLR is best characterized. As noted earlier, TLR are a family of PAMP receptors that specifically bind numerous pathogen products typically characterized by repetitive structural elements (eg, lipopolysaccharide, CpG DNA) [32]. These microbial products are abundant in potent adjuvants such as complete Freund's or are part of the vaccine molecule in the case of "naked" DNA vaccines [33]. TLR binding results in DC activation as manifested by migration to lymph nodes, upregulation of MHC class II and costimulatory ligand expression, and induction of immunomodulatory cytokines. Importantly from a vaccine standpoint, activation of different TLR (and other pattern recognition receptors such as the C-type lectins) results in activation of differing downstream signal transduction pathways and cytokine secretion (eg, interleukin-12, interleukin-10), resulting in differing Th1 versus Th2 versus Treg skewing during T cell activation. Thus, it not only is critical for a vaccine to activate DC, but also to activate them in the right way.

The second important aspect of DC biology relevant to tumor vaccines is antigen presentation. The traditional paradigm is that exogenous antigens are processed and presented on MHC class II (activating CD4$^+$ T cells), and endogenous antigens are processed and presented on MHC class I (activating CD8$^+$ lymphocytes), and never the twain shall meet. It would be a significant limitation for most vaccines (which except for the virally packaged variations are exogenous molecules) if the delivered antigen could not activate cytotoxic T cells. DC seem to have the unique ability, however, to cross-present antigen, whereby exogenous antigen is shuttled into the MHC class I processing pathway and presented to CD8$^+$ CTL. The mechanisms remain unresolved [34–36], but seem to involve the exogenous antigen gaining access to the endoplasmic reticulum (ER) compartment and undergoing retrograde translocation into the cytosol (where they undergo proteosome degradation to peptides and TAP [*t*ransporters *a*ssociated with antigen *p*rocessing]-mediated transport back into the ER for loading onto MHC class I molecules). Relevant to vaccine design, cross-presentation seems to be upregulated by specific DC activation stimuli [37] and is more efficient if antigen is taken up by receptor-mediated endocytosis (eg, antigen-antibody immune complexes taken up by Fcγ receptors [38,39]).

Researchers now are learning that the tumor is not an idle bystander, waiting around for the immune system to rise up and whack it. Rather, tumors actively inhibit immune responses at numerous different levels, one of which is inhibition of DC differentiation/activation. Although this inhibition is regarded as pathologic, it likely represents a normal physiologic response to a far more common form of neoplasia—wound healing after trauma. Robust adaptive immune responses at the sites of inflammatory but sterile trauma/wound healing would be a distinct evolutionary disadvantage for any species, and the mechanisms that exist to suppress these responses are also active in cancer (classically described as "the nonhealing wound"). One of these is via vascular endothelial growth factor. Vascular endothelial growth factor plays an important role in the neovascularization of normal wounds and tumors and suppresses DC differentiation and activation [40]; this seems to be mediated via modulation of STAT3 and NFκB signaling in the DC and DC progenitors [41]. Clinically, this is not a subtle effect, but leads to significant defects in T cell activation in patients with advanced disease [42]. Cancer vaccines must reopen the APC gateway into the immune system closed by tumor factors, only to be faced by the equally formidable hurdle of breaking T cell self-tolerance.

The Unresponsive T Cell

In addition to thymic deletion of self-reactive T cells (which is incomplete), other robust mechanisms exist to prevent T cell activation against self-proteins not presented in the thymus (eg, newly generated antibody idiotypes) and important exogenous antigens (eg, in food, fetuses). The early assumption in active specific immunotherapy was that peripheral tolerance to immunized self-antigens was due primarily to T cell–autonomous anergy. In the basic paradigm, autoreactive T cells are rendered persistently unresponsive when their T cell receptor (TCR) engages cognate peptide/MHC complexes (signal 1) without activation of a costimulatory receptor (signal 2), such as CD28 [43]. Because costimulatory ligands, such as CD80 and CD86 (previously B7.1 and B7.2), are primarily limited to professional APC, autoreactive naive T cells that encounter MHC-expressing normal and malignant nonimmune cells would be sent into hibernation. The correlate to this is that if costimulation (or the downstream effect of costimulation, such as immunostimulatory cytokine production) could be provided exogenously in a vaccine setting, self-reactive antitumor T cells could be brought out of their hibernation. Because effector and memory T cells seem to require little to no costimulation [44], when activated these T cells would be able destroy tumor cells regardless of whether these targets were expressing costimulatory ligands. This finding led to numerous strategies in which costimulatory ligands or cytokines were incorporated directly into the vaccine itself [45], which showed great promise in preclinical models and possible efficacy in clinical trials [46].

Although supplying exogenous costimulation may break self-tolerance in some settings, the simple observation that immune responses do not develop spontaneously against B cell lymphomas (which are typically laden with MHC class I/II and costimulatory ligands) and other "APC" hematologic malignancies points to the presence of other mechanisms that "externally" regulate effector T cell activation. Two important mechanisms have been resurrected from the dustbin of discarded theories—tumor immunosurveillance and regulatory/suppressor T cells. The concept that the immune system played an important surveillance role in eradicating mutated neoplastic cells originally was proposed by Burnet in 1970 [47] and fell out of favor with the rise of cell-autonomous mechanisms (p53 being the prototypic example) that eliminated cells with significant DNA damage. More recent studies [48,49] have found, however, that γ-interferon-dependent responses (involving innate immunity) play an important role in preventing endogenous tumor progression. Importantly from an immunotherapy standpoint, this immunologic selection pressure results in "immunoediting" [18], such that the tumors that do grow are significantly less immunogenic. On top of normal tolerance to self-proteins, endogenous immunosurveillance further shapes the cancers that oncologists see to be even less immunogenic. Whether endogenously arising tumors (which have been far less well studied in experimental systems) are less immunogenic or induce tolerance [50] is unsettled, but nonetheless both mechanisms are not conducive to cancer vaccine efficacy.

As if multiple mechanisms to obscure the immunogenicity of the tumor were not bad enough, active suppression of effector T cell responses by regulatory T cells represent another barrier to the induction of sustained antiself/antitumor immunity. Initially described as "antigen-nonspecific" immunosuppressive $CD4^+$ and $CD25^+$ T cells, it is now clear that there are natural and induced regulatory T cells that prevent effector T cell activation against global to specific antigens [50–53] and inhibit pathogenic autoimmunity responses and rejection of established tumors in experimental models [54]. In contrast to tolerance, in which it can be envisioned that immune responses persist when the initial unresponsiveness is overcome, inhibition by regulatory T cells is ongoing. So any fires that do get lit would get doused.

CHARACTERISTICS OF A GOOD TUMOR VACCINE
Rather than serve as a source of hopelessness, understanding the obstacles to inducing sustained antitumor immune responses points the way to better cancer vaccine strategies. Sustained endogenous antiself autoimmune responses have been described for almost all normal tissues of the body (albeit in the pathologic context of autoimmune syndromes), clearly showing that anergy and immunosuppression can be overcome. The characteristics of effective tumor vaccines would include the following:

1. Delivery of many potential antigens (polyvalency), which is likely to generate a broader immune response that is more difficult to escape from. Additionally, vaccines that can deliver a spectrum of tumor-derived antigens are essential in settings where defined tumor-specific/associated antigens are unknown. Finally, given that MHC class I seems to present immunogenic peptides encoded by all six reading frames of a single gene (cryptic translation products) [55], vaccines that nonselectively sample the entire cell peptide repertoire may elicit immune responses against targets that would never be present in synthetic peptide or defined protein formulations.
2. Targeted delivery to professional APC.
3. Directly activate APC/DC.
4. Ready access of vaccine/antigen to cross-presentation pathways.
5. Can induce effector T cell responses without significant reliance on multiple components of the immune system (eg, generation of $CD8^+$ CTL without $CD4^+$ help).
6. Activate components of innate immune system (eg, NK, macrophages).
7. Can be generated from public/universal antigens instead of having to be derived from each individual tumor for individual patients. Although this is not a consideration for vaccine efficacy, the constraint of having to make

personal/private vaccines represents a significant logistical barrier to general clinical application and large clinical trial testing.
8. Does not generate horrific autoimmunity. It seems likely, however, that some degree of autoimmune sequelae would be clinically manifest in the setting of sustained immunity against self-proteins.

HSP-based cancer vaccines fulfill many of these criteria.

HEAT SHOCK PROTEINS

In 1962, Ritossa [56] noted that thermal stress of *Drosophila* larvae resulted in chromosomal "puffs" at discrete locations, suggesting that heat was inducing transcription of specific genes. Subsequent characterization and cloning of these regions identified the first HSP, which now comprise a large family of evolutionarily conserved proteins (from microbes to mammals) that are most commonly subgrouped by molecular weight: high-molecular weight HSP (≥ 100 kd), HSP90 (81–99 kd), HSP70 (65–80 kd), HSP60 (55–64 kd), HSP40 (35–54 kd), and small HSP (sHSP) (≤ 34 kd) [57]. Although HSP vary in size, cytosolic localization, and inducibility by heat [58], they all share the common function of chaperoning their client proteins within the intracellular environment. Similar to high school prom chaperones, this function is essentially to ensure their charges get to where they are going and behave the way they are supposed to. In the context of proteins, this latter function is help newly translated polypeptides to fold correctly and under cellular conditions that cause protein denaturation (eg, heat, but also other stresses, such as inflammation, pH changes, oxidative stress) to help the denatured proteins refold correctly. This refolding is crucial in the molecularly jam-packed environment of the cell. Unfolded proteins expose motifs that are normally hidden (not unlike unchaperoned teenagers), including hydrophobic domains, which can interact with other proteins to cause aggregation and precipitation. Within the ER, this interaction occurs has part of the unfolded protein response, and if HSP (and other mechanisms) are unable to rescue these proteins, the cell undergoes apoptosis [57,59–61]. This apoptosis may be especially critical in cells that are producing high levels of secreted protein, such as plasma cells, and there is evidence that the activity of agents, such as the proteosome inhibitor bortezomib in myeloma, is via induction of the cell death aspect of the unfolded protein response [61a]. Additionally, it has been found that specific HSP (eg, HSP90) chaperone numerous client proteins that are involved in signal transduction important for tumor cell survival. Drugs such as 17-allylamino, 17-demethoxygeldanamycin (17-AAG) that target HSP90 seem to be promising chemotherapeutic agents.

Heat Shock Proteins in Antigen Processing and Presentation

In addition to general chaperone function, specific HSP seem to be directly in the stream of peptides headed for loading onto MHC class I and II complexes for presentation to the immune system. For antigen processing and presentation on MHC class I, intracellular proteins (cytosolic, nuclear) first are degraded into peptides by a large (28 subunit) cytosolic multicatalytic protease complex called the *proteosome.* Interferon upregulates the expression of three inducible proteo-some subunits (B1i [LMP2], B5i [LMP 7], and B2i [MECL-1]) that displace constitutive proteosome subunits, and the resulting immunoproteosome now generates peptides that are better suited to bind to MHC class I (peptides that are 8–10 amino acids long, with basic/hydrophobic residues at the carboxy termi-nus). These cytosolic peptides are transported from the cytosol into the ER (where properly folded MHC class I/β_2-microglobulin heterodimers await) by ER membrane-spanning heterodimers of TAP1 and TAP2. The peptides are loaded on the peptide binding groove of the MHC molecule.

Because of their central role in binding to unfolded proteins, it is not surprising that HSP are involved in shuttling irreversibly damaged proteins to the front end of proteosome for degradation and shuttling peptides from the back end of the proteosome through the cytosol into the MHC class I processing pathway. It has been found that the co-chaperone CHIP (*c*arboxyl terminus of *H*sc70-*i*nteracting *p*rotein) binds to HSP90 heterocomplexes (and to the HSP70 family member HSC70 [62]), targeting the HSP-bound protein to ubiquitin-conjugating enzymes and shuttling the ubiquitinated protein (as a complex) to the proteosome for degradation into peptides [63]. HSP also seem to move these peptides into the MHC class I processing pathway; this is suggested by studies showing that HSP70 preferentially binds to peptides that also are favored by the TAP1/TAP2 transporters and MHC class I complexes—peptides of 7 to 15 residues with basic/hydrophobic anchor residues [64,65]. Because there is evidence that HSP70 physically associates with TAP1/TAP2 [66], it has been hypothesized that HSP70 binds to proteosome-generated peptides in the cytosol that are structur-ally preferred by MHC class I and chaperone these to the TAP transporters for MHC class I loading in the ER [67]. Similarly, the ER resident HSP gp96 (also called GRP94) has been shown to bind to ER peptides translocated by TAP1/TAP2 [68] that are identical to those found bound to MHC class I complexes [64,69].

HSP also have been implicated in MHC class II antigen processing and presentation. In this pathway, exogenous antigens traffic through endosomal into lysosomal compartments, where they undergo proteolytic cleavage into peptides by acid/cysteine proteases (eg, cathepsin B, D, S, L). These peptide-loaded vesicles fuse with MHC class II vesicles (MIIC) vesicles containing MHC class II heterodimers bound to invariant chain (Ii, which blocks the MHC peptide binding groove). Ii is cleaved by the lysosomal proteases, and the residual MHC class II–associated invariant chain peptide is popped out of the peptide binding groove when the class II heterodimers associate with HLA-DM, which also serves to catalyze exogenous peptide binding to MHC. HSC70 has been shown to bind to exogenous antigen and colocalize with MHC class II complexes, and its overexpression augments antigen processing and presentation to MHC class II–restricted T cells [70]. More recently, a role for HSC70 in shuttling cytoplasmic peptides and proteins into the MHC class II antigen processing pathway has been described via its association with the transmembrane lysosomal glycoprotein Lamp-2a [71].

Seminal studies by Srivastava and others showed that when purified HSP are used as tumor vaccines, it is the associated peptide (and not the HSP itself) that directs the antitumor immune response [71–74]. Similarly, DC-derived exosomes, membrane vesicles that can deliver intracellular antigens and elicit potent antitumor immunity when used as vaccines [75], have selective accumulation of HSC70 [76]. It can be envisioned that the efficacy of HSP-based vaccines is due to the "superior" immunogenicity of the MHC class I–destined and MHC class II–destined peptides that are bound by these complexes. Although this may be true, it also has been shown that immunization of whole proteins bound to HSP110 can elicit robust antitumor immunity [66,77,78]. This finding suggests that it is not just the quality of the antigens delivered by the HSP, but some property of the HSP itself that enhances immunogenicity. It is becoming increasingly clear that these properties are the ability of extracellular HSP to deliver these antigens directly into the MHC processing/presenting pathways of DC and potently induce DC activation.

Extracellular Heat Shock Protein as Quanta of Information for Professional Antigen Presenting Cells

As the gatekeepers of the adaptive immune response, DC serve as the prime integrators of two key pieces of environmental information—evidence for "danger" (eg, inflammatory cytokines or microbial PAMP) and the antigenic signature of the pathogen. Although these traditionally are thought of as two independent signals, in certain settings, extracellular HSP may package both signals efficiently into a single quantum of information that directly targets the DC.

The concept that exogenous HSP are actively captured by DC initially arose from the observation that incredibly small amounts of HSP-chaperoned peptide could elicit immune responses—subnanogram amounts in one study [79] and 10^4 to 10^6 fold less than whole protein in another [79a]. Given the diffusion/dilution of the injected HSP peptides in these experiments, it seemed highly unlikely that nonspecific mechanisms, such as pinocytosis, could capture sufficient antigen and pointed to receptor-mediated uptake. Binder et al [80] first identified CD91 as the receptor for gp96, and this group later showed that CD91 also binds HSP90, HSP70, and calreticulin [81]. CD91 originally was identified as the receptor for the serum glycoprotein α_2-macroglobulin (which itself binds numerous other proteins, including proteases and growth factors) and may serve to clear these plasma proteins by endocytosis [80]. CD91 does not seem to be ubiquitously expressed on all $CD11c^+$ DC, but is limited to a small subset [82], suggesting DC subset specialization. Similarly, a second scavenger receptor LOX-1 (which binds oxidized low-density lipoproteins) on DC also has been shown to bind to and endocytose HSP70 [83]. Also, it has been shown that HSP70 binds to lipid raft microdomains on macrophages, stimulating phagocytosis [84].

In addition to efficient capture of extracellular HSP, these receptors deliver the chaperoned antigen to the MHC class II pathway via the traditional endosome-lysosome pathway and cross over into the MHC class I pathway to be cross-presented to CD8$^+$ CTL [85–87]. How this occurs is still unclear; the previously reported mechanisms have been for phagocytosized particulate antigens [36] or soluble proteins [35] and not receptor-bound proteins. It also can be envisioned, however, that receptor-scavenged proteins may be targeted to the proteosome for more efficient degradation, gaining entrance into the cytosol for receptor-bound HSP. Also, given that HSP shuttle cytosolic proteins into the lysosome [71], it seems possible that they also traffic proteins in the other direction. Other studies have suggested there are TAP-dependent and TAP-independent pathways by which HSP-chaperoned peptides can be presented by MHC class I [88,89].

Although these receptors may explain the remarkable ease by which HSP-bound peptides can enter MHC class I and MHC class II processing/presentation pathways, it does not explain how extracellular HSP activate DC to get these antigens presented to T cells. It seems highly unlikely that a constitutive scavenger receptor also would transduce a danger signal to DC, given the disastrous potential for autoimmunity. It has been shown that LOX-1 (which does signal through NFκB in fibroblasts [90]) does not activate DC [83], whereas no signaling ability has been reported for CD91. Nonetheless, several lines of evidence indicate that HSP can deliver this second piece of "danger" information to DC. Although uptake of apoptotic cells results in tolerogenic DC [91], necrotic cells potently activated DC [92–94]. Because necrosis results in the extracellular release of HSP, whereas apoptosis does not [93], it has been proposed that extracellular HSP physiologically function to alert the immune system that something bad is happening (ie, cells are dying not of their own accord) that may require an immune response [80,95,96]. Consistent with this are the more direct observations that HSP can recruit DC to the site of injection [79a], elicit inflammatory cytokine secretion [97,98], upregulate MHC and costimulatory ligand expression [99–101], induce DC migration to draining lymph nodes [102], and result in the loss of T cell tolerance and induction of autoreactivity in vitro [101] and in vivo [95].

It follows that similar to other DC activation/maturation stimuli (cytokines, TLR ligands) that these HSP effects also are receptor mediated. Although still controversial, extracellular HSP have been reported to activate TLR2 and TLR4 [103–105], CD14 [106], and CD40 [107]—all receptors that are well described in their ability to induce DC activation/maturation. It is undoubtedly far more complex than this, given that thermal/radiation burns induce HSP expression and cause necrosis and yet do not result in clinically obvious activation of T cell responses against the burned tissue. In this regard, although gp96-complexed peptides are active in cross-presentation to CD8 at picogram quantities of complexed peptide (this system is ideal to detect minute quantities of antigen released during cell damage by infection or central tumor necrosis), conversely, milligram quantities of gp96 are highly immunosuppressive [108]. Large-scale tissue destruction by trauma burns and possibly surgery suppresses immune responses even if antigenic peptides are present. More recent evidence indicates that gp96 is translocated to the plasma membrane in the uterus during pregnancy, where its immunosuppressive effect may protect the fetus from immune rejection (Eckhard Podack, MD, PhD, personal communication, 2006). These immune-activating and immune-inhibiting properties of gp96 give it Janus-like two faces so typical for immune regulators.

Although it might be expected that the primary effector cell stimulated by exogenous HSP-activated DC are CD8$^+$ CTL, it seems that an equally essential component is NK activation. The authors have found that vaccination with tumor cells secreting gp96 genetically fused to an immunoglobulin tail (gp96-Ig, which mimics exogenous HSP released by necrosis [109]) recruits not only DC to the site of injection, but also NK cells [79a]. Perforin and γ-interferon are necessary to elicit sustained CD8$^+$ antitumor responses (but CD4$^+$ help was unnecessary), pointing to an initial involvement of NK cells [110]. The authors have proposed that HSP activate DC to activate NK cells, which then lyse the tumor targets to release more HSP-peptide complexes (Fig. 1). Simultaneously, gp96-Ig peptide complexes are activating DC via binding to TLR2/4 and are being taken up by the DC through CD91, where the chaperoned peptide is shunted into the MHC class I processing pathway for cross-presentation and activation of CD8$^+$ CTL (in a CD4$^+$ T helper–independent fashion). It can be readily envisioned how this self-amplifying loop of the *adjuvant* signal might drive maximal T cell responses, possibly constrained only by the number of DC in the vicinity (given that activated DC leave to emigrate to the lymph nodes, this may serve as the physiologic brake).

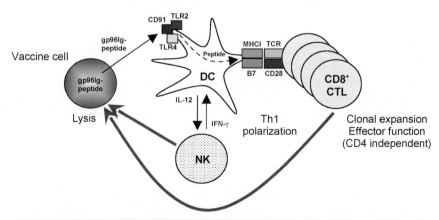

Fig. 1. Mechanism of gp96-Ig activation of antitumor immune responses. gp96-Ig molecules carrying tumor-associated peptides are secreted from the transfected tumor cell. The HSP-peptide complexes are taken up by CD91 on the DC and activate TLR2/4. The chaperoned peptide is cross-presented on MHC I molecules to induce CD8$^+$ CTL clonal expansion and effector function in a CD4 T helper–independent fashion. Activation of DC also activates NK cells, which lyse the target tumor cells, releasing more gp96-Ig-peptide complexes in a self-amplify loop. DC/NK cytokine secretion also results in Th1 polarization.

HEAT SHOCK VACCINES FOR CANCER

Given the biology of HSP, it is not a great leap to see their potential as tumor vaccines. HSP-peptide complexes have many of the previously listed characteristics of a good tumor vaccine: (1) They can deliver many potential antigens (and are known to bind to tumor-specific antigens [111]). (2) There is targeted delivery of HSP-peptides to APC. (3) The delivered peptides are readily cross-presented. (4) HSP directly activate APC/DC. (5) $CD8^+$ antitumor responses are generated without $CD4^+$ help. (6) Elements of the innate immune system (NK, macrophages) also are activated. As alluded to previously, numerous studies have shown the efficacy of HSP-based vaccines in generating antitumor immunity [112], including established disease [113].

The major challenge for HSP-based cancer vaccines is essentially their formulation, which is inextricably linked to their clinical testing. There are two basic problems: (1) It generally is believed (although not universally [114]) that exogenous HSP are not immunogenic in the absence of bound antigen [72]. HSP bind peptides noncovalently with relatively low affinity [67], however, and purification of intact HSP-peptide complexes from whole cells has been technically challenging. In clinical settings, although it is straightforward to determine the relative purity of the HSP in the final vaccine preparation [115], it is far more difficult to determine which and how many peptides remain bound to the HSP. Because only the carrier and not the antigens themselves can assayed for, from a "quality control" standpoint, this may result in significant batch-to-batch and trial-to-trial variability. (2) HSP vaccines generally are believed to be "private" vaccines—they deliver antigens unique to the individual's tumor [116] and would not be effective in another patient (in contrast to public or shared tumor antigens). Although individual efficacy may be greater, the logistics of having to make a clinical grade personalized vaccine for every patient is daunting, and is likely to be a significant impediment to large-scale clinical trials. Although HSP are abundant intracellular proteins, in many patients there is insufficient accessible tumor tissue (2–5 g to generate 250 μg of purified HSP [3]) from which to purify them. The HSP-vaccine formulations detailed subsequently discuss some of the strategies to overcome these obstacles and move these vaccines into the clinical arena.

In Vivo Tumor-Targeted Hyperthermia

In vivo tumor-targeted hyperthermia is not a vaccine approach per se, but attempts to induce endogenous HSP in tumors via whole-body hyperthermia (which is undergoing clinical evaluation for numerous diseases including cancer [117]) [118]. Hyperthermia elicits many physiologic changes in the tumor and the immune system [119,120], and a potential role for released or cell surface HSP is only beginning to be evaluated. A limitation of whole-body hyperthermia alone is that it is unlikely to result in significant tumor necrosis and release of endogenous HSP without cooking the patient. Ito et al [121] developed a novel strategy of "heat-controlled necrosis" using tumor-targeted magnetic nanoparticles that are internalized by the cells and generate intracellular hyperthermia when exposed to an alternating magnetic field. This strategy leads to HSP induction and release via necrosis, and in preclinical models it eradicates established tumors and elicits antitumor immunity [122].

Chaperone-Enriched Tumor Lysates
Because purification of individual HSP from tumor lysates is complex and inefficient, Katsanis' group [123–125] developed an approach of enriching tumor lysates for all chaperones using a relatively simple free-solution/isoelectric focusing technique [58]. This approach yields 1 to 2 mg of chaperone-rich cell lysates (CRCL) per gram of starting tissue compared with 100 µg/g of purified HSP from the same tumors. CRCL seem to have the same potency as purified HSP in eliciting antitumor immunity in preclinical models. Given that CRCL are mixtures of known and unknown proteins, however, it is possible that other immunostimulatory or inhibitory factors would generate "unexplained" variability in clinical testing.

Purified Endogenous Tumor Heat Shock Proteins
As detailed earlier, purified endogenous tumor HSP have been the most extensively tested in preclinical models and are the first to be tested clinically (see subsequently). In these studies, sufficient amounts of HSP (gp96, HSP70) could be routinely purified from tumor specimens by two-step ammonium sulfate precipitation/conA-affinity chromatography (gp96 [126]) or adenosine diphosphate–affinity chromatography (HSP70 [115]), followed by diethylaminoethyl anion exchange chromatography.

It was asserted earlier that HSP-based tumor vaccines are private vaccines. This statement may not be entirely accurate, however. Several studies suggested that HSP derived from nonautologous cell lines can deliver shared antigens that elicit antiautologous tumor immune responses [101,127,128] (Luis Raez, MD, Eckhard Podack, MD, PhD, unpublished findings, 2005). This suggestion raises the possibility of manufacturing tumor-specific/patient-independent HSP vaccine formulations that would be more amenable to large-scale production and testing.

Secreted gp96-Ig
The possibility of HSP-chaperoned shared tumor antigens raises the prospect of using cell lines to produce HSP vaccines, which raises the possibility of manipulating the HSP through genetic/molecular biology approaches. Using this approach, the authors showed that gp96 (deleted for the ER retention signal) genetically fused to the Fc portion of IgG1 (gp96-Ig) and transfected into tumor cells is readily secreted into the media, is easily purified by protein G affinity chromatography, and elicits potent antigen-specific antitumor immunity [129]. Similarly, vaccination with whole tumor cells transfected with gp96-Ig (a strategy that would allow additional manipulation of the tumor's immunogenicity) resulted in potent antitumor responses [109,110]. These studies have formed the basis of an ongoing institutional phase I trial in non–small cell lung

Table 1
Clinical trials of heat shock protein–based vaccines in cancer

Clinical phase	Cancer type	HSP	Toxicity	Immune response	Clinical response	Reference
Pilot	Multiple solid	gp96	Grade I/II pain, hot flashes, renal failure, fever, neutropenia	6/12 patients positive CD8+ antitumor responses by γIFN ELISpot	Disease stabilization 3/7 patients, 1 patient with 50% reduction in 1 lesion (rest unchanged) 2 CR, 3 SD, MTP 29 d, DFS 117 d, OS 402 d	[126]
II	Melanoma (stage IV metastatic)	gp96	Mild induration at injection sites	11/23 patients γIFN ELISpot positive	Statistically significant correlation between immune response and response 24-mo OS 79%, 24-mo DFS 33%, MTP 210 d	[135]
II	Colon cancer (resected liver metastasis)	gp96	Grade I hypertension, flulike syndrome, fever, diarrhea, headache, abdominal pain	15/29 patients γIFN ELISpot positive	Statistically significant correlation between immune response and OS and DFS	[137]

II	Indolent NHL	gp96	Minor, but not detailed	Not described	Not described	[138]
II	CML (chronic phase, on imatinib)	HSP70 + imatinib	Grade I injection site soreness, erythema, and pruritus; pruritic rash; flu-like symptoms	11/20 patients γIFN ELISpot positive 10/16 patients increased NK activity	7/20 CCR, 1 major response, 1 minor response.	[115]
II	Melanoma (stage IV metastatic)	gp96 + GM-CSF + IFN-α	Grade I induration at injection site, nausea, vertigo, fatigue, vomiting, malaise, fever, pain, itching	5/17 patients γIFN ELISpot positive 12/18 patients increased NK activity	Statistically significant correlation between immune response and clinical response 11/18 pt SD, MTP 145 d OS 583 d	[136]

Abbreviations: CCR, clinical complete response; CML, chronic myelocytic leukemia; CR, complete response; DFS, disease-free survival; MTP, median time to progression; NHL, non-Hodgkin lymphoma; OS, overall survival (median); SD, stable disease.

cancer using a non–small cell lung cancer cell line transfected with gp96-Ig and HLA-A1 [130].

Heat Shock Protein–Defined Protein Complexes

An alternative approach to purifying endogenous HSP-peptide complexes is to bind recombinant HSP with synthetic peptides or recombinant proteins in a cell free system. Although the diversity of antigens is less than with endogenously purified HSP-peptide complexes, in the setting of a known tumor-specific/associated antigen, this approach greatly simplifies vaccine production. Additionally, the amount of HSP that is bound to peptide/protein can be readily calculated, allowing standardization of antigen delivery that cannot be achieved currently with endogenously derived HSP complexes. This approach has been used successfully in preclinical models with peptides from a model tumor antigen [79] and larger protein domains of melanoma-associated gp100 and HER2/neu [77,131]. Similarly, genetic fusions of HSP and tumor-associated antigens can be generated [132,133]. As for gp96-Ig, these strategies allow for direct manipulation and modification of the HSP.

CLINICAL TRIALS OF HEAT SHOCK PROTEIN–BASED VACCINES IN CANCER

Although numerous HSP-based vaccine trials are currently under way [58,134], the results from only six therapeutic trials have been reported in the literature since the initial studies were begun in 1995. The results of these trials are summarized in Table 1. Most of these trials have been conducted with autologous gp96-peptide complexes (the first introduced into clinical trials was HSPPC-96 [vitespen, OncoPhage]). As can be seen, toxicity has been generally mild without any evidence for autoimmunity. The percent of patients who developed CD8$^+$ antitumor T cell responses (as measured by γIFN ELISpot) is low, around 50% across all studies. The high frequency of patients who had augmentation of the NK responses (typically assayed by the killing of the MHC class I–negative cell line K562, not by actual NK killing of autologous tumor cells) also is surprising, but consistent with observations made in murine models.

Overall, the clinical responses have been modest, with two complete responses seen in the first melanoma trial [135], but less promising results from the second trial from the same group adding additional immunomodulators (GM-CSF + interferon-α) to the HSP vaccination [136]. More impressive results were seen in chronic myelocytic leukemia patients, with the caveat made by the authors that clinical use of imatinib still was being refined at the time of the trial, so how much of the therapeutic effect was due to the vaccine and how much to the drug is unclear [115]. Nonetheless, the statistical correlation between the immunologic responses and better clinical outcome in several trials suggests a real effect of these vaccines. At this early stage, the clinical experience with autologous HSP-based vaccines is similar to other tumor vaccine approaches–little toxicity, evidence for induction of antitumor CD8$^+$ T cell responses in a significant percentage of patients, and modest clinical responses.

SUMMARY

Even for HSP-based vaccines, the chasm between preclinical hope and clinical reality remains great. Nonetheless, the potential of HSP vaccines is firmly grounded in well-established immunologic mechanisms, and it is only a matter of implementation. Most importantly in this regard are the exponentially increasing avenues for innovation in vaccine design and strategies that can fulfill the promise of HSP-based tumor vaccines.

References

[1] Harris G. New drug points up problems in developing cancer cures. New York Times. December 21, 2005.

[2] Achievements in public health, 1900–1999 impact of vaccines universally recommended for children—United States, 1900–1998. MMWR Mortal Morbid Wkly Rep 1999; 48:243–8.

[3] Srivastava PK. Immunotherapy of human cancer: lessons from mice. Nat Immunol 2000; 1:363–6.

[4] Stone RM, O'Donnell MR, Sekeres MA. Acute myeloid leukemia. Hematology (Am Soc Hematol Educ Program) 2004;98–117.

[5] Arya M, Chao D, Patel HR. Allogeneic hematopoietic stem-cell transplantation: the next generation of therapy for metastatic renal cell cancer. Nat Clin Pract Oncol 2004; 1:32–8.

[6] Hsu FJ, Caspar CB, Czerwinski D, et al. Tumor-specific idiotype vaccines in the treatment of patients with B-cell lymphoma—long-term results of a clinical trial. Blood 1997;89: 3129–35.

[7] Bergenbrant S, Yi Q, Osterborg A, et al. Modulation of anti-idiotypic immune response by immunization with the autologous M-component protein in multiple myeloma patients. Br J Haematol 1996;92:840–6.

[8] Marshall JL, Hawkins MJ, Tsang KY, et al. Phase I study in cancer patients of a replication-defective avipox recombinant vaccine that expresses human carcinoembryonic antigen. J Clin Oncol 1999;17:332–7.

[9] Thurner B, Haendle I, Roder C, et al. Vaccination with mage-3A1 peptide-pulsed mature, monocyte-derived dendritic cells expands specific cytotoxic T cells and induces regression of some metastases in advanced stage IV melanoma. J Exp Med 1999;190: 1669–78.

[10] Jager E, Gnjatic S, Nagata Y, et al. Induction of primary NY-ESO-1 immunity: CD8+ T lymphocyte and antibody responses in peptide-vaccinated patients with NY-ESO-1+ cancers. Proc Natl Acad Sci U S A 2000;97:12198–203.

[11] Rasmussen T, Hansson L, Osterborg A, Johnsen HE, Mellstedt H. Idiotype vaccination in multiple myeloma induced a reduction of circulating clonal tumor B cells. Blood 2003; 101:4607–10.

[12] Massaia M, Borrione P, Battaglio S, et al. Idiotype vaccination in human myeloma: generation of tumor-specific immune responses after high-dose chemotherapy. Blood 1999;94:673–83.

[13] Osterborg A, Yi Q, Henriksson L, et al. Idiotype immunization combined with granulocyte-macrophage colony-stimulating factor in myeloma patients induced type I, major histocompatibility complex-restricted, CD8- and CD4-specific T-cell responses. Blood 1998; 91:2459–66.

[14] Yee C, Thompson JA, Byrd D, et al. Adoptive T cell therapy using antigen-specific CD8+ T cell clones for the treatment of patients with metastatic melanoma: in vivo persistence,

migration, and antitumor effect of transferred T cells. Proc Natl Acad Sci U S A 2002; 99:16168–73.

[15] Malmberg KJ. Effective immunotherapy against cancer: a question of overcoming immune suppression and immune escape? Cancer Immunol Immunother 2004;53:879–92.

[16] Knutson KL, Schiffman K, Cheever MA, Disis ML. Immunization of cancer patients with a HER-2/neu, HLA-A2 peptide, p369–377, results in short-lived peptide-specific immunity. Clin Cancer Res 2002;8:1014–8.

[17] Dhodapkar MV, Geller MD, Chang DH, et al. A reversible defect in natural killer T cell function characterizes the progression of premalignant to malignant multiple myeloma. J Exp Med 2003;197:1667–76.

[18] Dunn GP, Old LJ, Schreiber RD. The immunobiology of cancer immunosurveillance and immunoediting. Immunity 2004;21:137–48.

[19] Corthay A, Skovseth DK, Lundin KU, et al. Primary antitumor immune response mediated by CD4+ T cells. Immunity 2005;22:371–83.

[20] Ikeda H, Chamoto K, Tsuji T, et al. The critical role of type-1 innate and acquired immunity in tumor immunotherapy. Cancer Sci 2004;95:697–703.

[21] Mesa C, Fernandez LE. Challenges facing adjuvants for cancer immunotherapy. Immunol Cell Biol 2004;82:644–50.

[22] Hawiger D, Inaba K, Dorsett Y, et al. Dendritic cells induce peripheral T cell unresponsiveness under steady state conditions in vivo. J Exp Med 2001;194:769–79.

[23] Steinman RM, Nussenzweig MC. Avoiding horror autotoxicus: the importance of dendritic cells in peripheral T cell tolerance. Proc Natl Acad Sci U S A 2002;99:351–8.

[24] Pulendran B. Modulating vaccine responses with dendritic cells and Toll-like receptors. Immunol Rev 2004;199:227–50.

[25] Mellman I, Steinman RM. Dendritic cells: specialized and regulated antigen processing machines. Cell 2001;106:255–8.

[26] Steinman RM, Hawiger D, Nussenzweig MC. Tolerogenic dendritic cells. Annu Rev Immunol 2003;21:685–711.

[27] Banchereau J, Briere F, Caux C, et al. Immunobiology of dendritic cells. Annu Rev Immunol 2000;18:767–811.

[28] Fernandez NC, Lozier A, Flament C, et al. Dendritic cells directly trigger NK cell functions: cross-talk relevant in innate anti-tumor immune responses in vivo. Nat Med 1999;5:405–11.

[29] Kharfan-Dabaja MA, Ayala E, Lindner I, et al. Differentiation of acute and chronic myeloid leukemic blasts into the dendritic cell lineage: analysis of various differentiation-inducing signals. Cancer Immunol Immunother 2005;54:25–36.

[30] Bonifaz L, Bonnyay D, Mahnke K, et al. Efficient targeting of protein antigen to the dendritic cell receptor DEC-205 in the steady state leads to antigen presentation on major histocompatibility complex class I products and peripheral CD8+ T cell tolerance. J Exp Med 2002;196:1627–38.

[31] Matzinger P. Tolerance, danger, and the extended family. Annu Rev Immunol 1994;12:991–1045.

[32] Iwasaki A, Medzhitov R. Toll-like receptor control of the adaptive immune responses. Nat Immunol 2004;5:987–95.

[33] Krieg AM. CpG motifs in bacterial DNA and their immune effects. Annu Rev Immunol 2002;20:709–60.

[34] Guermonprez P, Amigorena S. Pathways for antigen cross presentation. Springer Semin Immunopathol 2005;26:257–71.

[35] Ackerman AL, Kyritsis C, Tampe R, Cresswell P. Access of soluble antigens to the endoplasmic reticulum can explain cross-presentation by dendritic cells. Nat Immunol 2005;6:107–13.

[36] Guermonprez P, Saveanu L, Kleijmeer M, et al. ER-phagosome fusion defines an MHC class I cross-presentation compartment in dendritic cells. Nature 2003;425:397–402.

[37] Delamarre L, Holcombe H, Mellman I. Presentation of exogenous antigens on major

histocompatibility complex (MHC) class I and MHC class II molecules is differentially regulated during dendritic cell maturation. J Exp Med 2003;198:111–22.

[38] Nagata Y, Ono S, Matsuo M, et al. Differential presentation of a soluble exogenous tumor antigen, NY-ESO-1, by distinct human dendritic cell populations. Proc Natl Acad Sci U S A 2002;99:10629–34.

[39] Regnault A, Lankar D, Lacabanne V, et al. Fcgamma receptor-mediated induction of dendritic cell maturation and major histocompatibility complex class I-restricted antigen presentation after immune complex internalization. J Exp Med 1999;189:371–80.

[40] Gabrilovich DI, Chen HL, Girgis KR, et al. Production of vascular endothelial growth factor by human tumors inhibits the functional maturation of dendritic cells [published erratum appears in Nat Med 1996;2(11):1267]. Nat Med 1996;2:1096–103.

[41] Gabrilovich D. Mechanisms and functional significance of tumour-induced dendritic-cell defects. Nat Rev Immunol 2004;4:941–52.

[42] Gabrilovich DI, Corak J, Ciernik IF, et al. Decreased antigen presentation by dendritic cells in patients with breast cancer. Clin Cancer Res 1997;3:483–90.

[43] Lee KP, Harlan DM, June CH. Role of co-stimulation in the host response to infection. In: Gallin JI, Synderman R, editors. Inflammation: basic principles and clinical correlates. Philadelphia: Lippincott Williams & Wilkins; 1999. p. 191–206.

[44] Liebowitz DN, Lee KP, June CH. Costimulatory approaches to adoptive immunotherapy. Curr Opin Oncol 1998;10:533–41.

[45] Horspool JH, Perrin PJ, Woodcock JB, et al. Nucleic acid vaccine-induced immune responses require CD28 costimulation and are regulated by CTLA4. J Immunol 1998; 160:2706–14.

[46] Raez LE, Cassileth PA, Schlesselman JJ, et al. Allogeneic vaccination with a B7.1 HLA-A gene-modified adenocarcinoma cell line in patients with advanced non-small-cell lung cancer. J Clin Oncol 2004;22:2800–7.

[47] Burnet FM. The concept of immunological surveillance. Prog Exp Tumor Res 1970;13: 1–27.

[48] Shankaran V, Ikeda H, Bruce AT, et al. IFNgamma and lymphocytes prevent primary tumour development and shape tumour immunogenicity. Nature 2001;410:1107–11.

[49] Dunn GP, Bruce AT, Sheehan KC, et al. A critical function for type I interferons in cancer immunoediting. Nat Immunol 2005;6:722–9.

[50] Willimsky G, Blankenstein T. Sporadic immunogenic tumours avoid destruction by inducing T-cell tolerance. Nature 2005;437:141–6.

[51] Bluestone JA, Tang Q. How do CD4+ CD25+ regulatory T cells control autoimmunity? Curr Opin Immunol 2005;17:638–42.

[52] Nomura T, Sakaguchi S. Naturally arising CD25+ CD4+ regulatory T cells in tumor immunity. Curr Top Microbiol Immunol 2005;293:287–302.

[53] Thompson C, Powrie F. Regulatory T cells. Curr Opin Pharmacol 2004;4:408–14.

[54] Yu P, Lee Y, Liu W, et al. Intratumor depletion of CD4+ cells unmasks tumor immunogenicity leading to the rejection of late-stage tumors. J Exp Med 2005;201:779–91.

[55] Schwab SR, Li KC, Kang C, et al. Constitutive display of cryptic translation products by MHC class I molecules. Science 2003;301:1367–71.

[56] Ritossa F. Discovery of the heat shock response. Cell Stress Chaperones 1996;1:97–8.

[57] Macario AJ, Conway DM. Sick chaperones, cellular stress, and disease. N Engl J Med 2005;353:1489–501.

[58] Gullo CA, Teoh G. Heat shock proteins: to present or not, that is the question. Immunol Lett 2004;94:1–10.

[59] Schroder M, Kaufman RJ. The mammalian unfolded protein response. Annu Rev Biochem 2005;74:739–89.

[60] Brewer JW, Hendershot LM. Building an antibody factory: a job for the unfolded protein response. Nat Immunol 2005;6:23–9.

[61] Ma Y, Hendershot LM. The role of the unfolded protein response in tumour development: friend or foe? Nat Rev Cancer 2004;4:966–77.

[61a] Obeng EA, Carlson LM, Gutman DM, et al. Proteasome inhibitors induce a terminal unfolded protein response in multiple myeloma cells. Blood 2006; in press.

[62] Meacham GC, Patterson C, Zhang W, et al. The Hsc70 co-chaperone CHIP targets immature CFTR for proteasomal degradation. Nat Cell Biol 2001;3:100–5.

[63] Connell P, Ballinger CA, Jiang J, et al. The co-chaperone CHIP regulates protein triage decisions mediated by heat-shock proteins. Nat Cell Biol 2001;3:93–6.

[64] Breloer M, Marti T, Fleischer B, et al. Isolation of processed, H-2Kb-binding ovalbumin-derived peptides associated with the stress proteins HSP70 and gp96. Eur J Immunol 1998;28:1016–21.

[65] Fourie AM, Sambrook JF, Gething MJ. Common and divergent peptide binding specificities of hsp70 molecular chaperones. J Biol Chem 1994;269:30470–8.

[66] Chen D, Androlewicz MJ. Heat shock protein 70 moderately enhances peptide binding and transport by the transporter associated with antigen processing. Immunol Lett 2001; 75:143–8.

[67] Calderwood SK, Theriault JR, Gong J. Message in a bottle: role of the 70-kDa heat shock protein family in anti-tumor immunity. Eur J Immunol 2005;35:2518–27.

[68] Lammert E, Arnold D, Nijenhuis M, et al. The endoplasmic reticulum-resident stress protein gp96 binds peptides translocated by TAP. Eur J Immunol 1997;27:923–7.

[69] Nieland TJ, Tan MC, Monne-van Muijen M, et al. Isolation of an immunodominant viral peptide that is endogenously bound to the stress protein GP96/GRP94. Proc Natl Acad Sci U S A 1996;93:6135–9.

[70] Panjwani N, Akbari O, Garcia S, et al. The HSC73 molecular chaperone: involvement in MHC class II antigen presentation. J Immunol 1999;163:1936–42.

[71] Zhou D, Li P, Lin Y, et al. Lamp-2a facilitates MHC class II presentation of cytoplasmic antigens. Immunity 2005;22:571–81.

[72] Udono H, Srivastava PK. Heat shock protein 70-associated peptides elicit specific cancer immunity. J Exp Med 1993;178:1391–6.

[73] Li Z, Srivastava PK. Tumor rejection antigen gp96/grp94 is an ATPase: implications for protein folding and antigen presentation. EMBO J 1993;12:3143–51.

[74] Srivastava PK, Maki RG. Stress-induced proteins in immune response to cancer. Curr Top Microbiol Immunol 1991;167:109–23.

[75] Zitvogel L, Regnault A, Lozier A, et al. Eradication of established murine tumors using a novel cell-free vaccine: dendritic cell-derived exosomes. Nat Med 1998;4: 594–600.

[76] Thery C, Regnault A, Garin J, et al. Molecular characterization of dendritic cell-derived exosomes: selective accumulation of the heat shock protein hsc73. J Cell Biol 1999; 147:599–610.

[77] Wang XY, Chen X, Manjili MH, et al. Targeted immunotherapy using reconstituted chaperone complexes of heat shock protein 110 and melanoma-associated antigen gp100. Cancer Res 2003;63:2553–60.

[78] Manjili MH, Henderson R, Wang XY, et al. Development of a recombinant HSP110-HER-2/neu vaccine using the chaperoning properties of HSP110. Cancer Res 2002;62: 1737–42.

[79] Blachere NE, Li Z, Chandawarkar RY, et al. Heat shock protein-peptide complexes, reconstituted in vitro, elicit peptide-specific cytotoxic T lymphocyte response and tumor immunity. J Exp Med 1997;186:1315–22.

[79a] Oizumi, Podack, in press.

[80] Binder RJ, Han DK, Srivastava PK. CD91: a receptor for heat shock protein gp96. Nat Immunol 2000;1:151–5.

[81] Basu S, Binder RJ, Ramalingam T, et al. CD91 is a common receptor for heat shock proteins gp96, hsp90, hsp70, and calreticulin. Immunity 2001;14:303–13.

[82] Hart JP, Gunn MD, Pizzo SV. A CD91-positive subset of CD11c+ blood dendritic cells: characterization of the APC that functions to enhance adaptive immune responses against CD91-targeted antigens. J Immunol 2004;172:70–8.

[83] Delneste Y, Magistrelli G, Gauchat J, et al. Involvement of LOX-1 in dendritic cell-mediated antigen cross-presentation. Immunity 2002;17:353–62.

[84] Wang R, Kovalchin JT, Muhlenkamp P, et al. Exogenous heat shock protein-70 binds macrophage-lipid raft-microdomain and stimulates phagocytosis, processing and MHC-II presentation of antigens. Blood 2006;107(4):1636–42.

[85] Suto R, Srivastava PK. A mechanism for the specific immunogenicity of heat shock protein-chaperoned peptides. Science 1995;269:1585–8.

[86] Arnold-Schild D, Hanau D, Spehner D, et al. Cutting edge: receptor-mediated endocytosis of heat shock proteins by professional antigen-presenting cells. J Immunol 1999;162: 3757–60.

[87] Binder RJ, Srivastava PK. Peptides chaperoned by heat-shock proteins are a necessary and sufficient source of antigen in the cross-priming of CD8+ T cells. Nat Immunol 2005; 6:593–9.

[88] Arnold D, Faath S, Rammensee H, et al. Cross-priming of minor histocompatibility antigen-specific cytotoxic T cells upon immunization with the heat shock protein gp96. J Exp Med 1995;182:885–9.

[89] Castellino F, Boucher PE, Eichelberg K, et al. Receptor-mediated uptake of antigen/heat shock protein complexes results in major histocompatibility complex class I antigen presentation via two distinct processing pathways. J Exp Med 2000;191:1957–64.

[90] Cominacini L, Pasini AF, Garbin U, et al. Oxidized low density lipoprotein (ox-LDL) binding to ox-LDL receptor-1 in endothelial cells induces the activation of NF-kappaB through an increased production of intracellular reactive oxygen species. J Biol Chem 2000;275:12633–8.

[91] Steinman RM, Turley S, Mellman I, et al. The induction of tolerance by dendritic cells that have captured apoptotic cells. J Exp Med 2000;191:411–6.

[92] Gallucci S, Lolkema M, Matzinger P. Natural adjuvants: endogenous activators of dendritic cells. Nat Med 1999;5:1249–55.

[93] Basu S, Binder RJ, Suto R, et al. Necrotic but not apoptotic cell death releases heat shock proteins, which deliver a partial maturation signal to dendritic cells and activate the NF-kappa B pathway. Int Immunol 2000;12:1539–46.

[94] Sauter B, Albert ML, Francisco L, Larsson M, Somersan S, Bhardwaj N. Consequences of cell death: exposure to necrotic tumor cells, but not primary tissue cells or apoptotic cells, induces the maturation of immunostimulatory dendritic cells. J Exp Med 2000;7:423–34.

[95] Millar DG, Garza KM, Odermatt B, et al. Hsp70 promotes antigen-presenting cell function and converts T-cell tolerance to autoimmunity in vivo. Nat Med 2003;9:1469–76.

[96] Melcher A, Todryk S, Hardwick N, et al. Tumor immunogenicity is determined by the mechanism of cell death via induction of heat shock protein expression. Nat Med 1998; 4:581–7.

[97] Singh-Jasuja H, Scherer HU, Hilf N, et al. The heat shock protein gp96 induces maturation of dendritic cells and down-regulation of its receptor. Eur J Immunol 2000;30: 2211–5.

[98] Moroi Y, Mayhew M, Trcka J, et al. Induction of cellular immunity by immunization with novel hybrid peptides complexed to heat shock protein 70. Proc Natl Acad Sci U S A 2000;97:3485–90.

[99] Cho BK, Palliser D, Guillen E, et al. A proposed mechanism for the induction of cytotoxic T lymphocyte production by heat shock fusion proteins. Immunity 2000;12:263–72.

[100] Kuppner MC, Gastpar R, Gelwer S, et al. The role of heat shock protein (hsp70) in dendritic cell maturation: hsp70 induces the maturation of immature dendritic cells but reduces DC differentiation from monocyte precursors. Eur J Immunol 2001;31:1602–9.

[101] Qian J, Wang S, Yang J, et al. Targeting heat shock proteins for immunotherapy in multiple myeloma: generation of myeloma-specific CTLs using dendritic cells pulsed with tumor-derived gp96. Clin Cancer Res 2005;11:8808–15.

[102] Binder RJ, Anderson KM, Basu S, et al. Cutting edge: heat shock protein gp96 induces maturation and migration of CD11c+ cells in vivo. J Immunol 2000;165:6029–35.

[103] Vabulas RM, Braedel S, Hilf N, et al. The endoplasmic reticulum-resident heat shock protein Gp96 activates dendritic cells via the Toll-like receptor 2/4 pathway. J Biol Chem 2002;277:20847–53.

[104] Ohashi K, Burkart V, Flohe S, Kolb H. Cutting edge: heat shock protein 60 is a putative endogenous ligand of the toll-like receptor-4 complex. J Immunol 2000;164: 558–61.

[105] Asea A, Rehli M, Kabingu E, et al. Novel signal transduction pathway utilized by extracellular HSP70: role of toll-like receptor (TLR) 2 and TLR4. J Biol Chem 2002;277: 15028–34.

[106] Asea A, Kraeft SK, Kurt-Jones EA, et al. HSP70 stimulates cytokine production through a CD14-dependent pathway, demonstrating its dual role as a chaperone and cytokine. Nat Med 2000;6:435–42.

[107] Becker T, Hartl FU, Wieland F. CD40, an extracellular receptor for binding and uptake of Hsp70-peptide complexes. J Cell Biol 2002;158:1277–85.

[108] Chandawarkar RY, Wagh MS, Kovalchin JT, et al. Immune modulation with high-dose heat-shock protein gp96: therapy of murine autoimmune diabetes and encephalomyelitis. Int Immunol 2004;16:615–24.

[109] Strbo N, Yamazaki K, Lee K, et al. Heat shock fusion protein gp96-Ig mediates strong CD8 CTL expansion in vivo. Am J Reprod Immunol 2002;48:220–5.

[110] Strbo N, Oizumi S, Sotosek-Tokmadzic V, et al. Perforin is required for innate and adaptive immunity induced by heat shock protein gp96. Immunity 2003;18:381–90.

[111] Srivastava P. Interaction of heat shock proteins with peptides and antigen presenting cells: chaperoning of the innate and adaptive immune responses. Annu Rev Immunol 2002;20: 395–425.

[112] Parmiani G, Testori A, Maio M, et al. Heat shock proteins and their use as anticancer vaccines. Clin Cancer Res 2004;10:8142–6.

[113] Tamura Y, Peng P, Liu K, et al. Immunotherapy of tumors with autologous tumor-derived heat shock protein preparations. Science 1997;278:117–20.

[114] Baker-LePain JC, Sarzotti M, Fields TA, et al. GRP94 (gp96) and GRP94 N-terminal geldanamycin binding domain elicit tissue nonrestricted tumor suppression. J Exp Med 2002;196:1447–59.

[115] Li Z, Qiao Y, Liu B, et al. Combination of imatinib mesylate with autologous leukocyte-derived heat shock protein and chronic myelogenous leukemia. Clin Cancer Res 2005; 11:4460–8.

[116] Liu B, DeFilippo AM, Li Z. Overcoming immune tolerance to cancer by heat shock protein vaccines. Mol Cancer Ther 2002;1:1147–51.

[117] Kraybill WG, Olenki T, Evans SS, et al. A phase I study of fever-range whole body hyperthermia (FR-WBH) in patients with advanced solid tumours: correlation with mouse models. Int J Hyperthermia 2002;18:253–66.

[118] Kraybill WG, Olenki T, Evans SS, et al. A phase I study of fever-range whole body hyperthermia (FR-WBH) in patients with advanced solid tumours: correlation with mouse models. Int J Hyperthermia 2002;18:253–66.

[119] van der ZJ. Heating the patient: a promising approach? Ann Oncol 2002;13:1173–84.

[120] Hildebrandt B, Wust P, Ahlers O, et al. The cellular and molecular basis of hyperthermia. Crit Rev Oncol Hematol 2002;43:33–56.

[121] Ito A, Honda H, Kobayashi T. Cancer immunotherapy based on intracellular hyperthermia using magnetite nanoparticles: a novel concept of "heat-controlled necrosis" with heat shock protein expression. Cancer Immunol Immunother 2006;55:320–8.

[122] Ito A, Tanaka K, Honda H, et al. Complete regression of mouse mammary carcinoma with a size greater than 15 mm by frequent repeated hyperthermia using magnetite nanoparticles. J Biosci Bioeng 2003;96:364–9.

[123] Zeng Y, Graner MW, Feng H, et al. Imatinib mesylate effectively combines with chaperone-rich cell lysate-loaded dendritic cells to treat bcr-abl + murine leukemia. Int J Cancer 2004;110:251–9.

[124] Graner MW, Zeng Y, Feng H, et al. Tumor-derived chaperone-rich cell lysates are effective therapeutic vaccines against a variety of cancers. Cancer Immunol Immunother 2003;52:226–34.

[125] Graner M, Raymond A, Akporiaye E, et al. Tumor-derived multiple chaperone enrichment by free-solution isoelectric focusing yields potent antitumor vaccines. Cancer Immunol Immunother 2000;49:476–84.

[126] Janetzki S, Palla D, Rosenhauer V, et al. Immunization of cancer patients with autologous cancer-derived heat shock protein gp96 preparations: a pilot study. Int J Cancer 2000; 88:232–8.

[127] Todryk SM, Eaton J, Birchall L, et al. Heated tumour cells of autologous and allogeneic origin elicit anti-tumour immunity. Cancer Immunol Immunother 2004;53:323–30.

[128] Casey DG, Lysaght J, James T, et al. Heat shock protein derived from a non-autologous tumour can be used as an anti-tumour vaccine. Immunology 2003;110:105–11.

[129] Yamazaki K, Nguyen T, Podack ER. Cutting edge: tumor secreted heat shock-fusion protein elicits CD8 cells for rejection. J Immunol 1999;163:5178–82.

[130] Raez LE, Fein S, Podack ER. Lung cancer immunotherapy. Clin Med Res 2005;3:221–8.

[131] Manjili MH, Wang XY, Chen X, et al. HSP110–HER2/neu chaperone complex vaccine induces protective immunity against spontaneous mammary tumors in HER-2/neu transgenic mice. J Immunol 2003;171:4054–61.

[132] Ma JH, Sui YF, Ye J, et al. Heat shock protein 70/MAGE-3 fusion protein vaccine can enhance cellular and humoral immune responses to MAGE-3 in vivo. Cancer Immunol Immunother 2005;54:907–14.

[133] Wu Y, Wan T, Zhou X, et al. Hsp70-like protein 1 fusion protein enhances induction of carcinoembryonic antigen-specific CD8+ CTL response by dendritic cell vaccine. Cancer Res 2005;65:4947–54.

[134] Lewis JJ. Therapeutic cancer vaccines: using unique antigens. Proc Natl Acad Sci U S A 2004;101(Suppl 2):14653–6.

[135] Belli F, Testori A, Rivoltini L, et al. Vaccination of metastatic melanoma patients with autologous tumor-derived heat shock protein gp96-peptide complexes: clinical and immunologic findings. J Clin Oncol 2002;20:4169–80.

[136] Pilla L, Patuzzo R, Rivoltini L, et al. A phase II trial of vaccination with autologous, tumor-derived heat-shock protein peptide complexes Gp96, in combination with GM-CSF and interferon-alpha in metastatic melanoma patients. Cancer Immunol Immunother 2005;1–11.

[137] Mazzaferro V, Coppa J, Carrabba MG, et al. Vaccination with autologous tumor-derived heat-shock protein gp96 after liver resection for metastatic colorectal cancer. Clin Cancer Res 2003;9:3235–45.

[138] Younes A. A phase II study of heat shock protein-peptide complex-96 vaccine therapy in patients with indolent non-Hodgkin's lymphoma. Clin Lymphoma 2003;4:183–5.

Hematol Oncol Clin N Am 20 (2006) 661–687

HEMATOLOGY/ONCOLOGY CLINICS
OF NORTH AMERICA

ELSEVIER
SAUNDERS

Viral Vaccines for Cancer Immunotherapy

Andrew Eisenberger, Brian M. Elliott, Howard L. Kaufman, MD*

Divisions of Surgical Oncology and The Tumor Immunology Laboratory, Department of Surgery, Columbia University, New York, NY, USA

The development of vaccines for cancer has been supported by significant "proof of principle" data from animal models and critical observations in patients who have cancer [1]. Powerful evidence has emerged from knockout mice to suggest that tumor surveillance is a normal function of the immune system, and occurs in a T-lymphocyte– and interferon (IFN)-γ–dependent manner [2]. Further data, using a variety of vaccine strategies aimed at activating T cells, demonstrated antitumor responses in animal models [3,4]. Although the translation of these findings to the clinic has been disappointing, there have been significant observations to support the role of the immune system in eradicating human tumors [5,6]. Patients who have melanoma or renal cell carcinoma and receive high doses of interleukin (IL)-2 exhibit a small, but durable, clinical benefit from immunotherapy [7]. The identification of tumor-associated antigens suggests that there are highly specific targets for immune recognition, and provides a mechanism whereby the immune system can detect subtle differences in neoplastic cells [8]. Early-phase clinical studies demonstrated long-term immunity that was induced by vaccines, and occasional objective clinical responses have been reported [9,10]. In the past few years we have gained a better understanding of how tumors escape immune detection; this has led to more innovative strategies that combine vaccines with methods that are designed to block immune inhibitory factors [11]. Thus, tumors clearly possess immunogenic properties; continued efforts are needed to define the optimal vaccine candidates and regimens for use in cancer immunotherapy.

Viruses have long been recognized as disease pathogens and as important vectors for preventing infectious disease. The process of preventing disease, termed vaccination, generally uses pre-exposure to small fragments or attenuated forms of live viruses to initiate long-term immunity against the pathogen [12]. Vaccination makes use of the natural host immune response against viral

* Corresponding author. Columbia-Presbyterian Medical Center, 177 Fort Washington Avenue, MHB-7SK, New York, NY 10032. *E-mail address:* hlk2003@columbia.edu (H.L. Kaufman).

0889-8588/06/$ – see front matter
doi:10.1016/j.hoc.2006.02.006

particles to induce protection against disease. Applying this principle to patients who have cancer, viruses can be used as vectors for induction of antitumor immunity by exploiting the natural pathogenesis of viral infections and introducing tumor specificity to the vector by directly injecting tumor cells or expressing tumor antigens through viral genomes. Because viral infection is naturally immunogenic and initiates a cascade of immunomodulatory cytokines and chemokines, this can be used to help generate strong immune responses against tumor cells. In the simplest form, the genes that encode tumor-associated antigens can be inserted into the viral genome [13]. More recently, viruses also have been used to encode immunomodulatory molecules which can help to orchestrate the type and acuity of immune response [14]. Alternatively, viruses can be engineered to deliver destructive agents to tumor cells or induce direct lysis of tumor cells following intratumoral or tumor-targeted administration. Viruses also are constructed easily and generally do not require patient-derived tumor cells or other individualized materials that can limit successful vaccine preparation.

Several potentially useful viruses are available for vaccine development, and the literature is replete with examples from nearly every major virus family. This ranges from large DNA viruses, such as poxviruses, to the small RNA retroviruses. Each has distinct advantages and disadvantages as vectors for use in tumor vaccine development (Table 1). Despite the intense interest in viruses as vectors for tumor vaccines, only a few have entered into clinical trials; these include the poxviruses, adenoviruses, adeno-associated viruses (AAVs), herpesviruses (HPVs), and retroviruses. This article focuses on the general properties and mechanism of action for these viral vaccines and discusses the current status of clinical trials in patients who have cancer. The next several years likely will witness the completion of pivotal phase III studies using these agents alone and in combination with other cancer therapeutics, while continued research efforts will refine and improve their immunogenicity and therapeutic potential.

THE IMMUNE RESPONSE TO VACCINE IMMUNOTHERAPY

Before considering specific examples of viral-based vaccines, it is important to understand how such vectors can be used to mediate therapeutic responses in patients who have cancer. Tumor rejection by the immune system is an intricate process that is orchestrated by numerous cells, including T lymphocytes, B cells, natural killer (NK) cells, NK T cells, dendritic cells, and macrophages. The role of these cells is confounded by the presence of a complex regulatory network that is designed to control immune responses and prevent autoimmunity, which is only now beginning to be understood [15]. Nevertheless, most viral vaccines have focused on activating CD8$^+$ T cells, because these often are found infiltrating tumors and their presence is associated frequently with tumor regression [16].

The initiation of a CD8$^+$ T-cell response is dependent on the interplay of many other factors, most notably dendritic cells (DCs) and CD4$^+$ T cells that provide critical helper functions for CD8$^+$ T-cell activation. DCs are the most potent professional antigen-presenting cells, and avidly engulf and process

Table 1

Characteristics of commonly used viral vectors in tumor vaccines

Vector	Advantages of use	Disadvantages of use
Poxviruses	Large genomes allow insertion of large or multiple eukaryotic genes Elicits strong humoral and cell-mediated immunity Multiple strains permit prime-boost immunization Cytoplasmic replication prevents insertional mutagenesis and cell transformation Recombinant particles are stable and replicate accurately Good safety record	Neutralizing antibodies with replicating viruses reduces efficacy of boosters Vaccinia virus has toxicity in immunocompromised hosts and those who have eczema
Adenoviruses	Elicits strong immune response that can promote tumor immunity Infects proliferating and quiescent cells Can encode 8000+ nucleotides after deletion of some or all nonessential genes Absence of chromosomal integration precludes insertional mutagenesis and cell transformation Infection is highly efficient	Earlier generation viruses have small genomes High prevalence of previous exposure and neutralizing antibodies which reduces efficacy of subsequent booster vaccinations Rare incidence of acute hepatitis Lack of integration leads to transient gene expression
Adeno-associated viruses	Less immunogenic Site-specific integration results in long-term expression without potential for insertional mutagenesis Can infect proliferating and quiescent cells High level expression possible	Small vector with limitation on gene sequences that can be expressed Require helper viruses for packaging Most of population is sero-positive
Herpesviruses	Large genome allows expression of large gene segments Strongly cytolytic in cancer cells Presence of preexisting neutralizing antibodies less problematic when given by intratumoral administration	Need to be injected directly into tumor Safety not documented
Retroviruses and Lentiviruses	Long-term expression of heterologous genes through stable integration into host Transduced cells pass gene on to progeny cells Efficient process when conditions are favorable Can engineer systems with self-activating and self-inactivating genes of interest	Narrow host range Limited insert size (8 kb) Only infect actively dividing cells (except lentiviruses) Potential for cell transformation and insertional mutagenesis

exogenous antigens from their local environments. The DCs display processed peptides by surface major histocompatibility complex class I and II molecules, which activate CD8$^+$ effector T cells and CD4$^+$ helper T cells, respectively [17]. DCs are important regulators of immunity because they also express several accessory, or costimulatory, molecules that are required for complete T-cell activation [18]. The interactions that are necessary for activation of CD8$^+$ T cells generally are believed to occur predominantly in secondary lymphoid tissue where naive CD8$^+$ T cells encounter antigen-bearing DCs that were recruited from the periphery. Following activation, CD8$^+$ T cells are able to home back to sites of antigen expression in a chemokine-dependent manner [19]. Upon encountering an antigen, these CD8$^+$ T cells release local perforins and granzymes, or by direct intercellular contact (eg, *fas-FasL*), that destroys target cells. This cycle can be initiated by viral infections of peripheral tissue and, to a lesser extent, by early tumors [12,16].

Although this discussion is highly simplified, an understanding of how T-cell responses are generated is important because viral vaccines are designed to manipulate all aspects of this process. Thus, the benefits of any particular vaccine depends on how well the virus can enhance T-cell priming and activation. Similarly, the limitations of any particular viral vaccine depend to a great degree on how the host immune response contains the virus and, in turn, how particular viruses prevent activation of T-cell responses. The nature of the antigens that are used for targeting the T-cell responses is a critical difference in developing vaccines for cancer compared with infectious disease. In the case of infectious diseases, most antigens are prokaryotic and foreign to the immune system. This greatly facilitates the potency and strength of the immune response. In contrast, patients who have cancer generally do not express prokaryotic genes as part of the malignant process, and thus, initiation of immune responses can be more difficult and the responses less robust when they do occur. Despite these differences, the last decade witnessed the identification of more than 100 tumor-associated antigens (TAAs).

TUMOR-ASSOCIATED ANTIGENS

The recognition that some proteins are expressed uniquely or aberrantly by malignant cells, and are not expressed or are expressed minimally by normal host cells, has been crucial to the development of vaccine immunotherapy. These TAAs include a variety of antigens that have been classified into several convenient categories. The viral proteins, which may be the most promising for tumor vaccine development, may be perceived as foreign by the tumor-bearing host immune system. Perhaps this is best exemplified by the human papillomavirus (HPV) E6 and E7 proteins that are expressed in cervical cancer [20]. Other TAAs are mutated proteins that yield unique amino acid sequences that are not found in cells that express the normal counterpart; for example, the *ras* proto-oncogene, which is found in several tumors, provides a mechanism for the immune system to distinguish normal and malignant cells [21]. Most TAAs, however, are normal, nonmutated self proteins that may be recognized because they are expressed at the wrong time (eg, differentiation antigens, such as tyrosinase), the wrong place (eg, cancer-testis antigens, such as NY-ESO-1), or at the wrong concentration (eg, embryonic antigens, such as the carcinoembryonic antigen [CEA]) [22]. Although tolerance may exist to TAAs, especially when they are proteins in their normal form, this often can be overcome through expression by highly immunogenic vectors or by the inclusion of strong adjuvants in vaccine regimens.

The earliest iteration of viral vaccines used viruses that expressed TAAs as a method for inducing stronger immune responses against known antigens that typically exhibit weak immunity [23]. Although this approach garnered significant support in animal models, there has been little evidence of therapeutic responses in early-phase clinical trials [5]. Further refinements to the vaccine approach, including consideration of vaccine dose, route of administration, booster vaccinations, inclusion of immunomodulatory accessory molecules, and vaccine adjuvants, has improved the potency of current vaccine candidates markedly. The ability to monitor antigen-specific immune responses carefully in clinical trials also has revealed clues about how such vaccines work, and has guided the rational design of prospective randomized studies of vaccines alone and in combination with other forms of cancer treatment.

POXVIRUSES

The poxviruses have been the most extensively studied viruses for tumor vaccine development. This is based, in part, on the recognition of poxviruses as disease-causing agents more than 200 years ago, and from knowledge gained through the world-wide smallpox eradication program of the twentieth century [24]. Smallpox is caused by the variola virus, and it is believed to have first infected the human population approximately 10,000 years ago. Similar to most poxviruses, the host range for variola is highly restricted, in this case to humans, which is one of the reasons why smallpox eventually could be contained [25]. The poxviruses are among the largest known viruses and can be seen under light microscopy, which no doubt aided in their recognition as disease pathogens. Smallpox also represents an important disease; it was recognized in many cultures that individuals who were pre-exposed to pox lesions often were protected from the disease during subsequent smallpox outbreaks or at least experienced less severe forms of the disease. This formal observation usually is credited to Edward Jenner, who, in 1798, described in detail that British milkmaids who were exposed to cowpox virus were protected later against smallpox [26]. Jenner also generated the virus—initially believed to be cowpox—for smallpox vaccination, and strongly espoused the practice of immunization. The exact origin of the Jenner virus is not clear, and modern molecular biology techniques suggest that vaccinia is neither cowpox nor variola, but rather is a distinct poxvirus strain. Vaccinia virus differs from most poxviruses in having a wider host range, including mammals and rodents, and serves as a minor human pathogen, particularly in the immunocompromised host [27]. Vaccinia virus has been given to millions of people through the highly successful smallpox eradication program of the World Health Organization, which declared the complete elimination of smallpox from the human population in the early 1980s [28].

Interest in vaccinia virus was renewed when it became clear that vaccinia could be used to generate recombinant vectors that express foreign transgenes [29]. This knowledge has been used to adapt poxviruses as potential vectors for immunotherapy in cancer [14,23,34]. Several inherent characteristics of poxviruses make them excellent candidates as tumor vaccines. Poxviruses have large double-stranded DNA genomes, with an average of 200 kilobase (kb) pairs, and can be manipulated easily in the laboratory to express recombinant prokaryotic and eukaryotic genes [13]. The life cycle of the poxviruses also confers certain advantages as vaccine candidates, because they replicate entirely within the cytoplasm of infected cells, which eliminates the potential for latent infection or insertional mutagenesis. Poxvirus DNA replication is highly accurate and allows reliable gene expression, which includes normal host cell posttranslational modifications of expressed transgenes. The replicative process is mediated by proteins that are carried by poxvirus particles, whereas infection of mammalian cells by vaccinia virus results in an inhibition of host cell transcription and translation [27].

Poxviruses are especially useful as tumor vaccines because they elicit pronounced humoral and cell-mediated immunity against the virus and expressed transgenes [30]. The details of how poxviruses elicit immune responses are not understood completely; however, poxviruses encode several cytokine- and chemokine-binding genes, which suggests that IFN-γ and related cytokines are important in viral clearance and escape [27]. The best information comes from studies of vaccinia virus during the smallpox eradication program. Strong neutralizing antibody responses occur following vaccinia vaccination, and these antibodies are protective against smallpox and subsequent vaccinia virus exposure [31]. This may be helpful for tumor immunotherapy but also limits the ability to immunize patients with the same virus repeatedly, because high titers of neutralizing antibodies significantly attenuate replication of virus after further booster vaccinations [32].

Vaccination also induces T-cell responses, and these can be sufficient to protect individuals, because patients who had agammaglobulinemia and were vaccinated with vaccinia virus were immune to smallpox in the absence of antibody titers [25]. Although the contribution of humoral and cellular immunity to subsequent protection is debated among virologists, vaccination likely induces both, and this may be especially useful for tumor vaccines [33,34]. The effects of vaccinia virus infection on DCs also is controversial, with early evidence supporting DC dysfunction and apoptosis after vaccinia infection; however, recent data demonstrate that DCs that are infected with recombinant poxviruses can direct cytotoxic T-cell responses against TAAs [35–37]. Further research is needed to better understand the interaction of the poxviruses with DCs and the contribution of T cells following exposure to vaccinia virus.

The difference in host range between vaccinia virus and other poxvirus family members has important implications for viral infectivity, pathogenicity, and immunogenicity [27]. The avipoxviruses, for example, typically infect birds but also can enter human cells without causing further infection, because these viruses are unable to replicate in mammalian cells. Thus, the levels of neutralizing antibodies are lower in mammals that are infected with avipoxviruses but persist longer, which allows the initiation of potent T-cell responses [38]. Viral replication also is inhibited in specialized strains of vaccinia virus—most notably the modified vaccinia virus Ankara (MVA), which was generated after more than 500 serial passages in tissue culture cells [39]. Similar to avipoxviruses, MVA does not replicate in mammalian cells, and therefore, it can be administered repeatedly to mammals without inducing high levels of neutralizing antibody titers. The nonreplicating viruses have been used alone and in combination with vaccinia virus in a prime-boost strategy that permits repeated vaccination without generating viral resistance [40].

The first recombinant poxvirus to express a relevant TAA was vaccinia-CEA, which demonstrated therapeutic responses in a murine CEA colon cancer model [41]. The vaccinia-CEA vaccine was well tolerated in early phase I clinical trials, but no clinical responses were observed [42,43]. To diminish the role of neutralizing antivaccinia antibody titers, a recombinant canarypox virus (ALVAC) that expressed CEA was generated and tested in a phase I clinical trial that used a dose-escalation study design [44]. This trial determined that vaccination was well tolerated but failed to induce objective responses; however, induction of CEA-specific T cells that were evaluated by enzyme-linked immunospot (ELISPOT) assay demonstrated a postvaccination increase in 7 of the patients tested. The ALVAC-CEA vaccine was used in a randomized prime-boost clinical trial that compared patients who received a single vaccinia-CEA vaccine followed by three ALVAC-CEA booster immunizations with patients who were given three ALVAC-CEA vaccines followed by one vaccinia-CEA vaccine [45]. This trial established the superiority of the vaccinia prime followed by ALVAC, because nearly all such treated patients developed increased CEA-specific T cell responses, although again, clinical responses were not seen.

A further refinement to the poxvirus vaccine system occurred when it was demonstrated that the coexpression of TAAs with potent costimulatory molecules improved the activation of T-cell responses and increased the therapeutic effects of the vaccines in animal models [14,46]. An ALVAC virus that expressed CEA and the B7.1 costimulatory molecule, which specifically activates $CD4^+$ and $CD8^+$ T cells through ligation of the CD28 molecule, was tested in a series of phase I clinical trials [47,48]. These trials enrolled patients who had metastatic CEA-expressing tumors, and documented the safety of the vaccine. Furthermore, CEA-specific T-cell responses were induced in a minority of patients, but these responses correlated with disease stabilization. Additional data from murine studies suggested that the inclusion of multiple costimulatory molecules and cytokines could enhance T-cell activation [49,50]. A particular triad of costimulatory molecules, including B7.1, the intracellular adhesion molecule (ICAM-1), and the lymphocyte function-associated antigen (LFA-3), was designated as the triad of costimulatory molecules (TRICOM), and was found to be especially powerful when compared with poxviruses that expressed only a single costimulatory molecule [46].

In a cohort of 58 heavily pretreated patients who had metastatic CEA-expressing cancers, Marshall and colleagues [51] used a prime-boost strategy that involved vaccinia and avipox vectors that expressed CEA and the TRICOM costimulatory molecules given with or without local granulocyte-macrophage colony-stimulating factor (GM-CSF). Most patients had colorectal or other gastrointestinal cancers, and no major toxicities occurred. Although 1 patient had an enduring complete pathologic response, 40% of the participants achieved stable disease at 4 months, although half of these people progressed during the first 2 months and stabilized during months 3 and 4. Overall, 25% of the study population had stable disease for greater than 6 months. Several patients (6 of 12) who achieved stable disease on a monthly vaccination schedule progressed when they were switched to a quarterly vaccination regimen; they achieved stable disease again when their vaccinations were changed back to monthly boosters. A correlation was seen between CEA-specific T-cell response and 1-year survival. These studies demonstrate nicely how combining new knowledge in immunology can be used to improve the effectiveness of vaccines; the ultimate test of the usefulness of this approach will depend on results from randomized phase III clinical trials.

Poxviruses also have been investigated for the treatment of prostate cancer, the most common cancer of men in the United States. The prostate-specific antigen (PSA) is a kallikrein protein, which is released by prostate cancer cells, that can be used to detect occult disease in patients [52]. The PSA gene has been identified and cloned with evidence that human T cells can recognize HLA-restricted peptides that are contained within the coding sequences of the PSA protein [53]. A recombinant vaccinia virus that expressed the human PSA gene was generated and tested in a series of phase I clinical trials. In one study, 33 men with elevated PSA levels following radical prostatectomy, radiation treatment, or both were treated with three monthly vaccinations of vaccinia-PSA in a dose-escalation trial [54]. Ten patients on the highest vaccine dose also received adjuvant GM-CSF. The vaccine regimen was well tolerated with only grade I cutaneous reactions reported following vaccination. The PSA levels were stable for 6 months in 14 of the 33 men, and 9 patients' levels were stable for 11 to 25 months. Overall, 6 patients remained free from PSA progression at 21 months of follow-up. This trial also reported the appearance of PSA-specific T-cell responses following vaccination. In a related trial, 42 men who had androgen-independent metastatic prostate cancer were treated with vaccinia-PSA using a similar dose-escalation study design [55]. This study supported the safety of the vaccine and again reported only mild cutaneous reactions that were related to the vaccination. This trial also reported the identification of PSA-specific T cells following immunization, and documented the ability of these T cells to lyse PSA-expressing tumor cells in vitro.

To avoid the neutralizing antibody response that is elicited against vaccinia virus, a fowlpox virus that expressed PSA was generated and tested in a prime-boost strategy in a prospective, randomized phase 2 clinical trial [56]. In this trial, 64 men who had hormone-dependent prostate cancer and who had elevated PSA levels following primary treatment of their cancer without evidence of metastatic disease, were eligible for participation. Patients were assigned randomly to one of three groups. Group A received four immunizations with fowlpox-PSA every 6 weeks. Group B received three fowlpox-PSA vaccines followed by a single vaccinia-PSA vaccine given at 6-week intervals. The patients in Group C received one vaccinia-PSA and three fowlpox-PSA vaccines also at 6-week intervals and represented the prime-boost experimental cohort. All vaccination schedules were tolerated well. There was no difference between the three arms with respect to the primary end point; at 6 months, only 16% of participants had PSA progression. Overall, nearly half of the participants did not experience PSA progression at a median follow-up of 19.1 months. The median time to PSA and clinical progression was 9.2 and 9.0 months for Groups A and B, respectively, but was not reached for Group C. Although this trend was not statistically significant, it has persisted for up to 45 months of follow-up [57].

In an effort to improve the effectiveness of the vaccines, a recombinant vaccinia virus that expressed PSA and the B7.1 costimulatory molecules was tested with fowlpox-PSA booster vaccines in men with an increasing PSA after failing hormone therapy. In this trial, 42 men were randomized to vaccination or antiandrogen treatment with nilutamide [58]. The median time to treatment failure was 9.9 months in men who received vaccine, compared with 7.6 months in men who were on nilutamide ($P=.28$). Based on preclinical models that demonstrated the benefit of combining poxvirus vaccines with radiation [59], a clinical trial was conducted in men who were eligible for radiation treatment of localized prostate cancer [60]. In this study, 30 men were randomized in a 2:1 fashion to vaccine plus radiotherapy or standard radiotherapy alone. In this trial, the vaccine included priming with vaccinia viruses that expressed PSA and B7.1, which was followed by seven monthly booster vaccinations with fowlpox-PSA. Patients also were treated with local GM-CSF and low-dose IL-2 after each vaccine. Radiation was administered per routine protocol between the fourth and sixth vaccine. Of 17 patients who completed all scheduled vaccinations, 13 exhibited an increase in PSA-specific T-cell responses compared with no increase in the group that received radiation alone ($P<.0005$). The only toxicities that were related to the vaccine were low-grade injection site reactions, although several grade 3 events were related to cytokine administration and radiation treatment. The sample size was too small to draw meaningful conclusions about clinical end points.

The mucin gene, MUC-1, is overexpressed in a large number of adenocarcinomas, including pancreatic, breast, colon, and prostate cancers. A recombinant vaccinia virus that was engineered to express MUC-1 and IL-2 was tested in a phase I clinical trial in patients who had advanced prostate cancer [61]. A standard dose-escalation trial design was used, and vaccine was administered by intramuscular injection. The vaccine was well tolerated with only low-grade vaccine-related adverse events. There was one objective clinical response in a patient who received the intermediate dose of vaccine; this patient also had evidence of a strong immune response induced by the vaccine. A related approach that used the modified vaccinia virus MVA, expressing MUC-1 and IL-2, was tested in 13 patients who had various solid tumors that were known to express MUC-1 [62]. The vaccine was well tolerated, and 4 patients showed disease stabilization for 6 to 9 months; 1 patient who had lung carcinoma demonstrated tumor regression that lasted for 14 months.

Another strategy to improve responses with poxviruses has been to use these vectors in a prime-boost regimen with recombinant peptides or proteins. Several recent studies used this approach in HPV-associated malignancies (eg, cervical cancer) or premalignant conditions (eg, vulvar intraepithelial neoplasia). Davidson and colleagues [63] enrolled 11 women who had vulvar intraepithelial neoplasia—most of whom had had a clinical (>50% shrinkage) or symptomatic response to immunization with a recombinant vaccinia vector that expressed the HPV type 16 and 18 E6 and E7 proteins—into a follow-up study. In this trial, participants received three booster immunizations of a recombinant HPV-16 L2E6E7 fusion protein [64]. Of 10 evaluable patients, all but 1 demonstrated HPV 16-specific proliferative T-cell or serologic responses following the booster vaccination. Three patients experienced regression of their lesions, although no direct correlation between clinical and immunologic responses was observed. In a related phase II study, Smyth and colleagues [65] enrolled 29 women who had high-grade vulvar or vulvo-anal intraepithelial neoplasia to receive three successive doses of the fusion protein followed by a single dose of vaccinia-HPV. Following immunization, 11 out of 25 evaluable patients had demonstrable T-cell responses to HPV-16–associated antigens (greater than threefold increase in HPV-antigen–specific T cells), and more than half of the participants had significant increases in antibodies specific to HPV-16 antigens. Nineteen of 29 patients had stable disease, 6 had objective responses (including a single complete response), and 4 had progressive lesions. Similar to the first trial, there was no correlation between clinical response and immunologic response. The investigators speculated that the lack of correlation might be because regression of vulvar lesions depends on infiltrating T cells, rather than on T cells that are found in peripheral blood. They further suggested that vaccine-mediated immune responses to vulvar intraepithelial neoplasia may not be related to an absolute increase in the numbers of T cells, but rather to qualitative changes, such as increases in effector $CD8^+$ T cells that are able to infiltrate target lesions.

Poxviruses also have been used as intratumoral vaccines to alter the local tumor microenvironment. A phase I trial used recombinant vaccinia virus that expressed the B7.1 costimulatory molecule in patients who had metastatic melanoma [66]. Twelve patients who had at least one lesion accessible for vaccination received three monthly injections. Only low-grade constitutional and injection site reactions were reported as side effects. Two patients had objective partial responses, one of which lasted for more than 59 months and was associated with new-onset vitiligo. Three additional patients had stable disease for 3 months. Vaccination was associated with an increase in gp100 and the melanoma antigen recognized by T-cells (MART-1)–specific T-cell responses. Examination of the tumor microenvironment confirmed that responding lesions were correlated more positively with local IFN-γ and were correlated negatively with IL-10 release.

ADENOVIRUSES

In contrast to the long history of poxviruses, the adenoviruses were recognized as distinct agents only in 1953 [67]. There are more than 50 serotypes of adenoviruses, and they are responsible for the common cold and ocular, respiratory, and intestinal illnesses in humans. The adenoviruses contain a small, double-stranded DNA genome that is composed of approximately 36 kb. The genome is divided into two overlapping regions that contain six early (E) and five late (L) genes based on the timing of gene transcription after infection. The E1a and E1b genes are transcribed early after infection, and include proteins that are involved in the regulation of other early functions [68]. The E2 genes encode proteins that are involved in viral replication [69]. The E3 genes help to mediate the host antiviral immune response and block tumor necrosis factor (TNF)-α–mediated apoptosis of infected cells [70]. The E4 genes encode proteins that are involved in regulation of DNA transcription and replication, and also down-regulate host cell protein synthesis. Generally, the late genes are involved in structural maturation of new viral particles [69]. The adenoviruses enter cells through specific receptors, such as the Coxsackie virus and adenovirus receptor, and exist in endocytic vesicles. Cell entry can be facilitated by certain integrins, including the $\alpha_v\beta_3$ and $\alpha_v\beta_5$ integrins [71]. After the pH within the endosome is lowered, viral particles are transferred to the nucleus where viral transcription is initiated, although chromosomal integration does not occur [72].

The broad host range of adenoviral vectors and their ability to infect proliferating and quiescent cells have made them useful for expressing foreign proteins and for gene delivery. This is offset by their highly immunogenic nature and rapid clearance from hosts that were exposed previously to adenoviruses, which is a significant issue because of the high prevalence of adenovirus infection in the general population. Nonetheless, adenoviruses have been useful in vaccine development, because they can be optimized by careful selection of specific serotypes and through generation of vectors with deletions of specific viral genes, which renders the viruses less immunogenic. The most commonly used vectors have been the type 5 adenoviruses with deletions of the E1, E3, and E4 genes, which result in replication-deficient vectors [73]. A further advantage of deleting portions of the E1 and E3 genes is that this allows the introduction of up to 8000 nucleotides that encode foreign transgenes. Newer recombinant vectors include selected deletions in E2 genes, which have resulted in prolonged transgene expression and further diminished immunogenicity [74]. More recently, complete eradication of nonessential genes, or so-called "gutless" adenovirus vectors, have been generated that allow longer sequences of recombinant DNA to be expressed [75]. Thus, through selected engineering, adenoviral vectors can be designed to express variable lengths of foreign DNA and exhibit different degrees of vector-specific immunity following vaccination.

Recombinant adenovirus vectors have been studied extensively in animal models and in veterinary medicine where they have induced protection against numerous infectious diseases, including rabies, swine fever, foot and mouth disease, and others [73]. Similar to poxviruses, adenovirus infection serves as a natural adjuvant for the immune system. Recent data demonstrate that adenoviruses promote maturation of DCs, and thereby, can potentiate antitumor cytotoxic T-cell responses [76–78]. Conversely, the world-wide prevalence of adenovirus infection has been an impediment to its use as immunotherapy, because many patients have preexisting neutralizing antibody titers. A novel approach that is being developed to circumvent this problem is to use serotypes with a low global prevalence, such as adenovirus type 35 (Group B) [79,80]. Prime-boost approaches that are similar to those used with poxvirus vectors also have been used with adenovirus vectors to prevent the rapid clearance of vaccine that is due to preexisting antibodies [81]. The potentially severe toxicity that is associated with native adenoviruses, specifically the development of acute or even fulminant hepatitis, has been subverted by the use of less immunogenic constructs [82].

In 2004, Dummer and colleagues [83] demonstrated the potency of a recombinant adenoviral vector that expressed a single cytokine. Nine heavily pretreated patients who had refractory cutaneous lymphoma received successive intralesional vaccinations with TG1042, a nonreplicative adenovirus vector that contained the IFN-γ gene sequence. The immunizations had an excellent safety profile; the main side effects were low-grade local cutaneous responses, headache, malaise, and fever. Three of the 9 study participants had complete responses in the inoculated lesions, and 2 of these patients had systemic complete responses as well. Two other patients had partial responses in their target lesion. Of the 4 remaining patients, 3 had stable disease and 1 had progressive disease. The median duration of response was 3 months (range, 1–6 months). Immunohistochemical analysis revealed that all patients had increased numbers of CD8$^+$ T cells in vaccinated lesions. Also, 4 of 8 patients tested had significant titers of antiviral antibodies before the start of the study, and 7 of 8 had higher titers after being immunized with TG1042. The investigators did not evaluate the relationship between preexisting antibody titers and clinical responses, but of the 4 patients who had elevated adenovirus-specific titers at study entry, 2 had a complete response and 1 had a partial response. The investigators speculated that the presence of preexisting antibodies against adenovirus may prevent the vaccine from entering the circulation and increasing the neutralizing antibody titers. A similar dose-escalation phase I trial, which used adenovirus that expressed IFN-γ, was conducted in patients who had advanced or locally recurrent melanoma [84]. Eleven patients received three weekly intratumoral vaccinations, and 1 patient achieved stable disease. The most frequent toxicities were grade 1 injection site erythema and fatigue, and 1 patient developed grade 3 fever and deep venous thrombosis.

Another phase I trial was conducted using a subcutaneous vaccine, which was composed of autologous plasma cells infected with adenovirus that expressed IL-2, in 8 patients who had multiple myeloma [85]. In this trial, vaccine production was successful for 6 patients, and only mild systemic side effects were observed. Although the vaccine site was infiltrated with $CD8^+$ T cells, no myeloma-specific immune or clinical response was demonstrated. The same vector was used in a separate trial of 12 men who had localized prostate cancer and a Gleason score greater than 7 or a PSA level greater than 10 [86]. In this study, the vaccine was injected 4 weeks before prostatectomy, and side effects included hematuria, perineal discomfort, flulike symptoms, and urinary hesitancy. Examination of resected tumors revealed a predominant $CD8^+$ T-cell infiltrate and areas of tumor necrosis.

More recently, preliminary results were reported for a multi-institutional trial that used a nonreplicating adenovirus that expressed TNF-α under control of the early growth response 1 promoter, which is activated by ionizing radiation [87]. In this study, patients who had solid tumors were injected over 5 weeks, and radiation was initiated 3 days after the sixth-week injection. Four patients had complete regression of their tumors, and three patients were alive more than 2 years from the time of treatment.

The ONYX-015 adenovirus is a type 2/5 chimeric virus that was modified genetically by disruption of the E1B protein, which binds to and inactivates cellular *p53* [88]. Thus, ONYX-015 is a replication-selective virus that is designed to replicate preferentially in tumors with defects in the *p53* pathway [89]. The vector demonstrated antitumor effects in vitro against a wide range of human tumor cells, including numerous carcinoma lines with mutated and normal *p53* gene sequences; this suggested that the mechanism of action may be more complex [90]. The virus was administered to 40 patients who had relapsed head and neck squamous cell carcinomas by intratumoral injection [91]. Thirty patients received vaccine once a day for five consecutive days and 10 patients received two daily dosages for two consecutive weeks in a 21-day treatment cycle. The cohort that received daily administration had a 14% objective response rate (and 41% stable disease), compared with the objective response of 10% in the other cohort (and 62% stable disease). In another trial, ONYX-015 was delivered to 11 patients by injection into the hepatic artery [92]. In this trial, most patients had gastrointestinal tumors, and the vaccine was used with 5-fluorouracil (5-FU) in selected patients. Toxicity was mild, and 1 patient who was refractory to 5-FU had an objective response to treatment with combined virus and 5-FU. Another phase I trial used this virus in 16 women who had recurrent ovarian cancer [93]. Although no clinical response was seen, the virus generally was well tolerated; adverse events included flu-like symptoms, abdominal pain, and vomiting. The virus also was delivered by endoscopic ultrasound to 21 patients who had localized pancreatic cancer [94]. In this trial there was no evidence of pancreatitis, and 2 patients had a partial response, 2 had a minor response, and 6 had stable disease. Some patients, however, also received gemcitabine chemotherapy. ONYX-015 was tested in 19 patients who had tumors of the liver, gall bladder, or bile ducts. It was administered by CT-guided injection or by intraperitoneal injection in patients who had malignant ascites [95]. In this trial, 1 patient had an objective partial response, 1 patient had prolonged disease stabilization for 49 weeks, and 8 patients had a greater than 50% reduction in tumor markers. The virus also was administered to patients who had glioma, colorectal cancer, or sarcoma with similar results, although large randomized trials have not been reported [96–98].

ADENO-ASSOCIATED VIRUS

AAV is a small single-stranded DNA parvovirus, and although it is not known to cause human disease, 50% to 90% of the adult population is seropositive, which indicates previous AAV exposure [99]. There are six serotypes; type 2 has been studied the most extensively for gene therapy and vaccine development. The heparin sulfate proteoglycan is the attachment receptor for AAV, and cell entry is facilitated by several accessory molecules, including fibroblast growth factor receptor 1 and the $\alpha_v\beta_5$ integrin, which mediates entry of the viral particle into the endocytic pathway. Following endosome acidification, AAV gradually accumulates within the nucleus of infected cells, where replication depends on the presence of helper viruses, typically adenovirus or HPV [100]. In the absence of helper viruses, the single-stranded DNA AAV genome is converted into double-stranded DNA and integrates into a specific locus (q13.3) on chromosome 19 [101]. Recombinant AAV vectors can be generated by cotransfecting permissive cells with AAV plasmids and helper plasmids that support packaging of recombinant AAV vectors [73]. Like adenovirus, AAV has a broad host range and can infect proliferating and quiescent cells, which makes these good vectors for gene delivery. The efficiency of gene transduction depends on the status of receptors and mediators of AAV cell entry and processing. The integration of AAV can result in long-term gene expression, and the site-specific nature of this integration avoids the potential problem of random integration and insertional mutagenesis. Another advantage of AAV vectors is the limited host immune response against them, which also may promote long-term gene expression [102]. There is accumulating evidence that neutralizing antibody and T-cell responses can be generated against AAV, and further studies are needed to define how and to what extent this occurs [73]. In addition, different serotypes may exhibit different tropism for tumor cells, although the type 2 AAV has been used the most widely and is supported by high transduction efficiency of cell lines in vitro [103].

Although AAV has not been used widely in the clinic there are many examples of its potential usefulness in preclinical models. AAV that expressed the extracellular domain of the TNF-related apoptosis-inducing ligand (TRAIL) resulted in secretion of soluble TRAIL and apoptosis following introduction into the A549 lung adenocarcinoma cell line [104]. AAV-TRAIL–transduced tumor cells also were inhibited from growing in a murine system, and improved the survival of tumor-bearing mice. In another study, subcutaneous establishment of gliomas, renal cell carcinomas, and melanoma could be prevented by liver-targeted delivery of AAV that expressed IFN-β [105]. In a different study that used a similar treatment approach, liver-derived IFN-β following AAV delivery significantly restricted the growth of a murine neuroblastoma tumor, and induced complete regression when combined with low-dose cyclophosphamide treatment [106]. These encouraging preclinical results await confirmation in clinical trials.

HERPESVIRUS

Herpes simplex virus type 1 (HSV-1) is a double-stranded DNA virus with a genome of approximately 150 kb that has been studied predominantly as a mediator of viral oncolysis. Typically, wild-type HSV-1 is cytolytic in many human tissues, but through recombinant DNA technology it can be engineered to destroy malignant cells without damaging nearby normal cells. The disruption or deletion of HSV-1 genes, such as thymidine kinase, ribonucleotide reductase, and $\gamma_1 34.5$, abrogates replication and subsequent cytolysis in noncancerous cells, but does not affect viral growth in malignant cells [107–109]. HSV-1 with one or more of these gene deletions can replicate effectively only in cells with high mitotic rates [110]. These "replication-conditional" viruses also are less neurotropic, and hence, are safer for vaccine development. These vectors were shown to infect several tumor cell lines and released progeny viruses after infection of malignant cells, which provided a continued source of new virus, such that direct infection of every cell within a tumor mass is not necessary. The effects of wild-type HSV-1 infection on immune responses are complex and are incompletely understood. Although HSV-1 infection inhibits the ability of DCs to migrate to lymphoid tissue and induces DC apoptosis, there is evidence that HSV-1 also induces maturation and cross-presentation by noninfected DCs [111–113]. Because oncolytic HSVs exert direct effects on tumor cells, the resultant inflammatory mediators—secondary to tumor lysis—can stimulate additional DC presentation of in situ tumor cells [114].

The large HSV-1 genome allows insertion of foreign genes, including TAAs and cytokine genes, that can upregulate oncolysis or promote antitumor immunity (ie, IL-12, PM2, GM-CSF). HSV-1–mediated oncolysis has been studied in a broad array of cell lines (prostate, lung, cholangiocarcinoma, bladder, ovarian), but it is closest to reaching clinical translation in malignant glioma and melanoma. Markert and colleagues reported the results of a phase I trial using a single intratumoral injection of a replication-conditional HSV-1 in 21 patients who had radiologically demonstrated recurrent malignant primary brain tumors [109]. The patients had been pretreated heavily; all had received radiotherapy, 17 had surgical debulking, and about half had received chemotherapy. The investigators concluded that the vaccine was safe and well tolerated. No episodes of herpes encephalitis were reported, and although several individuals had neurologic complications, these were attributed to progressive glioma. Eight of 20 patients had decreases in tumor volume 1 month after injection, but these were not measured quantitatively and no data was provided that correlated responses with survival or immunologic variables. In a recent phase I study, Harrow and colleagues studied the effects of the replication-competent HSV-1 strain

HSV1716 on newly diagnosed or recurrent high-grade gliomas [114]. This group had published two previous trials of HSV1716 in this population, which demonstrated that HSV1716 was tolerated well and could replicate in high-grade gliomas, but no clinical responses were seen [115,116]. In a more recent study of 12 patients (10 had glioblastoma multiforme), HSV1716 was injected into the brain next to residual tumor, following debulking surgery. Patients were permitted to receive adjuvant chemotherapy or radiotherapy following resection and HSV1716 administration. No significant toxicities that were attributable to HSV1716 were seen. Although 8 patients died from progressive disease and another died from unrelated causes, 1 patient who received no adjuvant therapy was alive without evidence of disease progression 22 months after surgery. A second patient who received only adjuvant radiotherapy was alive without evidence of disease progression 15 months after surgery. A final patient who progressed at 3 months had a second debulking operation and received adjuvant 1-(2-Chloroethyl)-3-cyclohexyl-1-nitrosourea (CCNU) and was alive 18 months after the initial surgery. The investigators did not find a consistent trend in any of the immunologic data (eg, anti-HSV IgM and IgG titers or the presence of HSV DNA in serum) to explain why certain patients may have responded to HSV1716 injection. Although HSV1716 could be cultured in vitro in tissue samples that were taken at the time of debulking treatment from 4 patients, all of these patients experienced disease progression. Collectively, these data illustrate the feasibility of oncolytic HSVs in a tumor that normally has a poor prognosis, although initial clinical responses generally were poor.

HSV1716 also showed activity against melanoma cell lines in vitro, and a pilot study in five patients who had melanoma was reported in 2001 [117]. In one patient, a flattening of palpable tumor nodules was seen 21 days after two intralesional injections. Three patients received two or more injections, and all had evidence of tumor necrosis on histologic analysis. A related HSV-2 vector that expresses human GM-CSF has been generated and is awaiting clinical testing [118].

RETROVIRUSES AND LENTIVIRUSES

Retroviruses encompass any virus that contains two plus-stranded, single-strand RNA molecules per virion and the enzyme reverse transcriptase. These viruses infect cells through an interaction between the virally encoded envelope protein that is embedded in their lipid membrane and host cell receptors. Once inside a cell, they are capable of reverse transcribing their RNA genome into double-stranded proviral DNA, which inserts into the host cell genome through the action of virally encoded integrases. Thus, latency is a hallmark of retroviral infection. The proviral DNA can be transcribed into mRNA by host cell transcriptional machinery. Spliced mRNA is translated to form viral protein, whereas unspliced proviral mRNA is packaged into new retroviral particles [119].

The retroviruses were classified previously into oncovirus, lentivirus, and spumavirus subfamilies, but current classification systems separate them into seven distinct genera. Oncoviruses, such as human T-cell leukemia virus (*Delta-retrovirus*) and murine leukemia virus (*Gammaretrovirus*) carry oncogenes that, when inserted into the host genome, transform permissive cells into cancer cells. In general, most retroviruses require actively proliferating cells to generate stable integration into the host cell genome; however, members of the genus *Lentivirus*, including HIV-1 and simian immunodeficiency virus (SIV), are able to infect cells that are not dividing actively, and may offer an advantage for vaccine development. Advantages of retroviruses are their ability to integrate into the host genome, and therefore, provide long-term expression of heterologous genes. This is tempered by limitations that are imposed by their narrow host range and, with the exception of the lentiviruses, their inability to infect cells that are not dividing actively (see Table 1).

Because in most gene therapy applications it is desirable to prevent spread of virus beyond the targeted tissue, retrovirus vectors normally contain one or more deletions of viral protein coding sequences so that they are not replication competent [120]. Therefore, helper constructs, most commonly in the form of engineered culture cells, are designed to express viral genes that are lacking in these vectors and to support production of recombinant viruses. Moreover, retroviral systems can be engineered to include an inactivated gene of interest that is activated upon delivery and incorporation into target cells. Through the introduction of repeated sequences within the gene of interest, which are deleted subsequently through an inherent property of reverse transcriptase, these systems self-activate the gene and self-inactivate the vector during transcription within the host [120].

A major concern with the use of retroviruses is the potential for insertional mutagenesis; recent studies suggested that they tend to insert into active transcriptional sites [121,122]. As a result, these vectors present a significant risk for activating growth-promoting genes or inactivating tumor-suppressor genes. Clinical trials of retroviral therapy using modified lentivirus for X-linked severe combined immunodeficiency revealed the development of leukemia in patients from vector-associated insertional mutagenesis [123]. Therefore, limiting expression of the incorporated retroviral genome to specifically targeted cells is critical for the development of safe retroviral vaccines. Tumor-specific targeting has been reported by displaying anti-CEA antibodies on the surface of retroviruses [124]. Pseudotyping is another method of retroviral targeting whereby the envelope structure is modified by incorporating glycoproteins that are derived from other enveloped viruses. Pseudotyped retroviruses exhibit an expanded host range [125] and may enhance viral transduction efficiency [126]. The most popular protein for this has been the G envelope glycoprotein of the vesicular stomatitis virus. Additionally, the generation of truncated virus like particles has been used to provide transient gene expression without the potential for long-term chromosomal integration [127]. Although there have been some promising reports of retroviruses in murine tumor studies, clinical trials of retroviral vectors that express TAAs or cytokines have not been reported.

The lentiviruses have received significant interest recently because they possess several unique features that support their ability to generate vaccines for cancer. For example, the protein transduction domain of the HIV-1 Tat protein has been used to facilitate intercellular spreading as a part of fusion proteins [128]. Thus, Tat has been incorporated into a fusion protein with the HSV thymidine kinase (HSV-TK), a suicide gene that is used in cancer gene therapy that renders cells susceptible to the antiviral drug ganciclovir. Although when cloned into a lentivirus vector, the fusion protein did not provoke translocation between glioma cells in vitro, it made these and a human ovarian carcinoma cell line more sensitive to ganciclovir than did a fusion protein that lacked Tat [129]. Lentiviruses also have been used to transduce DCs, because they do not induce major changes in DC maturation status or antigen-presenting function. In a murine melanoma model, lentivirus-transduced DCs induced significant antitumor effects and generated antigen-specific T-cell responses [130].

Despite these promising preclinical studies, the use of lentivirus vectors in clinical trials is limited by safety concerns and because of difficulties in producing high-titer virus stocks. The development of replication-deficient lentivirus vectors has begun to address these concerns, as exemplified by the equine infectious anemia virus [131]. The use of tissue-specific promoters is another method that is under investigation for controlling lentiviral gene expression. A lentivirus that encoded a probasin-derived, prostate-specific probasin gene promoter, ARR_2PB, achieved differential expression of the enhanced green fluorescent protein reporter gene in prostate cancer cells in vitro and in vivo [132]. Furthermore, when an additional DNA sequence that is recognized by eIF4E—a translation initiation factor that is overexpressed in many cancers—was added in front of the HSV-TK suicide gene, the killing effects of ganciclovir were restricted to prostate cancer cells [133]. Another approach for tumor-selective targeting was developed using the human telomere reverse transcriptase promoter (hTERTp), because more than 85% to 90% of primary tumors display high telomerase activity [134]. A self-inactivating HIV-based lentiviral vector was generated with the HSV-TK gene under transcriptional control of the hTERTp [135]. Because hTERTp was active only in tumor cells, HSV-TK expression was targeted and selectively eradicated tumor cells in vitro and in vivo. This concept also was tested, using a self-inactivating lentivirus that expressed B7.1 and IL-2, in acute myeloid leukemia (AML) blasts [136]. Infected AML blasts generated increased stimulation of allogeneic and autologous T cells with a greater level of T helper 1 cytokine release.

Another safeguard that is being investigated is a system to regulate the amount of therapeutic protein that is expressed by the viral vectors. In the tetracycline regulatory (Tet-On) system, target gene expression can be turned on in the presence of doxycycline, and gene expression can be switched off by withdrawal of the antibiotic. Thus, when two pseudoviruses—one expressing Tet-On (RevTet-On) and the other expressing HSV-TK (RevTRE/HSVtk)—were administered simultaneously to human breast cancer MCF-7 cells and followed by doxycycline and ganciclovir treatment, the cells were arrested at S phase and their growth was suppressed in vitro and in vivo [137]. These novel techniques have addressed many of the safety concerns that are related to insertional mutagenesis, unrestricted protein production, and spread of virus to normal tissue, and clinical trials are likely in the near future.

NOVEL APPROACHES USING VIRAL VECTORS

The use of viral vaccines to initiate antitumor immune responses or to deliver therapeutic gene products to tumors has been discussed. These vectors, however, also can be used in novel ways to enhance treatment of cancer. For example, viral vectors can be used to infect DCs directly, and then the infected DCs are used as a vaccine. Autologous DCs are obtained easily by leukapheresis, infected ex vivo, and then reinfused or injected into the patient. This approach allows DCs to be manipulated in a more controlled fashion and away from the potentially suppressive tumor environment. In a proof of concept study, Meyer and colleagues [138] infected ex vivo DCs from patients who had stage II resected melanoma with MVA expressing the tyrosinase melanoma antigen. Although the study demonstrated strong $CD4^+$ and $CD8^+$ T-cell responses against MVA, no response was detected against tyrosinase. In contrast, Di Nicola and colleagues [139] reported positive responses when they vaccinated six patients who had metastatic melanoma with autologous DCs that were infected by the same MVA-tyrosinase vector. Two patients had vitiligo in response to vaccination and four of five patients tested had significant increases in tyrosinase-specific T cells, but not in gp100-specific T cells. One patient who had vitiligo following immunization survived for more than 40 months. Another patient had partial regression of a subcutaneous nodule after immunization, which was then resected, and the patient has had no evidence of disease 29 months later. The reason for the differences in these trials may relate to the methods that were used for generating DCs, the patient population, or the selection of immune monitoring assays.

In a similar approach, Morse and colleagues [140] reported the results of a phase I study of 14 patients who had CEA-expressing cancers. They received intradermal injections of autologous DCs that were infected ex vivo with a recombinant fowlpox virus that expressed CEA and TRICOM. Patients had a median of two metastatic sites, and had received a median of two previous chemotherapy regimens. No grade 3 or 4 adverse effect was attributed to therapy. Five patients had stable disease after one cycle of vaccination, and one of these patients continued to have stable disease after a second cycle of treatment. Thirteen of 14 patients had increases in CEA-specific T cells after vaccination, and the extent of this increase was highest in patients who had a measurable clinical response.

SUMMARY AND FUTURE DIRECTIONS

Viruses are a diverse group of pathogenic agents that are responsible for a multitude of human disease and suffering. These same viruses, however, also have been used to prevent disease, and can be manipulated genetically to provide potent vaccines and gene delivery vehicles to alleviate disease. A better understanding of the immune system and how it mediates tumor surveillance and rejection has helped to guide the rational design of modern tumor vaccines. The selection of an appropriate viral vector depends on careful consideration of many factors, including the availability of strong tumor antigens, the stage of disease at the time of vaccination, and the desired endpoint, which may include establishing tumor-reactive immune effectors or stable expression of transgenes within established tumors. Among the many viruses that are used for vaccine development, the poxviruses and adenoviruses have been studied the most widely. Other viral candidates include AAV, HPVs, and retroviruses (including lentiviruses). Early clinical trials have established the safety profile of these vectors, and occasional clinical responses have been observed; however, these studies were not designed to determine clinical response, and the usefulness of viral vaccines must wait for results from larger prospective, randomized clinical trials.

The future of viral vaccines will include continued efforts to refine the viral genomes and test new immunomodulatory molecules and combinations. Additional investigation on the optimal route of administration, the selection of adjuvants, and the appropriate timing of vaccination with respect to disease stage and combinations with other treatment modalities will help to refine when and how viral vaccines will be helpful. The development of validated surrogate assays for vaccine trials in patients who have cancer—similar to the assays that are used for evaluation of infectious disease vaccines—remains another important goal. An effort to recommend participation in clinical trials of viral vaccines also will be critical to the evaluation of their full potential in the treatment and prevention of cancer.

References

[1] Disis ML, Lyerly HK. Global role of the immune system in identifying cancer initiation and limiting disease progression. J Clin Oncol 2005;23:8923–5.
[2] Dunn GP, Bruce AT, Ikeda H, et al. Cancer immunoediting: from immunosurveillance to tumor escape. Nat Immunol 2002;3:991–8.
[3] Kaufman HL, Flanagan K, Lee CS, et al. Insertion of interleukin-2 (IL-2) and interleukin-12 (IL-12) genes into vaccinia virus results in effective anti-tumor responses without toxicity. Vaccine 2002;20:1862–9.
[4] Flanagan K, Glover RT, Horig H, et al. Local delivery of recombinant vaccinia virus expressing secondary lymphoid chemokine (SLC) results in a CD4 T-cell dependent anti-tumor response. Vaccine 2004;22:2894–903.
[5] Rosenberg SA, Yang JC, Restifo NP. Cancer immunotherapy: moving beyond current vaccines. Nat Med 2004;10:909–15.
[6] Timmerman JM, Levy R. Cancer vaccines: pessimism in check. Nat Med 2004;10:1279.
[7] Spanknebel K, Cheung KY, Stoutenburg J, et al. Initial clinical response predicts outcome and is associated with dose schedule in metastatic melanoma and renal cell carcinoma patients treated with high-dose interleukin-2. Ann Surg Oncol 2005;12:381–90.
[8] Yang F, Yang XF. New concepts in tumor antigens: their significance in future immunotherapies for tumors. Cell Mol Immunol 2005;2:331–41.
[9] Disis ML, Schiffman K, Guthrie K, et al. Effect of dose on immune response in patients vaccinated with an her-2/neu intracellular domain protein-based vaccine. J Clin Oncol 2004;22:1916–25.

[10] Levy B, Deeken JF, Holt G, et al. Immunologic therapies for gastrointestinal cancers. Clin Colorectal Cancer 2005;5:37–49.
[11] Pure E, Allsion P, Schreiber RD. Breaking down the barriers to cancer immunotherapy. Nat Immunol 2005;6:1207–10.
[12] Arvin AM, Greenberg HB. New viral vaccines. Virology 2006;344(1):240–9.
[13] Moss B. Genetically engineered poxviruses for recombinant gene expression, vaccination, and safety. Proc Natl Acad Sci U S A 1996;93:11341–8.
[14] Hodge JW, McLaughlin JP, Abrams SI, et al. Admixture of a recombinant vaccinia virus containing the gene for the costimulatory molecule B7 and a recombinant vaccinia virus containing a tumor-associated antigen gene results in enhanced specific T-cell responses and antitumor immunity. Cancer Res 1995;55:3598–603.
[15] Shevach EM. CD4+ CD25+ suppressor T cells: more questions than answers. Nat Rev Immunol 2002;2:389–400.
[16] Pages F, Berger A, Camus M, et al. Effector memory T cells, early metastasis, and survival in colorectal cancer. N Engl J Med 2005;353(25):2654–66.
[17] Mellman I, Steinman RM. Dendritic cells: specialized and regulated antigen processing machines. Cell 2001;106:255–8.
[18] Hodge JW, Greiner JW, Tsang KY, et al. Costimulatory molecules as adjuvants for immunotherapy. Front Biosci 2006;11:788–803.
[19] Sallusto F, Lanzavecchia A. Understanding dendritic cell and T-lymphocyte traffic through the analysis of chemokine receptor expression. Immunol Rev 2000;177:134–40.
[20] Mahdavi A, Monk BJ. Vaccines against human papillomavirus and cervical cancer: promises and challenges. Oncologist 2005;10(7):528–38.
[21] Bristol JA, Schlom J, Abrams SI. Persistence, immune specificity, and functional ability of murine mutant ras epitope-specific CD4(+) and CD8(+) T lymphocytes following in vivo adoptive transfer. Cell Immunol 1999;194(1):78–89.
[22] Scanlan MJ, Simpson AJ, Old LJ. The cancer/testis genes: review, standardization, and commentary. Cancer Immunol 2004;4:1.
[23] Kaufman H, Schlom J, Kantor J. A recombinant vaccinia virus expressing human carcino-embryonic antigen (CEA). Int J Cancer 1991;48(6):900–7.
[24] Cono J, Casey CG, Bell DM. Smallpox vaccination and adverse reactions. Guidance for clinicians. MMWR Recomm Rep 2003;52(RR-4):1–28.
[25] Fenner F, Wittek R, Dumbell KR. The orthopoxviruses. San Diego (CA): Academic Press; 1989.
[26] Jenner E. An inquiry into the causes and effects of the variolae vaccinae, a disease discovered in some of the western counties of England, particularly near Gloucestershire, and known by the name of the Cow Pox. New York: Dover; 1798.
[27] Shen Y, Nemunaitis J. Fighting cancer with vaccinia virus: teaching new tricks to an old dog. Mol Ther 2005;11:180–95.
[28] World Health Organization. The global eradication of smallpox: final report of the Global Commission for the Certification of Smallpox Eradication, Geneva, December, 1979. Geneva (Switzerland): World Health Organization; 1980.
[29] Smith GL, Moss B. Infectious poxvirus vectors have capacity for at least 25,000 base pairs of foreign DNA. Gene 1983;25(1):21–8.
[30] Zhu MZ, Marshall J, Cole D, et al. Specific cytolytic T-cell responses to human CEA from patients immunized with recombinant avipox-CEA vaccine. Clin Cancer Res 2000; 6:24–33.
[31] Belshe RB, Newman FK, Frey SE, et al. Dose-dependent neutralizing-antibody responses to vaccinia. J Infect Dis 2004;189:493–7.
[32] Belyakov IM, Moss B, Strober W, et al. Mucosal vaccination overcomes the barrier to recombinant vaccinia immunization caused by preexisting poxvirus immunity. Proc Natl Acad Sci U S A 1999;96:4512–7.
[33] Kass E, Panicali DL, Mazzara G, et al. Granulocyte/macrophage-colony stimulating factor produced by recombinant avian poxviruses enriches the regional lymph nodes

with antigen-presenting cells and acts as an immunoadjuvant. Cancer Res 2001;61: 206–14.

[34] Kaufman HL. Integrating bench with bedside: the role of vaccine therapy in the treatment of solid tumors. J Clin Oncol 2005;23(4):659–61.

[35] Engelmayer J, Larsson M, Subklewe M, et al. Vaccinia virus inhibits the maturation of human dendritic cells: a novel mechanism of immune evasion. J Immunol 1999;163: 6762–8.

[36] Jenne L, Hauser C, Arrighi JF, et al. Poxvirus as a vector to transduce human dendritic cells for immunotherapy: abortive infection but reduced APC function. Gene Ther 2000;7: 1575–83.

[37] Larsson M, Fonteneau JF, Somersan S, et al. Efficiency of cross presentation of vaccinia virus-derived antigens by human dendritic cells. Eur J Immunol 2001;31:3432–42.

[38] Paoletti E. Applications of pox virus vectors to vaccination: an update. Proc Natl Acad Sci U S A 1996;93:11349–53.

[39] Mayr A, Stickl H, Muller HK, et al. [The smallpox vaccination strain MVA: marker, genetic structure, experience gained with the parenteral vaccination and behavior in organisms with a debilitated defence mechanism]. Zentralbl Bakteriol [B] 1978;167:375–90. [in German].

[40] Hodge JW, McLaughlin JP, Kantor JA, et al. Diversified prime and boost protocols using recombinant vaccinia virus and recombinant non-replicating avian pox virus to enhance T-cell immunity and antitumor responses. Vaccine 1997;15:759–68.

[41] Kantor J, Irvine K, Abrams S, et al. Anti-tumor activity and immune responses induced by a recombinant vaccinia-carcinoembryonic antigen (CEA) vaccine. J Natl Cancer Inst 1992;84:1084–91.

[42] McAneny D, Ryan CA, Beazley RM, et al. Results of a phase I trial of a recombinant vaccinia virus that expresses carcinoembryonic antigen in patients with advanced colorectal cancer. Ann Surg Oncol 1996;3:495–500.

[43] Conry RM, Khazaeli MB, Saleh MN, et al. Phase I trial of a recombinant vaccinia virus encoding carcinoembryonic antigen in metastatic adenocarcinoma: comparison of intra-dermal versus subcutaneous administration. Clin Cancer Res 1999;5:2330–7.

[44] Kantor J, Irvine K, Abrams S, et al. Anti-tumor activity and immune responses induced by a recombinant vaccinia-carcinoembryonic antigen (CEA) vaccine. J Natl Cancer Inst 1992;84:1084–91.

[45] Marshall JL, Hoyer RJ, Toomey MA, et al. Phase I study in advanced cancer patients of a diversified prime-and-boost vaccination protocol using recombinant vaccinia virus and recombinant nonreplicating avipox virus to elicit anti-carcinoembryonic antigen immune responses. J Clin Oncol 2000;18:3964–73.

[46] Hodge JW, Sabzevari H, Yafal AG, et al. a triad of costimulatory molecules synergize to amplify T-cell activation. Cancer Res 1999;59:5800–7.

[47] Horig H, Lee DS, Conkright W, et al. Phase I clinical trial of a recombinant canary-poxvirus (ALVAC) vaccine expressing human carcinoembryonic antigen and the B7.1 co-stimulatory molecule. Cancer Immunol Immunother 2000;49:504–14.

[48] von Mehren M, Arlen P, Tsang KY, et al. Pilot study of a dual gene recombinant avipox vaccine containing both carcinoembryonic antigen (CEA) and B7.1 transgenes in patients with recurrent CEA-expressing adenocarcinomas. Clin Cancer Res 2000;6:2219–28.

[49] Grosenbach DW, Barrientos JC, et al. Synergy of vaccine strategies to amplify antigen-specific immune responses and antitumor effects. Cancer Res 2001;61:4497–505.

[50] Greiner JW, Zeytin H, Anver MR, et al. Vaccine-based therapy directed against carcino-embryonic antigen demonstrates antitumor activity on spontaneous intestinal tumors in the absence of autoimmunity. Cancer Res 2002;62:6944–51.

[51] Marshall JL, Gulley JL, Arlen PM, et al. Phase I study of sequential vaccinations with fowlpox-CEA(6D)-TRICOM alone and sequentially with vaccinia-CEA(6D)-TRICOM, with and without granulocyte-macrophage colony-stimulating factor, in patients with carci-noembryonic antigen-expressing carcinomas. J Clin Oncol 2005;23:720–31.

[52] Oesterling JE. Prostate specific antigen: a critical assessment of the most useful tumor marker for adenocarcinoma of the prostate. J Urol 1991;145:907–23.

[53] Correale P, Walmsley K, Zaremba S, et al. Generation of human cytolytic T lymphocyte lines directed against prostate-specific antigen (PSA) employing a PSA oligoepitope peptide. J Immunol 1998;161:3186–94.

[54] Eder JP, Kantoff PW, Roper K, et al. A phase I trial of a recombinant vaccinia virus expressing prostate-specific antigen in advanced prostate cancer. Clin Cancer Res 2000; 6:1632–8.

[55] Gulley J, Chen AP, Dahut W, et al. Phase I study of a vaccine using recombinant vaccinia virus expressing PSA (rV-PSA) in patients with metastatic androgen-independent prostate cancer. Prostate 2002;53(2):109–17.

[56] Kaufman HL, Wang W, Manola J, et al. Phase II randomized study of vaccine treatment of advanced prostate cancer (E7897): a trial of the Eastern Cooperative Oncology Group. J Clin Oncol 2004;22:2122–32.

[57] Kaufman HL, Wang W, Manola J, et al. Phase II prime/boost vaccination using poxviruses expressing PSA in hormone dependent prostate cancer: Follow-up clinical results from ECOG 7897. Am Soc Clin Oncol 2005;23:378s [abstract].

[58] Arlen PM, Gulley JL, Todd N, et al. Antiandrogen, vaccine and combination therapy in patients with nonmetastatic hormone refractory prostate cancer. J Urol 2005;174: 539–46.

[59] Chakraborty M, Abrams SI, Coleman CN, et al. External beam radiation of tumors alters phenotype of tumor cells to render them susceptible to vaccine-mediated T-cell killing. Cancer Res 2004;64:4328–37.

[60] Gulley JL, Arlen PM, Bastian A, et al. Combining a recombinant cancer vaccine with standard definitive radiotherapy in patients with localized prostate cancer. Clin Cancer Res 2005;11:3353–62.

[61] Pantuck AJ, van Ophoven A, Gitlitz BJ, et al. Phase I trial of antigen-specific gene therapy using a recombinant vaccinia virus encoding MUC-1 and IL-2 in MUC-1-positive patients with advanced prostate carcinoma. J Immunother 2004;27:240–53.

[62] Rochlitz C, Figlin R, Squiban P, et al. Phase I immunotherapy with a modified vaccinia virus (MVA) expressing human MUC1 as antigen-specific immunotherapy in patients with MUC1-positive advanced cancer. J Gene Med 2003;5:690–9.

[63] Davidson EJ, Boswell CM, Sehr P, et al. Immunological and clinical responses in women with vulval intraepithelial neoplasia vaccinated with a vaccinia virus encoding human papillomavirus 16/18 oncoproteins. Cancer Res 2003;63:6032–41.

[64] Davidson EJ, Faulkner RL, Sehr P, et al. Effect of TA-CIN (HPV 16 L2E6E7) booster immunisation in vulval intraepithelial neoplasia patients previously vaccinated with TA-HPV (vaccinia virus encoding HPV 16/18 E6E7). Vaccine 2004;22:2722–9.

[65] Smyth LJ, Van Poelgeest MI, Davidson EJ, et al. Immunological responses in women with human papillomavirus type 16 (HPV-16)-associated anogenital intraepithelial neoplasia induced by heterologous prime-boost HPV-16 oncogene vaccination. Clin Cancer Res 2004;10:2954–61.

[66] Kaufman HL, DeRaffele G, Mitcham J, et al. Targeting the local tumor microenvironment with vaccinia virus expressing B7.1 for the treatment of melanoma. J Clin Invest 2005; 115:1903–12.

[67] Rowe WP, Heubner RJ, Gilmore LK, et al. Isolation of a cytopathogenic agent from human adenoids undergoing spontaneous degeneration in tissue culture. Proc Soc Exp Biol Med 1953;84:570–3.

[68] Jones N, Shenk T. An adenovirus type 5 early gene function regulates expression of other early viral genes. Proc Natl Acad Sci U S A 1979;76:3665–9.

[69] Babiss LE, Ginsberg HS. Adenovirus type 5 early region 1b gene product is required for efficient shutoff of host protein synthesis. J Virol 1984;50:202–12.

[70] Tollefson AE, Hermiston TW, Lichtenstein DL, et al. Forced degradation of Fas inhibits apoptosis in adenovirus-infected cells. Nature 1998;392:726–30.

[71] Wickham TJ, Carrion ME, Kovesdi I. Targeting of adenovirus penton base to new receptors through replacement of its RGD motif with other receptor-specific peptide motifs. Gene Ther 1995;2:750–6.

[72] Greber UF, Willetts M, Webster P, et al. Stepwise dismantling of adenovirus 2 during entry into cells. Cell 1993;75:477–86.

[73] Lai CM, Lai YK, Rakoczy PE. Adenovirus and adeno-associated virus vectors. DNA Cell Biol 2002;21:895–913.

[74] Engelhardt JF, Litzky L, Wilson JM. Prolonged transgene expression in cotton rat lung with recombinant adenoviruses defective in E2a. Hum Gene Ther 1994;5:1217–29.

[75] Fisher KJ, Choi H, Burda J, et al. Recombinant adenovirus deleted of all viral genes for gene therapy of cystic fibrosis. Virology 1996;217:11–22.

[76] Zhang Y, Chirmule N, Gao GP, et al. Acute cytokine response to systemic adenoviral vectors in mice is mediated by dendritic cells and macrophages. Mol Ther 2001;3: 697–707.

[77] Cho HI, Kim HJ, Oh ST, et al. In vitro induction of carcinoembryonic antigen (CEA)-specific cytotoxic T lymphocytes by dendritic cells transduced with recombinant adeno-viruses. Vaccine 2003;22(2):224–36.

[78] Schumacher L, Ribas A, Dissette VB, et al. Human dendritic cell maturation by adenovirus transduction enhances tumor antigen-specific T-cell responses. J Immunother 2004;27: 191–200.

[79] Seshidhar Reddy P, Ganesh S, Limbach MP, et al. Development of adenovirus serotype 35 as a gene transfer vector. Virology 2003;311:384–93.

[80] Vogels R, Zuijdgeest D, van Rijnsoever R, et al. Replication-deficient human adenovirus type 35 vectors for gene transfer and vaccination: efficient human cell infection and bypass of preexisting adenovirus immunity. J Virol 2003;77:8263–71.

[81] Wang X, Wang JP, Rao XM, et al. Prime-boost vaccination with plasmid and adenovirus gene vaccines control HER2/neu + metastatic breast cancer in mice. Breast Cancer Res 2005;7:R580–8.

[82] Reid T, Warren R, Kirn D. Intravascular adenoviral agents in cancer patients: lessons from clinical trials. Cancer Gene Ther 2002;9:979–86.

[83] Dummer R, Hassel JC, Fellenberg F, et al. Adenovirus-mediated intralesional interferon-gamma gene transfer induces tumor regressions in cutaneous lymphomas. Blood 2004; 104(6):1631–8.

[84] Khorana AA, Rosenblatt JD, Sahasrabudhe DM, et al. A phase I trial of immunotherapy with intratumoral adenovirus-interferon-gamma (TG1041) in patients with malignant mela-noma. Cancer Gene Ther 2003;10:251–9.

[85] Trudel S, Li Z, Dodgson C, et al. Adenovector engineered interleukin-2 expressing autologous plasma cell vaccination after high-dose chemotherapy for multiple myeloma—a phase 1 study. Leukemia 2001;15:846–54.

[86] Trudel S, Trachtenberg J, Toi A, et al. A phase I trial of adenovector-mediated delivery of interleukin-2 (AdIL-2) in high-risk localized prostate cancer. Cancer Gene Ther 2003;10: 755–63.

[87] McLoughlin JM, McCarty TM, Cunningham C, et al. TNFerade, an adenovector carrying the transgene for human tumor necrosis factor alpha, for patients with advanced solid tumors: surgical experience and long-term follow-up. Ann Surg Oncol 2005;12:825–30.

[88] Heise C, Sampson-Johannes A, Williams A, et al. ONYX-015, an E1B gene-attenuated adenovirus, causes tumor-specific cytolysis and antitumoral efficacy that can be aug-mented by standard chemotherapeutic agents. Nat Med 1997;3:639–45.

[89] Heise C, Ganly I, Kim YT, et al. Efficacy of a replication-selective adenovirus against ovarian carcinomatosis is dependent on tumor burden, viral replication and p53 status. Gene Ther 2000;7:1925–9.

[90] McCormick F. Cancer-specific viruses and the development of ONYX-015. Cancer Biol Ther 2003;2:S157–60.

[91] Nemunaitis J, Khuri F, Ganly I, et al. Phase II trial of intratumoral administration of ONYX-

015, a replication-selective adenovirus, in patients with refractory head and neck cancer. J Clin Oncol 2001;19(2):289–98.

[92] Reid T, Galanis E, Abbruzzese J, et al. Intra-arterial administration of a replication-selective adenovirus (dl1520) in patients with colorectal carcinoma metastatic to the liver: a phase I trial. Gene Ther 2001;8:1618–26.

[93] Vasey PA, Shulman LN, Campos S, et al. Phase I trial of intraperitoneal injection of the E1B–55-kd-gene-deleted adenovirus ONYX-015 (dl1520) given on days 1 through 5 every 3 weeks in patients with recurrent/refractory epithelial ovarian cancer. J Clin Oncol 2002;20:1562–9.

[94] Hecht JR, Bedford R, Abbruzzese JL, et al. A phase I/II trial of intratumoral endoscopic ultrasound injection of ONYX-015 with intravenous gemcitabine in unresectable pancreatic carcinoma. Clin Cancer Res 2003;9:555–61.

[95] Makower D, Rozenblit A, Kaufman H, et al. Phase II clinical trial of intralesional administration of the oncolytic adenovirus ONYX-015 in patients with hepatobiliary tumors with correlative p53 studies. Clin Cancer Res 2003;9:693–702.

[96] Nemunaitis J, Cunningham C, Tong AW, et al. Pilot trial of intravenous infusion of a replication-selective adenovirus (ONYX-015) in combination with chemotherapy or IL-2 treatment in refractory cancer patients. Cancer Gene Ther 2003;10:341–52.

[97] Chiocca EA, Abbed KM, Tatter S, et al. A phase I open-label, dose-escalation, multi-institutional trial of injection with an E1B-Attenuated adenovirus, ONYX-015, into the peritumoral region of recurrent malignant gliomas, in the adjuvant setting. Mol Ther 2004;10:958–66.

[98] Galanis E, Okuno SH, Nascimento AG, et al. Phase I–II trial of ONYX-015 in combination with MAP chemotherapy in patients with advanced sarcomas. Gene Ther 2005; 12:437–45.

[99] Chirmule N, Propert K, Magosin S, et al. Immune responses to adenovirus and adeno-associated virus in humans. Gene Ther 1999;6:1574–83.

[100] Buller RM, Janik JE, Sebring ED, et al. Herpes simplex virus types 1 and 2 completely help adenovirus-associated virus replication. J Virol 1981;40:241–7.

[101] Ferrari FK, Samulski T, Shenk T, et al. Second-strand synthesis is a rate-limiting step for efficient transduction by recombinant adeno-associated virus vectors. J Virol 1996;70: 3227–34.

[102] Afione SA, Conrad CK, Kearns WG, et al. In vivo model of adeno-associated virus vector persistence and rescue. J Virol 1996;70:3235–41.

[103] Hacker UT, Wingenfeld L, Kofler DM, et al. Adeno-associated virus serotypes 1 to 5 mediated tumor cell directed gene transfer and improvement of transduction efficiency. J Gene Med 2005;7:1429–38.

[104] Shi J, Zheng D, Liu Y, et al. Overexpression of soluble TRAIL induces apoptosis in human lung adenocarcinoma and inhibits growth of tumor xenografts in nude mice. Cancer Res 2005;65:1687–92.

[105] Streck CJ, Dickson PV, Ng CY, et al. Antitumor efficacy of AAV-mediated systemic delivery of interferon-beta. Cancer Gene Ther 2006;13:99–106.

[106] Streck CJ, Dickson PV, Ng CY, et al. Adeno-associated virus vector-mediated systemic delivery of IFN-beta combined with low-dose cyclophosphamide affects tumor regression in murine neuroblastoma models. Clin Cancer Res 2005;11:6020–9.

[107] Chou J, Kern ER, Whitley RJ, et al. Mapping of herpes simplex virus-1 neurovirulence to gamma 134.5, a gene nonessential for growth in culture. Science 1990;250: 1262–6.

[108] Mineta T, Rabkin SD, Martuza RL. Treatment of malignant gliomas using ganciclovir-hypersensitive, ribonucleotide reductase-deficient herpes simplex viral mutant. Cancer Res 1994;54:3963–6.

[109] Markert JM, Medlock MD, Rabkin SD, et al. Conditionally replicating herpes simplex virus mutant, G207 for the treatment of malignant glioma: results of a phase I trial. Gene Ther 2000;7:867–74.

[110] Shah AC, Benos D, Gillespie GY, et al. Oncolytic viruses: clinical applications as vectors for the treatment of malignant gliomas. J Neurooncol 2003;65:203–26.

[111] Pollara G, Jones M, Handley ME, et al. Herpes simplex virus type-1-induced activation of myeloid dendritic cells: the roles of virus cell interaction and paracrine type I IFN secretion. J Immunol 2004;173:4108–19.

[112] Bosnjak L, Miranda-Saksena M, Koelle DM, et al. Herpes simplex virus infection of human dendritic cells induces apoptosis and allows cross-presentation via uninfected dendritic cells. J Immunol 2005;174:2220–7.

[113] Prechtel AT, Turza NM, Kobelt DJ, et al. Infection of mature dendritic cells with herpes simplex virus type 1 dramatically reduces lymphoid chemokine-mediated migration. J Gen Virol 2005;86:1645–57.

[114] Harrow S, Papanastassiou V, Harland J, et al. HSV1716 injection into the brain adjacent to tumour following surgical resection of high-grade glioma: safety data and long-term survival. Gene Ther 2004;11:1648–58.

[115] Papanastassiou V, Rampling R, Fraser M, et al. The potential for efficacy of the modified (ICP 34.5(-)) herpes simplex virus HSV1716 following intratumoural injection into human malignant glioma: a proof of principle study. Gene Ther 2002;9:398–406.

[116] Rampling R, Cruickshank G, Papanastassiou V, et al. Toxicity evaluation of replication-competent herpes simplex virus (ICP 34.5 null mutant 1716) in patients with recurrent malignant glioma. Gene Ther 2000;7:859–66.

[117] MacKie RM, Stewart B, Brown SM. Intralesional injection of herpes simplex virus 1716 in metastatic melanoma. Lancet 2001;357:525–6.

[118] Loudon PT, Blakeley DM, Boursnell ME, et al. Preclinical safety testing of DISC-hGMCSF to support phase I clinical trials in cancer patients. J Gene Med 2001;3:458–67.

[119] Galla M, Will E, Kraunus J, et al. Retroviral pseudotransduction for targeted cell manipulation. Mol Cell 2004;16:309–15.

[120] Hu WS, Pathak VK. Design of retroviral vectors and helper cells for gene therapy. Pharmacol Rev 2000;52:493–511.

[121] Schroder AR, Shinn P, Chen H, et al. HIV-1 integration in the human genome favors active genes and local hotspots. Cell 2002;110:521–9.

[122] Wu X, Li Y, Crise B, et al. Transcription start regions in the human genome are favored targets for MLV integration. Science 2003;300:1749–51.

[123] Hacein-Bey-Abina S, von Kalle C, Schmidt M, et al. A serious adverse event after successful gene therapy for X-linked severe combined immunodeficiency. N Engl J Med 2003;348:255–6.

[124] Khare PD, Liao S, Hirose Y, et al. Tumor growth suppression by a retroviral vector displaying scFv antibody to CEA and carrying the iNOS gene. Anticancer Res 2002;22: 2443–6.

[125] Cronin J, Zhang XY, Reiser J. Altering the tropism of lentiviral vectors through pseudotyping. Curr Gene Ther 2005;5:387–98.

[126] Burns JC, Friedmann T, Driever W, et al. Vesicular stomatitis virus G glycoprotein pseudotyped retroviral vectors: concentration to very high titer and efficient gene transfer into mammalian and nonmammalian cells. Proc Natl Acad Sci USA 1993;90:8033–7.

[127] Peretti S, Schiavoni I, Pugliese K, et al. Cell death induced by the herpes simplex virus-1 thymidine kinase delivered by human immunodeficiency virus-1-based virus-like particles. Mol Ther 2005;12:1185–96.

[128] Cascante A, Huch M, Rodriguez LG, et al. Tat8-TK/gcv suicide gene therapy induces pancreatic tumor regression in vivo. Hum Gene Ther 2005;16(12):1377–88.

[129] Merilainen O, Hakkarainen T, Wahlfors T, et al. HIV-1 TAT protein transduction domain mediates enhancement of enzyme prodrug cancer gene therapy in vitro: a study with TAT-TK-GFP triple fusion construct. Int J Oncol 2005;27:203–8.

[130] He Y, Zhang J, Mi Z, et al. Immunization with lentiviral vector-transduced dendritic cells induces strong and long-lasting T cell responses and therapeutic immunity. J Immunol 2005;174:3808–17.

[131] Ikeda Y, Collins MK, Radcliffe PA, et al. Gene transduction efficiency in cells of different species by HIV and EIAV vectors. Gene Ther 2002;9:932–8.

[132] Yu D, Jia WW, Gleave ME, et al. Prostate-tumor targeting of gene expression by lentiviral vectors containing elements of the probasin promoter. Prostate 2004;59:370–82.

[133] Yu D, Scott C, Jia WW, et al. Targeting and killing of prostate cancer cells using lentiviral constructs containing a sequence recognized by translation factor eIF4E and a prostate-specific promoter. Cancer Gene Ther 2006;13:32–43.

[134] Kim NW, Piatyszek MA, Prowse KR, et al. Specific association of human telomerase activity with immortal cells and cancer. Science 1994;266:2011–5.

[135] Painter RG, Lanson Jr NA, Jin Z, et al. Conditional expression of a suicide gene by the telomere reverse transcriptase promoter for potential post-therapeutic deletion of tumorigenesis. Cancer Sci 2005;96:607–13.

[136] Chan L, Hardwick N, Darling D, et al. IL-2/B7.1 (CD80) fusagene transduction of AML blasts by a self-inactivating lentiviral vector stimulates T cell responses in vitro: a strategy to generate whole cell vaccines for AML. Mol Ther 2005;11:120–31.

[137] Zeng ZJ, Li ZB, Luo SQ, et al. Retrovirus-mediated tk gene therapy of implanted human breast cancer in nude mice under the regulation of Tet-On. Cancer Gene Ther 2006; 13(3):290–7.

[138] Meyer H, Sutter G, Mayr A. Mapping of deletions in the genome of the highly attenuated vaccinia virus MVA and their influence on virulence. J Gen Virol 1991;72:1031–8.

[139] Di Nicola M, Carlo-Stella C, Mortarini R, et al. Boosting T cell-mediated immunity to tyrosinase by vaccinia virus-transduced, CD34(+)-derived dendritic cell vaccination: a phase I trial in metastatic melanoma. Clin Cancer Res 2004;10:5381–90.

[140] Morse MA, Nair SK, Mosca PJ, et al. Immunotherapy with autologous, human dendritic cells transfected with carcinoembryonic antigen mRNA. Cancer Invest 2003;21:341–9.

HEMATOLOGY/ONCOLOGY CLINICS
OF NORTH AMERICA

ELSEVIER
SAUNDERS

Dendritic Cell–Based Vaccination Against Cancer

Hiroaki Saito, MD, PhD, Davor Frleta, PhD,
Peter Dubsky, MD, A. Karolina Palucka, MD, PhD*

Baylor Institute for Immunology Research, 3434 Live Oak, Dallas, TX 75204, USA

L
ymphocytes (T cells, B cells, natural killer [NK] cells, and NK T [NKT] cells) and their products are controlled by dendritic cells (DC) [1,2]. DC sit in peripheral tissues where they are posed to capture antigens and process them for presentation to lymphocytes in secondary lymphoid tissues (Fig. 1). Antigen-loaded tissular DC migrate into the draining lymph nodes, where they present processed antigens to T cells via classic (MHC class I and class II) and nonclassic (CD1 family) antigen-presenting molecules. Immature (nonactivated) DC present self-antigens to T cells [3,4], which leads to tolerance. Mature, antigen-loaded DC are geared toward the launching of antigen-specific immunity [5] with T cell proliferation and differentiation into helper and effector cells with unique function and cytokine profiles. Mature DC also can expand regulatory/suppressor T cells. DC now are considered essential in central (ie, thymic [6]) and peripheral tolerance [7]. This article focuses on the basics of DC physiology, and how understanding of ways by which DC regulate immunity might affect the design of vaccines against cancer.

BIOLOGY OF DENDRITIC CELLS

DC encompass cells with (1) different anatomic localization, (2) distinct subsets, and (3) distinct functions. The anatomic localization often is linked to a specific function or distinct subset. Blood contains at least two subsets of DC precursors—$CD14^+$ $CD11c^+$ monocytes, which contain precursors of myeloid DC (mDC), and $LIN^{neg}CD11c^-IL-3R\alpha^+$ plasmacytoid DC (pDC). These precursor DC on pathogen recognition release high amounts of cytokines (eg, type I

This article was supported by grants from Baylor Health Care Systems Foundation and the National Institutes of Health (PO1 CA84512, U19 AIO57234, CA78846, CA085540, and CA89440). A.K. Palucka holds the Michael A. Ramsay Chair for Cancer Immunology Research.

A.K. Palucka is a scientific founder of ODC Therapy, Inc, a private company, and has stock options. ODC Therapy, Inc, is related to dendritic cell vaccines. ODC Therapy, Inc, has not in any way supported this article.

* Corresponding author. *E-mail address:* karolinp@baylorhealth.edu (A.K. Palucka).

0889-8588/06/$ – see front matter
doi:10.1016/j.hoc.2006.02.011

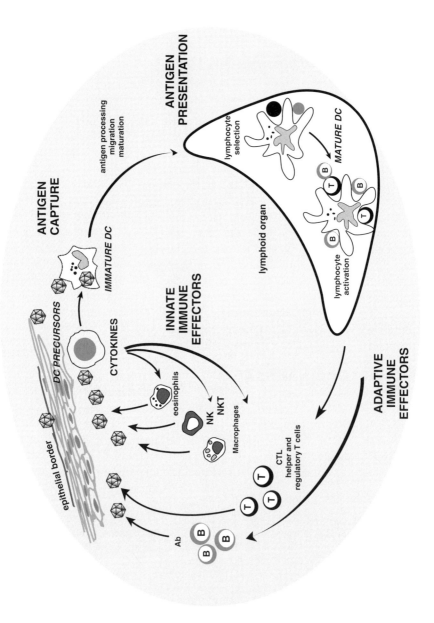

interferon [IFN]), limiting the spread of infection. Skin contains at least two subsets of mDC–epidermal Langerhans cells (LC) and dermal (interstitial) DC. These tissue-residing immature DC possess high endocytic and phagocytic capacity and are remarkably efficient in antigen capture. Mature DC, present within secondary lymphoid organs, express high levels of costimulatory molecules and are remarkably efficient in antigen presentation [8]. Lymphoid organs contain such a variety of DC as splenic marginal DC and T zone interdigitating cells, germinal center DC, and thymic DC, including those in Hassall's corpuscles, which drive differentiation of CD4$^+$ CD25$^+$ regulatory T cells [6]. These mature DC can be distinguished further based on their function particularly with regard to the regulation of B cell proliferation and differentiation of T cell responses toward type 1 or type 2, as discussed later.

Dendritic Cell Capture and Presenting Antigens

DC use several pathways to capture antigens, including (1) macropinocytosis; (2) receptor-mediated endocytosis via C-type lectins (eg, mannose receptor, DEC-205, DC-SIGN) [9,10] or Fcγ receptors type I (CD64) and type II (CD32) (uptake of immune complexes or opsonized particles) [11]; (3) phagocytosis of apoptotic and necrotic cells [12,13], viruses, bacteria [14,15], and intracellular parasites; and (4) internalization of heat shock proteins [16,17]. Captured antigens are processed in distinct intracellular compartments and loaded onto DC antigen-presenting molecules [18]. Protein antigens are presented by classic MHC class I [18] and class II molecules [19,20], whereas lipid antigens are presented through nonclassic CD1 antigen-presenting molecules [21,22]. Among CD1 molecules, CD1d is unique in that it is involved in the antigen presentation to NKT cells, a unique subset of T cells expressing a limited T-cell receptor repertoire mostly composed of Vα24Vβ11 [23]. These innate-like T cells contribute to the immune response against infection and malignancy. MHC class I presentation involves two pathways: (1) the classic presentation of endogenous peptides, originating from cellular and viral proteins that are made by a DC, and (2) the presentation of exogenous antigens via cross-priming/ presentation (ie, from proteins that are loaded onto DC) [3,24,25]. This pathway now is being exploited for loading antigens on DC vaccines as discussed later.

Fig. 1. The life cycle of DC. Circulating precursor DC enter tissues as immature DC. They can encounter pathogens (eg, viruses) directly, which induces secretion of cytokines (eg, IFN-α), or indirectly through pathogenic effect on stromal cells. Cytokines secreted by DC activate effector cells of innate immunity, such as eosinophils, macrophages, and NK cells. Microbial stimulation triggers DC migration toward secondary lymphoid organs and simultaneous maturation. Mature DC that enter lymphoid organs display pMHC complexes, which allow selection of rare circulating antigen-specific T lymphocytes. These activated T cells help DC in their terminal maturation, allowing for subsequent lymphocyte expansion and differentiation. Activated T lymphocytes traverse inflamed epithelia and reach the injured tissue, where they eliminate microbes or microbe-infected cells. B cells, activated by DC and T cells, and migrate into various areas where they mature into plasma cells that produce antibodies that neutralize the initial pathogen.

Dendritic Cell Migration and Maturation

DC control lymphocyte priming and the type of induced T cell immunity. This is important because the type of immune response can be a matter of life and death. In leprosy, the tuberculoid form of the disease is characterized by a "type 1" response and low morbidity, but the lepromatous form, which is characterized by a "type 2" response, often kills the host [26]. Type 1 response is associated with IFN-γ secretion by T cells, whereas type 2 response classically is associated with secretion of IL-4, IL-5, and IL-13 [27], as for example in allergy. Recent years witnessed the revival of regulatory/suppressor T cells that might protect humans from autoimmunity [28], but also represent a major obstacle to successful vaccination in cancer, as discussed later. Such determination of the type of immune response is intimately linked with several aspects of DC biology, including DC migration, maturation, and distinct DC subsets, as discussed later.

Dendritic cell migration

During their life span, DC traffic from the bone marrow throughout blood, peripheral tissues, and lymphoid tissues. DC migration to the periphery and from the periphery to lymphoid tissue represents two separate events that are regulated by distinct sets of molecules. DC circulating in the blood are attracted to tissues through MIP3-α (via CCR6) or MCP chemokines (via CCR2) as shown for LC in vitro [29] and in vivo [30]. Much less is known about how DC enter and traffic through the lymphatic vessels. The chemokine receptor CC-chemokine receptor 7 (CCR7) seems to be fundamental in this process [31]. More recent studies show that different DC subsets migrate to distinct sites in the lymphoid tissues. After skin immunization, dermal DC arrive in lymph nodes first and colonize areas distinct from slower migrating epidermal LC [32]. These results might contribute to understanding of how the immune response develops on cutaneous immunization, a classic route of vaccination.

Dendritic cell maturation

DC maturation is associated with several coordinated events, including (1) loss of endocytic/phagocytic receptors and diminished antigen capture; (2) changes in morphology that include the acquisition of high cellular motility [33]; (3) translocation of MHC class II antigen-presenting molecules to cell surface; (4) upregulation of costimulatory molecules, such as CD80, CD86, and several members of tumor necrosis factor (TNF)/TNF receptor family (eg, 4-1BB-L, and OX40-L) [34]; and (5) secretion of cytokines, including IL-12 and IL-23, which are important for the type 1 polarization of T cell immunity.

DC can receive maturation signals through three major pathways involving (1) DC surface molecules engaged in pathogen recognition including Toll-like receptors (TLR) [35] and C type lectins; (2) cell products, such as proinflammatory cytokines, including IL-1β, TNF, IL-6, and prostaglandin E_2 [36], or an apparently more potent combination of IL-1β and TNF with type I (IFN-α) and II (IFN-γ) interferons [37]; and (3) cells including T cell–derived CD40 ligand

[38] and signals from NK cells, NKT cells, and γ/δ T cells [39]. Most likely at any given time the DC are exposed to a combination of these signals, which influences the net result of T cell activation. TLR are differentially expressed by distinct human DC subsets. TLR9 (a receptor for unmethylated DNA–containing CpG motifs) is expressed only by pDC, whereas mDC preferentially express TLR2 and TLR4 (receptors for bacterial products, such as peptidogly-can and lipopolysaccharide [LPS]) [40]. Pathogens may contain several TLR agonists that could engage several TLR on the same DC or on two distinct DC subsets [41]. For human and mouse DC, TLR3 and TLR4 act in synergy with TLR7, TLR8, and TLR9 leading to increased production of IL-12 and IL-23 [42]. Another response scenario in which distinct TLR ligands induce polariza-tion of DC can be illustrated by TLR2 and TLR4 ligands. Minor structural differences in TLR ligands such as LPS may lead to the engagement of different TLR, as illustrated by *Escherichia coli* LPS, which induces a Th1 response via TLR4, whereas *Porphyromonas gingivalis* LPS, which triggers TLR2, induces a Th2 response [43,44]. Similarly, and as discussed later, different DC subsets express unique lectins [10], which may confer different maturation signals yielding distinct immune responses [45].

Dendritic Cells Determine the Type of T Cell Response

The current paradigm is that immature DC are tolerogenic, whereas mature DC are immunostimulatory [7]. This paradigm has been formally shown in vivo by the groups of Nussenzweig and Steinman, who have elegantly shown that fusion proteins targeted to immature DC lead to the induction of antigen-specific tolerance [46]. By contrast, concomitant activation of the DC via CD40 results in a potent immune response [47].

Immature steady-state DC are considered important in peripheral tolerance possibly because they present tissue antigens without appropriate costimulation. More recent studies suggest revisiting this paradigm because LC reaching lymph nodes under steady state were found to express similar levels of MHC class II, CD40, and CD86 as LC arriving under inflammatory conditions [32]. The determination of tolerance or priming might be related to the threshold of activation [48] or action of a unique set of inhibitory molecules, such as signaling through CD80/CD86 and CTLA-4 or PDL1/2 and PD-1 or immunoglobulin-like transcript 3 (ILT3) and ILT4 [49,50].

DC at distinct maturation stages can activate distinct regulatory/suppressor T cells. Two broad subsets of CD4$^+$ T cells with regulatory function have been characterized [51,52]. Naturally occurring CD4$^+$ CD25$^+$ T cells are produced in the thymus and mediate their suppressive effects in a cell contact–dependent, antigen-independent manner, without the requirement of suppressive cytokines, such as IL-10 or TGF. These cells are naturally "anergic" and require stimula-tion via their T-cell receptor for optimal suppressive function. Mature DC allow their expansion, which is partially dependent n the production of IL-2 by the T cell and B7 costimulation by the DC [53]. The induced T regulatory (T_R) cells are derived from CD4$^+$ 25$^-$ T cells and mediate their effects through the production of IL-10 and transforming growth factor (TGF)-β [54,55]. Two types have been described: T_R1 cells, which produce large amounts of IL-10 and low to moderate levels of TGF-β [54], and Th3 cells, which produce preferentially TGF-β [56] and provide help for IgA production [57]. Immature DC induce the differentiation of naive T cells into T_R cells [54,58,59]. Injection of immature DC pulsed with influenza-derived peptide into healthy adults leads to antigen-specific silencing of effector T cell function [60]. Murine pulmonary DC induce the development of T_R in an ICOS-ICOS-L–dependent fashion, which leads to the production of IL-10 by DC [61]. A population of "semimature" $CD45RB^{high}$ $CD11c^{low}$ murine DC located within the spleen and lymph nodes has been described. These cells secrete IL-10 after activation with LPS or CpG oligonucleotides, but do not upregulate MHC class II or costimulatory molecules under the same conditions. Most importantly, they are highly potent at inducing tolerance that is mediated through the differentiation of T_R cells in vivo [59,61].

Dendritic Cells Interact with Other Lymphocyte Types

DC regulate other lymphocytes as well, including naive [62] and memory [63] B cells, NK cells [64], and NKT cells [65].

Interaction with B cells

mDC can prime naive B cells [62]. Several molecules have been shown to be involved in this process, including IL-12, IL-6 [8], and, more recently BAFF/Blys [66], a molecule upregulated by IFN-α. IFN-αβ and IL-6 also are important in the differentiation of activated B cells into efficient immunoglobulin-secreting plasma cells on exposure to virus-triggered pDC [63]. There also may be an indirect contribution of IFN-α to plasma cell differentiation via activation of mDC [67,68]. Differential activation of $CD4^+$ T cells with B cell helper function by distinct DC subsets might play an important role in the induction of protective humoral immunity.

Cross-talk with innate lymphocytes

DC have a reciprocal interaction with NK, NKT, and γ/δ T cells. These innate immune effectors induce DC maturation through a combination of soluble and cell-mediated signals [39]. Mature DC also stimulate NK [64,69,70], NKT [71], and γ/δ T cells [72,73]. These reciprocal interactions occur largely in the secondary lymphoid organs and are important for the amplification of type 1 T cell immunity. They extend the classic ménage a trois [2]. It remains to be determined how DC conditioning by the innate effector cells affects humoral immunity. Distinct DC subsets seem to interact differentially with innate lymphocytes. Interstitial (dermal) DC derived from monocytes or from $CD34^+$ hematopoietic progenitor cells directly stimulate NK cell proliferation and cytotoxic function [74]. On the contrary, LC require exogenous cytokines to activate NK cells [74]. Such specialization may have an important impact for in vivo DC targeting for vaccination.

Dendritic Cells Are Composed of Subsets

In the early 1990s, culture systems were discovered that produced large amounts of mouse [75] and human DC, accelerating their characterization [76–78]. Classically, two main DC differentiation pathways from CD34$^+$ hematopoietic progenitor cells [76] are recognized [8,79]. One pathway generates pDC [80], which secrete large amounts of IFN-α/β after viral infection [81,82]. A myeloid pathway generates LC, which are found in stratified epithelia, such as the skin, and interstitial DC, which are found in all other tissues [83], as discussed earlier.

Distinct dendritic cell subsets are endowed with distinct functional properties

Each of these DC subsets has common and unique biologic functions, determined by a unique combination of cell surface molecules and cytokines. In vitro LC and interstitial DC generated from CD34$^+$ hematopoietic progenitors differ in their capacity to activate lymphocytes: Interstitial DC induce the differentiation of naive B cells into immunoglobulin-secreting plasma cells [62,83], whereas LC seem to be particularly efficient activators of cytotoxic CD8$^+$ T cells. They also differ in the cytokines that they secrete (ie, only interstitial DC produce IL-10) and in their enzymatic activity [62,83]. Such different enzymatic activity may be fundamental for antigen processing and selection of peptides that would be presented to T cells. Different enzymes are likely to degrade a given antigen into different peptide repertoires, as shown for HIV nef protein [84]; this would lead to different sets of pMHC complexes being presented and to distinct antigen-specific T cell repertoires.

DC subsets express unique lectins [10], which at least partially account for the biologic differences. LC express Langerin, which is crucial for the formation of Birbeck granules [85]. The role of these structures is not yet understood. The interstitial DC express DC-SIGN, involved in the interactions with T cells and DC migration, but also used by pathogens (eg, HIV) to hijack the immune system [86]. pDC express yet another lectin BDCA2 [87]. TLR also are differentially expressed. Such differential expression may permit specific in vivo targeting of DC subsets for induction of a desired type of immune responses, as shown in mice by targeting DEC-205 [46].

Monocytes yield distinct dendritic cells in vitro

Monocytes can differentiate into macrophages, which act as scavengers, or DC that induce specific immune responses [88,89]. Different cytokines skew the in vitro differentiation of monocytes into DC with different phenotypes and function. When activated (eg, by granulocyte-macrophage colony-stimulating factor [GM-CSF]) monocytes encounter IL-4, they yield IL4-DC [77,78,90]. By contrast, after an encounter with IFN-α/β, thymic stromal lymphopoietin (TSLP), TNF, or IL-15, activated monocytes differentiate into IFN-DC [91–94], TSLP-DC [95], TNF-DC [96], or IL15-DC [97]. This spectrum of DC represents immunostimulatory DC. A whole repertoire of DC exists, however, that exhibit immunoregulatory/tolerogenic functions (eg, DC generated by culturing monocytes with IL-10 in the presence of inflammatory cytokines such as GM-CSF or

IFN-α [50,98]). These are important in the context of the role of DC in maintaining peripheral tolerance. We view myeloid DC as central cells for priming T cell immunity (Fig. 2). mDC are polarized by other cells and their products, including IFN-α from pDC, IFN-γ from γ/δ T cells and NK cells, IL-4 and TNF from mast cells, IL-15 and TSLP from stromal cells, and IL-10 from lymphocytes. These distinct DC induce distinct types of T cell immunity. The challenge for years to come will be to link these distinct DC phenotypes in vitro with a specific type of immune response and immune pathology in vivo as exemplified by TNF and IFN-α [99,100] or by TSLP in allergic inflammation [95]. Currently, these distinct ex vivo–generated monocyte-derived DC can be used as vaccines in patients with cancer. More studies are needed, however, to

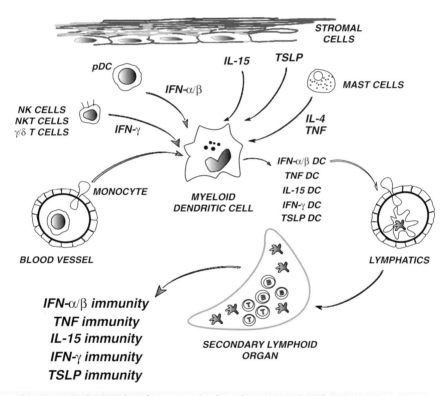

Fig. 2. Myeloid DC as the information relay from the innate to the adaptive immune system. A model is proposed in which the remarkable variety of observed T cell phenotypes could be explained by the plasticity of myeloid DC. Myeloid DC precursors yield different DC on encounter with different cells of the innate immune system and their products. Such imprinted DC convey this information to immune effectors, including T cells. Each DC triggers a unique type of T cell, permitting a broad functional repertoire. IL-15 DC are remarkably more efficient in priming and maturation of rare antigen-specific CTL compared with IL-4 DC. TSLP-DC induce CD4+ T cells to differentiate into proinflammatory type 2 cells secreting large amounts of IL-13 and TNF. Much remains to be done to establish the parameters of this model.

determine their value in the induction of therapeutic immunity in vivo as discussed in another article in this issue.

DENDRITIC CELLS IN VACCINATION AGAINST CANCER

Ex vivo–generated and antigen-loaded DC have now been used as vaccines to improve immunity in patients with cancer [101] and chronic HIV infection [102,103], providing a "proof-of-principle" that DC vaccines can work. Previous reviews by the authors and others have emphasized the shortcomings of current vaccination protocols [104–107]. The key issues of DC biology that need to be considered for improved vaccination have been discussed throughout this article. This section highlights a few points specific to vaccination in cancer.

Dendritic Cell Subsets

Several groups have used IL4-DC as vaccines [101] after pioneering clinical studies in patients with metastatic melanoma by Nestle et al [108] (using tumor lysate–loaded DC) and by Thurner et al [109] (using melanoma peptide–loaded DC). More recent discoveries point to some alternatives, however, to the classic way of generating DC. Melanoma peptide–pulsed IL15-DC are much more efficient than IL4-DC for the induction of antigen-specific CTL differentiation in vitro, whereas their ability to stimulate $CD4^+$ T cells is comparable [97]. Also, IFN-α-DC generated in 3-day cultures are efficient for the induction of specific immunity [93]. The immunogenicity of these distinct DC vaccines needs to be tested in vivo in clinical studies.

Monocytes are not the only source of DC precursors/progenitors that have been used in clinical studies. Blood DC loaded with specific idiotype protein have been used as vaccines in patients with follicular B cell lymphoma [110], and immune and clinical responses were observed. Similarly, blood DC loaded ex vivo with a recombinant fusion protein consisting of prostatic acid phosphatase linked to GM-CSF are being used in patients with prostate cancer [111]. Fong et al [112] used FLT3 ligand–mobilized blood DC and showed the induction of immune and some clinical responses in vaccinated patients. The authors have vaccinated patients with metastatic melanoma with antigen-loaded DC derived from $CD34^+$ hematopoietic progenitor cells (CD34-DC) [113]. CD34-DC vaccination elicited melanoma-specific immunity, and patients who survived longer were those who mounted immunity to more than two melanoma antigens [114]. These results justify the design of larger follow-up studies with a range of different DC vaccines to assess their immunologic and clinical efficacy. The proposal for standardization of DC vaccination protocols in cancer [115] might be premature because the optimal type of DC to be used for vaccination still remains to be determined.

Loading Dendritic Cell Vaccines with Antigen

Loading MHC class I and class II molecules on DC with peptides derived from defined antigens is the most commonly used strategy for DC vaccination [116,117]. Although this technique is important for "proof of concept" studies, the use of peptides has limitations, as follows: restriction to a given HLA type, limited number of well-characterized tumor-associated antigens, relatively rapid turnover of exogenous peptide-MHC complexes resulting in comparatively low antigen presentation at the time the DC arrive into draining lymph node after injection, and the induction of a restricted repertoire of T cell clones limiting the ability of the immune system to control tumor antigen variation. Loading DC with total antigen preparations and allowing "natural" processing and epitope selection is expected to improve efficacy and to allow the generation of a diverse immune response involving many clones of CD4$^+$ T cells and CTL. These strategies include loading DC with recombinant proteins, exosomes [118], viral vectors [119], plasmid DNA, RNA transfection [120], immune complexes [15], and antibodies specific for DC surface molecules [116,121]. Another technique involves exploiting the capacity of DC to cross-prime, discussed previously [3,122]. This approach can be applied to load DC vaccines to elicit immunity against multiple antigens regardless of patient HLA type. DC cultured with killed allogeneic melanoma, prostate cancer, and breast cancer cell lines prime naive CD8$^+$ T cells against tumor antigens in vitro [122,123]. The authors have now vaccinated 20 patients with metastatic melanoma with autologous monocyte-derived DC previously exposed to a killed allogeneic melanoma cell line (eight vaccines on a monthly basis). Vaccination has proved to be safe (no autoimmunity or other adverse events) and has led to the induction of melanoma-specific T cell immunity. In two patients, this vaccination has resulted in long-lasting tumor regression (unpublished observations). These results warrant larger clinical studies.

Dendritic Cell Migration

Monitoring the in vivo migration of labeled DC in patients showed that only a small fraction (<1%) of intradermally injected DC migrated rapidly to the regional lymphatics [124]. DC migration was improved in a mouse study by conditioning the injection site with TNF, which significantly increased DC migration to the draining lymph nodes and the magnitude of the CD4$^+$ T cell response [125]. Distinct maturation/activation signals (eg, prostaglandin E$_2$ [126,127]) may induce the preferential expression of CCR7 by DC, increasing the capacity of the DC to respond to appropriate ligands, such as CCL19 and CCL21 expressed in lymphatic vessels and secondary lymphoid organs [128].

Antigen-loaded DC may prime T cell responses regardless of the route of injection, but the quality of responses is affected, as shown by the induction of predominant Th1 responses after intradermal and intralymphatic administration, but unpolarized T cell and antibody responses after intravenous administration [129]. More recent studies in mice show that the induction of tissue-specific immunity is related to the tissue origin of DC [130,131]. Intravenous and subcutaneous immunization with peptide-pulsed DC in a mouse model of melanoma induced peptide-specific memory T cells in spleen and permitted the control of lung metastasis. Although subcutaneous immunization also induced memory T cells in the lymph nodes allowing subsequent protection against subcutaneously growing tumors, intravenous immunization failed to do so [131]. DC can prime T cells with different homing capacities. The consequence could be that intravenous administration of a DC vaccine for melanoma would be unlikely to induce skin-homing effector T cells.

Vaccination Frequency

The authors found in 18 patients with metastatic melanoma that four vaccinations over 6 weeks with melanoma peptide–loaded CD34-DC resulted in an increase in the number of melanoma-specific $CD8^+$ T cells in the blood as documented by IFN-γ ELISPOT [113,132] and CTL assay [133]. The melanoma-specific $CD8^+$ T cell immunity in the blood was short-lived, however. All analyzed patients lost specific T cells detectable by direct ELISPOT, and four of nine patients lost all recall responses by 2 months after the last vaccination. Several explanations might be considered. T cells might migrate from the blood to peripheral tissue (tumor site) [134]. Alternatively, the four biweekly vaccinations might have provided too-frequent antigen stimulation for optimal T cell differentiation. Mouse and human studies of vaccination against infectious agents [135,136] indicate that priming should be followed by a boost 4 to 6 weeks later for an optimal response. These rules may not apply to a chronic disease, however, such as cancer. By analogy, chronic viral infections are associated with exhausted T cells owing to chronic antigen presentation [137,138], and their reactivation through vaccination is likely to require different schedules. More recent studies show that DC vaccination stimulates a pathway of accelerated generation of memory T cells that undergo vigorous secondary expansion in response to a variety of booster immunizations, leading to increased numbers of effector and memory T cells and enhanced protective immunity [139].

Regulatory/Suppressor T Cells

A major obstacle to the success of cancer vaccines and possibly vaccines in chronic infections might be the presence of regulatory/suppressor T cells and the demonstration that DC regulate their expansion as discussed earlier. A large body of experimental evidence shows that these T cells suppress antitumor immunity, and that their removal allows tumor eradication [140,141]. An increased frequency of $CD4^+$ $CD25^+$ T cells has been observed in the blood and tissues of patients with cancer [142–144]. It is conceivable that distinct DC subsets or distinct DC maturation stimuli would have different capacities to induce regulatory T cells. This aspect needs to be explored further. Naturally occurring $CD4^+$ $CD25^+$ suppressor T cells may be controlled by pretreatment of patients with drugs that can eliminate or control these cells, meaning that DC vaccination may be more effective when combined with other therapies. Studies in the late 1970s and early 1980s showed that cytostatic drugs (eg, cyclophosphamide) facilitate adoptive immunotherapy for tumors in animal models [145]. The proposed mechanism was the elimination of suppressor T cells [145]. Data showing improved outcomes of vaccination with DC in myeloablated animals [146,147] reinforce this concept and indicate that controlled "immune ablation" may improve the clinical efficacy of DC vaccination trials in cancer. Besides the elimination of suppressor T cells, the mechanism also may involve the elimination of preexisting memory T cells, which might not be of the most effective phenotype (eg, Th2). Pretreatment of patients with metastatic cancer with cyclophosphamide before vaccination with DC is the best example of combination therapy and might improve DC vaccine efficacy significantly. In the late 1980s, clinical trials in patients with melanoma using whole tumor cells as vaccines showed improved immunity as a result of elimination of suppressor cells when vaccination was combined with cyclophosphamide [148,149].

Combining Dendritic Cell Vaccination with Other Therapies

Other combination therapies can be envisioned that would improve the vaccine itself, help the elicited T cells, and modulate the tumor environment [150]. As discussed earlier, studies in mice show that preinjection of TNF at the site of the DC vaccination greatly improves the migration of DC to the draining lymphoid tissue and the magnitude of induced immunity. This approach could be extrapolated to clinical studies in which the rate of DC migration could be measured using indium labeling. Concomitant administration of other cytokines (eg, IFN-α) could improve the performance of the DC vaccine [91–94] and possibly protect it from tumor-derived inhibitory factors (eg, VEGF or IL-10 [151]) and support induced T cells. Studies in mice have indicated that type I IFN support T cells in vivo directly, by sustaining their survival [152], or indirectly, by targeting antigen-presenting cells (possibly DC) to release IL-15, which enhances T cell growth [153]. The delivery of recombinant IFN-α or IL-2 after DC vaccination could protect the elicited T cells from the immunosuppressive tumor environment, improving vaccination efficacy. It will be important to determine, however, whether such strategies also yield concomitant expansion of regulatory T cells.

Assessing Immune Efficacy

The ultimate parameter of efficacy of DC vaccines is the rate of objective tumor regression and improved survival. A detailed measurement of elicited T cell and B cell responses in the blood can provide important clues as to the efficacy of a given DC vaccine.

Type of T cell immunity

Vaccine-specific T cell immunity classically has been measured by the quantity of tumor antigen–specific CD8$^+$ T cells [154]. There is no defined threshold, however, for how many T cells are sufficient to induce tumor regression. The elicited tumor antigen–specific T cells should be capable of cytokine production, proliferation on antigen re-exposure, migration to the tumor site, and CTL function [155]. Markers indicative of T cell migratory capacity include differential expression of CCR7 and CD45 isoforms: CCR7$^+$ CD45RO$^+$ T cells (central memory) are most likely migrate to lymph nodes, whereas the shift toward a CCR7$^-$ phenotype (effector memory) [156] should be associated with migration to the tissue.

Activation of other immune effectors

CD4$^+$ T cells, NKT cells, NK cells, and B cells also need to be taken into account when analyzing vaccine-specific immunity. In particular, CD4$^+$ T cells seem to be fundamental for priming long-lived CD8$^+$ T cell memory [157–159]. The lack of CD4$^+$ T cell activation in peptide-vaccination strategies might explain their limited efficacy in patients with cancer. Although such vaccines might elicit numerous circulating effector CD8$^+$ T cells, in the absence of CD4$^+$ T cell help, their quality might be compromised, and the establishment of specific CD8$^+$ T cell memory is unlikely [160]. The induction of NKT cells, which kill a wide spectrum of tumor cells [161], or NK cells, which recognize MHC class I–deficient tumor cells [162], could be desirable, yet caution must be taken with regard to the cytokines that they produce. IL-13-producing NKT cells may inhibit CTL-mediated tumor elimination and favor tumor progression [163].

Clinical Efficacy

Are DC vaccines better than other types of vaccine [104]? To address this question, the authors refer to a recently published critical assessment of clinical outcomes in several phase I/II vaccination trials, using peptides, tumor cells, tumor antigens expressed in viral vectors, and tumor antigens presented on DC in patients with various forms of metastatic cancer [164]. Because different types of cancer have unique challenges for successful vaccination, we selected from this review trials in patients with metastatic melanoma, which is a good model for vaccination because many tumor antigens have been well characterized, and tools to monitor immune responses are well developed. Vaccination with antigen-loaded DC showed 9.5% tumor regression–11 of 116 patients responded in six different clinical trials–compared with a maximum of 4.6% for other protocols. This rate of objective tumor regressions is still limited. These early outcomes warrant further exploration, however, to establish the therapeutic value of vaccination with DC.

The definition of clinical end points and the measures that are used to assess vaccine efficacy need to be revisited. Because cancer is a chronic disease, prolonged survival and good quality of life might be considered a therapeutic success and of benefit to the patient. When critically assessing different therapies, clinicians should be careful not to dismiss prematurely therapies that do not lead to a high rate of objective tumor regression [164]. It might be considered unrealistic to expect even the most efficient immune responses to eliminate the total tumor burden in a patient with advanced cancer. True analysis of improved survival requires randomized studies and long-term follow-up, however, which creates another set of logistic/regulatory difficulties, particularly for academic centers [150].

SUMMARY

DC are the crucial decision-making cells in the immune response. DC are an attractive target for therapeutic manipulation of the immune system to enhance

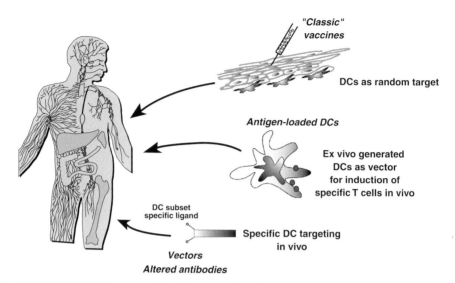

Fig. 3. DC as vectors for immunization. Classic vaccines target DC randomly. An intermediate approach is represented by vaccination with ex vivo–generated, antigen-pulsed DC subsets. The ultimate goal is to target DC subsets in vivo.

otherwise insufficient immune responses to tumor antigens. The complexity of the DC system requires rational manipulation of DC to achieve protective or therapeutic immunity and the move beyond random DC targeting as with classic vaccination strategies (Fig. 3). Further research is needed to analyze the immune responses induced in patients by distinct ex vivo–generated DC subsets activated via different pathways. The ultimate ex vivo–generated DC vaccine would be heterogeneous and composed of several subsets, each of which would target a specific immune effector. These ex vivo strategies should help to identify the parameters for DC targeting in vivo, which represents the next step in the development of DC-based vaccination.

Acknowledgments

The authors thank their patients for volunteering to participate in studies. The authors thank their colleagues and collaborators for their contributions. The authors are grateful to all former and current members of BIIR. The authors thank M. Ramsay and W. Duncan for support.

References

[1] Steinman RM. The dendritic cell system and its role in immunogenicity. Annu Rev Immunol 1991;9:271–96.

[2] Banchereau J, Steinman RM. Dendritic cells and the control of immunity. Nature 1998; 392:245–52.

[3] Albert ML, Sauter B, Bhardwaj N. Dendritic cells acquire antigen from apoptotic cells and induce class I- restricted CTLs. Nature 1998;392:86–9.

[4] Heath WR, Carbone FR. Cross-presentation, dendritic cells, tolerance and immunity. Annu Rev Immunol 2001;19:47–64.

[5] Finkelman FD, Lees A, Birnbaum R, et al. Dendritic cells can present antigen in vivo in a tolerogenic or immunogenic fashion. J Immunol 1996;157:1406–14.

[6] Watanabe N, Wang YH, Lee HK, et al. Hassall's corpuscles instruct dendritic cells to induce CD4+ CD25+ regulatory T cells in human thymus. Nature 2005;436:1181–5.

[7] Steinman RM, Hawiger D, Nussenzweig MC. Tolerogenic dendritic cells. Annu Rev Immunol 2003;21:685–711.

[8] Banchereau J, Briere F, Caux C, et al. Immunobiology of dendritic cells. Annu Rev Immunol 2000;18:767–811.

[9] Reis e Sousa C, Stahl PD, Austyn JM. Phagocytosis of antigens by Langerhans cells in vitro. J Exp Med 1993;178:509–19.

[10] Figdor CG, van Kooyk Y, Adema GJ. C-type lectin receptors on dendritic cells and Langerhans cells. Nat Rev Immunol 2002;2:77–84.

[11] Fanger NA, Wardwell K, Shen L, et al. Type I (CD64) and type II (CD32) Fc gamma receptor-mediated phagocytosis by human blood dendritic cells. J Immunol 1996; 157:541–8.

[12] Albert ML, Pearce SF, Francisco LM, et al. Immature dendritic cells phagocytose apoptotic cells via alphavbeta5 and CD36, and cross-present antigens to cytotoxic T lymphocytes. J Exp Med 1998;188:1359–68.

[13] Rubartelli A, Poggi A, Zocchi MR. The selective engulfment of apoptotic bodies by dendritic cells is mediated by the alpha(v)beta3 integrin and requires intracellular and extracellular calcium. Eur J Immunol 1997;27:1893–900.

[14] Inaba K, Inaba M, Naito M, et al. Dendritic cell progenitors phagocytose particulates, including bacillus Calmette-Guerin organisms, and sensitize mice to mycobacterial antigens in vivo. J Exp Med 1993;178:479–88.

[15] Regnault A, Lankar D, Lacabanne V, et al. Fcgamma receptor-mediated induction of dendritic cell maturation and major histocompatibility complex class I-restricted antigen presentation after immune complex internalization. J Exp Med 1999;189:371–80.

[16] Delneste Y, Magistrelli G, Gauchat J, et al. Involvement of LOX-1 in dendritic cell-mediated antigen cross-presentation. Immunity 2002;17:353–62.

[17] Asea A, Rehli M, Kabingu E, et al. Novel signal transduction pathway utilized by extracellular HSP70: role of toll-like receptor (TLR) 2 and TLR4. J Biol Chem 2002; 277:15028–34.

[18] Trombetta ES, Mellman I. Cell biology of antigen processing in vitro and in vivo. Annu Rev Immunol 2005;23:975–1028.

[19] Inaba K, Turley S, Iyoda T, et al. The formation of immunogenic major histocompatibility complex class II-peptide ligands in lysosomal compartments of dendritic cells is regulated by inflammatory stimuli. J Exp Med 2000;191:927–36.

[20] Turley SJ, Inaba K, Garrett WS, et al. Transport of peptide-MHC class II complexes in developing dendritic cells. Science 2000;288:522–7.

[21] Hava DL, Brigl M, van den Elzen P, et al. CD1 assembly and the formation of CD1-antigen complexes. Curr Opin Immunol 2005;17:88–94.

[22] Beckman EM, Porcelli SA, Morita CT, et al. Recognition of a lipid antigen by CD1-restricted alpha beta+ T cells. Nature 1994;372:691–4.

[23] Bendelac A, Rivera MN, Park SH, et al. Mouse CD1-specific NK1 T cells: development, specificity, and function. Annu Rev Immunol 1997;15:535–62.

[24] Carbone FR, Heath WR. The role of dendritic cell subsets in immunity to viruses. Curr Opin Immunol 2003;15:416–20.

[25] Sigal LJ, Crotty S, Andino R, et al. Cytotoxic T-cell immunity to virus-infected non-haematopoietic cells requires presentation of exogenous antigen. Nature 1999;398: 77–80.

[26] Pulendran B, Palucka K, Banchereau J. Sensing pathogens and tuning immune responses. Science 2001;293:253–6.

[27] Mosmann TR, Coffman RL. TH1 and TH2 cells: different patterns of lymphokine secretion lead to different functional properties. Annu Rev Immunol 1989;7:145–73.
[28] Bluestone JA, Tang Q. How do CD4+ CD25+ regulatory T cells control autoimmunity? Curr Opin Immunol 2005;17:638–42.
[29] Caux C, Vanbervliet B, Massacrier C, et al. Regulation of dendritic cell recruitment by chemokines. Transplantation 2002;73(1 Suppl):S7–11.
[30] Merad M, Manz MG, Karsunky H, et al. Langerhans cells renew in the skin throughout life under steady-state conditions. Nat Immunol 2002;3:1135–41.
[31] Kato H, Sato S, Yoneyama M, et al. Cell type-specific involvement of RIG-I in antiviral response. Immunity 2005;23:19–28.
[32] Kissenpfennig A, Henri S, Dubois B, et al. Dynamics and function of Langerhans cells in vivo: dermal dendritic cells colonize lymph node areas distinct from slower migrating Langerhans cells. Immunity 2005;22:643–54.
[33] Winzler C, Rovere P, Rescigno M, et al. Maturation stages of mouse dendritic cells in growth factor-dependent long-term cultures. J Exp Med 1997;185:317–28.
[34] Watts TH. TNF/TNFR family members in costimulation of T cell responses. Annu Rev Immunol 2005;23:23–68.
[35] Sporri R, Reis e Sousa C. Inflammatory mediators are insufficient for full dendritic cell activation and promote expansion of CD4+ T cell populations lacking helper function. Nat Immunol 2005;6:163–70.
[36] Jonuleit H, Kuhn U, Muller G, et al. Pro-inflammatory cytokines and prostaglandins induce maturation of potent immunostimulatory dendritic cells under fetal calf serum-free conditions. Eur J Immunol 1997;27:3135–42.
[37] Mailliard RB, Wankowicz-Kalinska A, Cai Q, et al. Alpha-type-1 polarized dendritic cells: a novel immunization tool with optimized CTL-inducing activity. Cancer Res 2004; 64:5934–7.
[38] Caux C, Massacrier C, Vanbervliet B, et al. Activation of human dendritic cells through CD40 cross-linking. J Exp Med 1994;180:1263–72.
[39] Munz C, Steinman RM, Fujii S. Dendritic cell maturation by innate lymphocytes: coordinated stimulation of innate and adaptive immunity. J Exp Med 2005;202:203–7.
[40] Kadowaki N, Ho S, Antonenko S, et al. Subsets of human dendritic cell precursors express different toll-like receptors and respond to different microbial antigens. J Exp Med 2001;194:863–9.
[41] Palucka K, Banchereau J. How dendritic cells and microbes interact to elicit or subvert protective immune responses. Curr Opin Immunol 2002;14:420–31.
[42] Napolitani G, Rinaldi A, Bertoni F, et al. Selected Toll-like receptor agonist combinations synergistically trigger a T helper type 1-polarizing program in dendritic cells. Nat Immunol 2005;6:769–76.
[43] Pulendran B, Kumar P, Cutler CW, et al. Lipopolysaccharides from distinct pathogens induce different classes of immune responses in vivo. J Immunol 2001;167:5067–76.
[44] Rogers NC, Slack EC, Edwards AD, et al. Syk-dependent cytokine induction by Dectin-1 reveals a novel pattern recognition pathway for C type lectins. Immunity 2005; 22:507–17.
[45] Boonstra A, Asselin-Paturel C, Gilliet M, et al. Flexibility of mouse classical and plasmacytoid-derived dendritic cells in directing T helper type 1 and 2 cell development: dependency on antigen dose and differential toll-like receptor ligation. J Exp Med 2003;197:101–9.
[46] Bonifaz L, Bonnyay DP, Mahnke K, et al. Efficient targeting of protein antigen to the dendritic cell receptor DEC-205 in the steady state leads to antigen presentation on major histocompatibility complex class I products and peripheral CD8+ T cell tolerance. J Exp Med 2002;196:1627–38.
[47] Bonifaz LC, Bonnyay DP, Charalambous A, et al. In vivo targeting of antigens to maturing dendritic cells via the DEC-205 receptor improves T cell vaccination. J Exp Med 2004; 199:815–24.

[48] Sallusto F, Lanzavecchia A. Mobilizing dendritic cells for tolerance, priming, and chronic inflammation. J Exp Med 1999;189:611–4.

[49] Walker LS, Abbas AK. The enemy within: keeping self-reactive T cells at bay in the periphery. Nat Rev Immunol 2002;2:11–9.

[50] Chang CC, Ciubotariu R, Manavalan JS, et al. Tolerization of dendritic cells by T(S) cells: the crucial role of inhibitory receptors ILT3 and ILT4. Nat Immunol 2002;3:237–43.

[51] O'Garra A, Vieira PL, Vieira P, et al. IL-10-producing and naturally occurring CD4+ Tregs: limiting collateral damage. J Clin Invest 2004;114:1372–8.

[52] Robinson DS, Larche M, Durham SR. Tregs and allergic disease. J Clin Invest 2004; 114:1389–97.

[53] Yamazaki S, Iyoda T, Tarbell K, et al. Direct expansion of functional CD25+ CD4+ regulatory T cells by antigen-processing dendritic cells. J Exp Med 2003;198:235–47.

[54] Groux H, O'Garra A, Bigler M, et al. A CD4+ T-cell subset inhibits antigen-specific T-cell responses and prevents colitis. Nature 1997;389:737–42.

[55] Roncarolo MG, Bacchetta R, Bordignon C, et al. Type 1 T regulatory cells. Immunol Rev 2001;182:68–79.

[56] Fukaura H, Kent SC, Pietrusewicz MJ, et al. Induction of circulating myelin basic protein and proteolipid protein-specific transforming growth factor-beta1-secreting Th3 T cells by oral administration of myelin in multiple sclerosis patients. J Clin Invest 1996;98:70–7.

[57] Weiner HL. Induction and mechanism of action of transforming growth factor-beta-secreting Th3 regulatory cells. Immunol Rev 2001;182:207–14.

[58] Jonuleit H, Schmitt E, Schuler G, et al. Induction of interleukin 10-producing, nonproliferating CD4(+) T cells with regulatory properties by repetitive stimulation with allogeneic immature human dendritic cells. J Exp Med 2000;192:1213–22.

[59] Wakkach A, Fournier N, Brun V, et al. Characterization of dendritic cells that induce tolerance and T regulatory 1 cell differentiation in vivo. Immunity 2003;18:605–17.

[60] Dhodapkar MV, Steinman RM, Krasovsky J, et al. Antigen-specific inhibition of effector T cell function in humans after injection of immature dendritic cells. J Exp Med 2001; 193:233–8.

[61] Akbari O, DeKruyff RH, Umetsu DT. Pulmonary dendritic cells producing IL-10 mediate tolerance induced by respiratory exposure to antigen. Nat Immunol 2001;2:725–31.

[62] Caux C, Massacrier C, Vanbervliet B, et al. CD34+ hematopoietic progenitors from human cord blood differentiate along two independent dendritic cell pathways in response to granulocyte-macrophage colony-stimulating factor plus tumor necrosis factor alpha: II. functional analysis. Blood 1997;90:1458–70.

[63] Jego G, Palucka AK, Blanck JP, et al. Plasmacytoid dendritic cells induce plasma cell differentiation through type I interferon and interleukin 6. Immunity 2003;19:225–34.

[64] Fernandez NC, Lozier A, Flament C, et al. Dendritic cells directly trigger NK cell functions: cross-talk relevant in innate anti-tumor immune responses in vivo. Nat Med 1999;5:405–11.

[65] Kadowaki N, Antonenko S, Ho S, et al. Distinct cytokine profiles of neonatal natural killer T cells after expansion with subsets of dendritic cells. J Exp Med 2001;193:1221–6.

[66] Schneider P, MacKay F, Steiner V, et al. BAFF, a novel ligand of the tumor necrosis factor family, stimulates B cell growth. J Exp Med 1999;189:1747–56.

[67] Dubois B, Vanbervliet B, Fayette J, et al. Dendritic cells enhance growth and differentiation of CD40-activated B lymphocytes. J Exp Med 1997;185:941–51.

[68] Litinskiy MB, Nardelli B, Hilbert DM, et al. DCs induce CD40-independent immunoglobulin class switching through BLyS and APRIL. Nat Immunol 2002;3:822–9.

[69] Gerosa F, Baldani-Guerra B, Nisii C, et al. Reciprocal activating interaction between natural killer cells and dendritic cells. J Exp Med 2002;195:327–33.

[70] Ferlazzo G, Tsang ML, Moretta L, et al. Human dendritic cells activate resting natural killer (NK) cells and are recognized via the NKp30 receptor by activated NK cells. J Exp Med 2002;195:343–51.

[71] Hermans IF, Silk JD, Gileadi U, et al. NKT cells enhance CD4+ and CD8+ T cell responses

to soluble antigen in vivo through direct interaction with dendritic cells. J Immunol 2003; 171:5140–7.

[72] Conti L, Casetti R, Cardone M, et al. Reciprocal activating interaction between dendritic cells and pamidronate-stimulated gammadelta T cells: role of CD86 and inflammatory cytokines. J Immunol 2005;174:252–60.

[73] Leslie DS, Vincent MS, Spada FM, et al. CD1-mediated gamma/delta T cell maturation of dendritic cells. J Exp Med 2002;196:1575–84.

[74] Munz C, Dao T, Ferlazzo G, et al. Mature myeloid dendritic cell subsets have distinct roles for activation and viability of circulating human natural killer cells. Blood 2005;105: 266–73.

[75] Inaba K, Inaba M, Romani N, et al. Generation of large numbers of dendritic cells from mouse bone marrow cultures supplemented with granulocyte/macrophage colony-stimulating factor. J Exp Med 1992;176:1693–702.

[76] Caux C, Dezutter-Dambuyant C, Schmitt D, et al. GM-CSF and TNF-alpha cooperate in the generation of dendritic Langerhans cells. Nature 1992;360:258–61.

[77] Romani N, Gruner S, Brang D, et al. Proliferating dendritic cell progenitors in human blood. J Exp Med 1994;180:83–93.

[78] Sallusto F, Lanzavecchia A. Efficient presentation of soluble antigen by cultured human dendritic cells is maintained by granulocyte/macrophage colony-stimulating factor plus interleukin 4 and downregulated by tumor necrosis factor alpha. J Exp Med 1994; 179:1109–18.

[79] Shortman K, Liu YJ. Mouse and human dendritic cell subtypes. Nat Rev Immunol 2002; 2:151–61.

[80] Liu YJ. IPC: professional type 1 interferon-producing cells and plasmacytoid dendritic cell precursors. Annu Rev Immunol 2005;23:275–306.

[81] Siegal FP, Kadowaki N, Shodell M, et al. The nature of the principal type 1 interferon-producing cells in human blood. Science 1999;284:1835–7.

[82] Cella M, Jarrossay D, Facchetti F, et al. Plasmacytoid monocytes migrate to inflamed lymph nodes and produce high levels of type I IFN. Nat Med 1999;5:919–23.

[83] Caux C, Vanbervliet B, Massacrier C, et al. CD34+ hematopoietic progenitors from human cord blood differentiate along two independent dendritic cell pathways in response to GM-CSF+ TNF alpha. J Exp Med 1996;184:695–706.

[84] Seifert U, Maranon C, Shmueli A, et al. An essential role for tripeptidyl peptidase in the generation of an MHC class I epitope. Nat Immunol 2003;4:375–9.

[85] Valladeau J, Duvert-Frances V, Pin JJ, et al. The monoclonal antibody DCGM4 recognizes Langerin, a protein specific of Langerhans cells, and is rapidly internalized from the cell surface. Eur J Immunol 1999;29:2695–704.

[86] Geijtenbeek TB, Torensma R, van Vliet SJ, et al. Identification of DC-SIGN, a novel dendritic cell-specific ICAM-3 receptor that supports primary immune responses. Cell 2000;100:575–85.

[87] Dzionek A, Fuchs A, Schmidt P, et al. BDCA-2, BDCA-3, and BDCA-4: three markers for distinct subsets of dendritic cells in human peripheral blood. J Immunol 2000;165: 6037–46.

[88] Randolph GJ, Inaba K, Robbiani DF, et al. Differentiation of phagocytic monocytes into lymph node dendritic cells in vivo. Immunity 1999;11:753–61.

[89] Chomarat P, Banchereau J, Davoust J, et al. IL-6 switches the differentiation of monocytes from dendritic cells to macrophages. Nat Immunol 2000;1:510–4.

[90] Peters JH, Xu H, Ruppert J, et al. Signals required for differentiating dendritic cells from human monocytes in vitro. Adv Exp Med Biol 1993;329:275–80.

[91] Paquette RL, Hsu NC, Kiertscher SM, et al. Interferon-alpha and granulocyte-macrophage colony-stimulating factor differentiate peripheral blood monocytes into potent antigen-presenting cells. J Leukoc Biol 1998;64:358–67.

[92] Luft T, Pang KC, Thomas E, et al. Type I IFNs enhance the terminal differentiation of dendritic cells. J Immunol 1998;161:1947–53.

[93] Santini SM, Lapenta C, Logozzi M, et al. Type I interferon as a powerful adjuvant for monocyte-derived dendritic cell development and activity in vitro and in Hu-PBL-SCID mice. J Exp Med 2000;191:1777–88.

[94] Blanco P, Palucka AK, Gill M, et al. Induction of dendritic cell differentiation by IFN-alpha in systemic lupus erythematosus. Science 2001;294:1540–3.

[95] Soumelis V, Reche PA, Kanzler H, et al. Human epithelial cells trigger dendritic cell mediated allergic inflammation by producing TSLP. Nat Immunol 2002;3:673–80.

[96] Chomarat P, Dantin C, Bennett L, et al. TNF skews monocyte differentiation from macrophages to dendritic cells. J Immunol 2003;171:2262–9.

[97] Mohamadzadeh M, Berard F, Essert G, et al. Interleukin 15 skews monocyte differentiation into dendritic cells with features of Langerhans cells. J Exp Med 2001;194: 1013–20.

[98] Pedersen AE, Gad M, Walter MR, et al. Induction of regulatory dendritic cells by dexamethasone and 1alpha,25-dihydroxyvitamin D(3). Immunol Lett 2004;91:63–9.

[99] Banchereau J, Pascual V, Palucka AK. Autoimmunity through cytokine-induced dendritic cell activation. Immunity 2004;20:539–50.

[100] Palucka AK, Blanck JP, Bennett L, et al. Cross-regulation of TNF and IFN-{alpha} in autoimmune diseases. Proc Natl Acad Sci U S A 2005;102:3372–7.

[101] Davis ID, Jefford M, Parente P, et al. Rational approaches to human cancer immunotherapy. J Leukoc Biol 2003;73:3–29.

[102] Lu W, Arraes LC, Ferreira WT, et al. Therapeutic dendritic-cell vaccine for chronic HIV-1 infection. Nat Med 2004;10:1359–65.

[103] Garcia F, Lejeune M, Climent N, et al. Therapeutic immunization with dendritic cells loaded with heat-inactivated autologous HIV-1 in patients with chronic HIV-1 infection. J Infect Dis 2005;191:1680–5.

[104] Banchereau J, Palucka AK. Dendritic cells as therapeutic vaccines against cancer. Nat Rev Immunol 2005;5:296–306.

[105] Schuler G, Schuler-Thurner B, Steinman RM. The use of dendritic cells in cancer immunotherapy. Curr Opin Immunol 2003;15:138–47.

[106] Finn OJ. Cancer vaccines: between the idea and the reality. Nat Rev Immunol 2003; 3:630–41.

[107] Steinman RM, Dhodapkar M. Active immunization against cancer with dendritic cells: the near future. Int J Cancer 2001;94:459–73.

[108] Nestle FO, Alijagic S, Gilliet M, et al. Vaccination of melanoma patients with peptide- or tumor lysate-pulsed dendritic cells. Nat Med 1998;4:328–32.

[109] Thurner B, Haendle I, Roder C, et al. Vaccination with mage-3A1 peptide-pulsed mature, monocyte-derived dendritic cells expands specific cytotoxic T cells and induces regression of some metastases in advanced stage IV melanoma. J Exp Med 1999; 190:1669–78.

[110] Hsu FJ, Benike C, Fagnoni F, et al. Vaccination of patients with B-cell lymphoma using autologous antigen- pulsed dendritic cells. Nat Med 1996;2:52–8.

[111] Small EJ, Fratesi P, Reese DM, et al. Immunotherapy of hormone-refractory prostate cancer with antigen-loaded dendritic cells. J Clin Oncol 2000;18:3894–903.

[112] Fong L, Hou Y, Rivas A, et al. Altered peptide ligand vaccination with Flt3 ligand expanded dendritic cells for tumor immunotherapy. Proc Natl Acad Sci U S A 2001; 98:8809–14.

[113] Banchereau J, Palucka AK, Dhodapkar M, et al. Immune and clinical responses in patients with metastatic melanoma to CD34(+) progenitor-derived dendritic cell vaccine. Cancer Res 2001;61:6451–8.

[114] Fay JW, Palucka AK, Paczesny S, et al. Long-term outcomes in patients with metastatic melanoma vaccinated with melanoma peptide-pulsed CD34(+) progenitor-derived dendritic cells. Cancer Immunol Immunother 2005;6:1–10.

[115] Figdor CG, de Vries IJ, Lesterhuis WJ, et al. Dendritic cell immunotherapy: mapping the way. Nat Med 2004;10:475–80.

[116] Gilboa E. The makings of a tumor rejection antigen. Immunity 1999;11:263–70.
[117] Wang RF, Wang X, Atwood AC, et al. Cloning genes encoding MHC class II-restricted antigens: mutated CDC27 as a tumor antigen. Science 1999;284:1351–4.
[118] Zitvogel L, Regnault A, Lozier A, et al. Eradication of established murine tumors using a novel cell-free vaccine: dendritic cell-derived exosomes. Nat Med 1998;4:594–600.
[119] Ribas A, Butterfield LH, Glaspy JA, et al. Cancer immunotherapy using gene-modified dendritic cells. Curr Gene Ther 2002;2:57–78.
[120] Boczkowski D, Nair SK, Snyder D, et al. Dendritic cells pulsed with RNA are potent antigen-presenting cells in vitro and in vivo. J Exp Med 1996;184:465–72.
[121] Fong L, Engleman EG. Dendritic cells in cancer immunotherapy. Annu Rev Immunol 2000;18:245–73.
[122] Berard F, Blanco P, Davoust J, et al. Cross-priming of naive CD8 T cells against melanoma antigens using dendritic cells loaded with killed allogeneic melanoma cells. J Exp Med 2000;192:1535–44.
[123] Neidhardt-Berard EM, Berard F, Banchereau J, et al. Dendritic cells loaded with killed breast cancer cells induce differentiation of tumor-specific cytotoxic T lymphocytes. Breast Cancer Res 2004;6:R322–8.
[124] Morse MA, Coleman RE, Akabani G, et al. Migration of human dendritic cells after injection in patients with metastatic malignancies. Cancer Res 1999;59:56–8.
[125] Martin-Fontecha A, Sebastiani S, Hopken UE, et al. Regulation of dendritic cell migration to the draining lymph node: impact on T lymphocyte traffic and priming. J Exp Med 2003;198:615–21.
[126] Scandella E, Men Y, Gillessen S, et al. Prostaglandin E2 is a key factor for CCR7 surface expression and migration of monocyte-derived dendritic cells. Blood 2002;100:1354–61.
[127] Luft T, Jefford M, Luetjens P, et al. Functionally distinct dendritic cell (DC) populations induced by physiologic stimuli: prostaglandin E(2) regulates the migratory capacity of specific DC subsets. Blood 2002;100:1362–72.
[128] Sallusto F, Schaerli P, Loetscher P, et al. Rapid and coordinated switch in chemokine receptor expression during dendritic cell maturation. Eur J Immunol 1998;28:2760–9.
[129] Fong L, Brockstedt D, Benike C, et al. Dendritic cells injected via different routes induce immunity in cancer patients. J Immunol 2001;166:4254–9.
[130] Mora JR, Bono MR, Manjunath N, et al. Selective imprinting of gut-homing T cells by Peyer's patch dendritic cells. Nature 2003;424:88–93.
[131] Mullins DW, Sheasley SL, Ream RM, et al. Route of immunization with peptide-pulsed dendritic cells controls the distribution of memory and efefctor T cells in lymphoid tissues and determines the pattern of regional tumor control. J Exp Med 2003;198:1–13.
[132] Palucka AK, Dhodapkar MV, Paczesny S, et al. Single injection of CD34+ progenitor-derived dendritic cell vaccine can lead to induction of T-cell immunity in patients with stage IV melanoma. J Immunother 2003;26:432–9.
[133] Paczesny S, Banchereau J, Wittkowski KM, et al. Expansion of melanoma-specific cytolytic CD8+ T cell precursors in patients with metastatic melanoma vaccinated with CD34+ progenitor-derived dendritic cells. J Exp Med 2004;199:1503–11.
[134] Masopust D, Vezys V, Marzo AL, et al. Preferential localization of effector memory cells in nonlymphoid tissue. Science 2001;291:2413–7.
[135] Kaech SM, Wherry EJ, Ahmed R. Effector and memory T-cell differentiation: implications for vaccine development. Nat Rev Immunol 2002;2:251–62.
[136] Zinkernagel RM. On natural and artificial vaccinations. Annu Rev Immunol 2003;21:515–46.
[137] Zajac AJ, Blattman JN, Murali-Krishna K, et al. Viral immune evasion due to persistence of activated T cells without effector function. J Exp Med 1998;188:2205–13.
[138] Wherry EJ, Blattman JN, Murali-Krishna K, et al. Viral persistence alters CD8 T-cell immunodominance and tissue distribution and results in distinct stages of functional impairment. J Virol 2003;77:4911–27.

[139] Badovinac VP, Messingham KA, Jabbari A, et al. Accelerated CD8+ T-cell memory and prime-boost response after dendritic-cell vaccination. Nat Med 2005;11:748–56.

[140] Steitz J, Bruck J, Lenz J, et al. Depletion of CD25(+) CD4(+) T cells and treatment with tyrosinase-related protein 2-transduced dendritic cells enhance the interferon alpha-induced, CD8(+) T-cell-dependent immune defense of B16 melanoma. Cancer Res 2001; 61:8643–6.

[141] Sutmuller RP, van Duivenvoorde LM, van Elsas A, et al. Synergism of cytotoxic T lymphocyte-associated antigen 4 blockade and depletion of CD25(+) regulatory T cells in antitumor therapy reveals alternative pathways for suppression of autoreactive cytotoxic T lymphocyte responses. J Exp Med 2001;194:823–32.

[142] Woo EY, Chu CS, Goletz TJ, et al. Regulatory CD4(+)CD25(+) T cells in tumors from patients with early-stage non-small cell lung cancer and late-stage ovarian cancer. Cancer Res 2001;61:4766–72.

[143] Viguier M, Lemaitre F, Verola O, et al. Foxp3 expressing CD4 + CD25(high) regulatory T cells are overrepresented in human metastatic melanoma lymph nodes and inhibit the function of infiltrating T cells. J Immunol 2004;173:1444–53.

[144] Wang HY, Lee DA, Peng G, et al. Tumor-specific human CD4+ regulatory T cells and their ligands: implications for immunotherapy. Immunity 2004;20:107–18.

[145] North RJ. The murine antitumor immune response and its therapeutic manipulation. Adv Immunol 1984;35:89–155.

[146] Ma J, Urba WJ, Si L, et al. Anti-tumor T cell response and protective immunity in mice that received sublethal irradiation and immune reconstitution. Eur J Immunol 2003;33: 2123–32.

[147] Asavaroengchai W, Kotera Y, Mule JJ. Tumor lysate-pulsed dendritic cells can elicit an effective antitumor immune response during early lymphoid recovery. Proc Natl Acad Sci U S A 2002;99:931–6.

[148] Berd D, Mastrangelo MJ. Effect of low dose cyclophosphamide on the immune system of cancer patients: depletion of CD4+, 2H4+ suppressor-inducer T-cells. Cancer Res 1988; 48:1671–5.

[149] Hoon DS, Foshag LJ, Nizze AS, et al. Suppressor cell activity in a randomized trial of patients receiving active specific immunotherapy with melanoma cell vaccine and low dosages of cyclophosphamide. Cancer Res 1990;50:5358–64.

[150] Pardoll D, Allison J. Cancer immunotherapy: breaking the barriers to harvest the crop. Nat Med 2004;10:887–92.

[151] Gabrilovich D. Mechanisms and functional significance of tumour-induced dendritic-cell defects. Nat Rev Immunol 2004;4:941–52.

[152] Marrack P, Kappler J, Mitchell T. Type I interferons keep activated T cells alive. J Exp Med 1999;189:521–30.

[153] Tough DF, Sun S, Zhang X, et al. Stimulation of naive and memory T cells by cytokines. Immunol Rev 1999;170:39–47.

[154] Phan GQ, Wang E, Marincola FM. T-cell-directed cancer vaccines: mechanisms of immune escape and immune tolerance. Expert Opin Biol Ther 2001;1:511–23.

[155] Stuge TB, Holmes SP, Saharan S, et al. Diversity and recognition efficiency of T cell responses to cancer. Plos Med 2004;1:149–60.

[156] Lanzavecchia A, Sallusto F. Regulation of T cell immunity by dendritic cells. Cell 2001; 106:263–6.

[157] Sun JC, Bevan MJ. Defective CD8 T cell memory following acute infection without CD4 T cell help. Science 2003;300:339–42.

[158] Shedlock DJ, Shen H. Requirement for CD4 T cell help in generating functional CD8 T cell memory. Science 2003;300:337–9.

[159] Janssen EM, Lemmens EE, Wolfe T, et al. CD4+ T cells are required for secondary expansion and memory in CD8+ T lymphocytes. Nature 2003;421:852–6.

[160] Northrop JK, Shen H. CD8+ T-cell memory: only the good ones last. Curr Opin Immunol 2004;16:451–5.

[161] Kronenberg M. Toward an understanding of NKT cell biology: progress and paradoxes. Annu Rev Immunol 2005;23:877–900.

[162] Cerwenka A, Lanier LL. Natural killer cells, viruses and cancer. Nat Rev Immunol 2001; 1:41–9.

[163] Terabe M, Matsui S, Noben-Trauth N, et al. NKT cell-mediated repression of tumor immunosurveillance by IL-13 and the IL-4R-STAT6 pathway. Nat Immunol 2000; 1:515–20.

[164] Rosenberg SA, Yang JC, Restifo NP. Cancer immunotherapy: moving beyond current vaccines. Nat Med 2004;10:909–15.

Hematol Oncol Clin N Am 20 (2006) 711–733

HEMATOLOGY/ONCOLOGY CLINICS
OF NORTH AMERICA

ELSEVIER
SAUNDERS

Adoptive T-Cell Therapy of Cancer

Cassian Yee, MD[a,b,*]

[a]Clinical Research Division, Fred Hutchinson Cancer Research Center, Seattle, WA, USA
[b]Department of Medicine, University of Washington Medical Center, Seattle, WA, USA

A doptive therapy involves the transfer of ex vivo expanded immune effector cells to patients as a means of augmenting the antitumor immune response. In general this transfer is accomplished by harvesting cells from the peripheral blood, tumor sites, or draining lymph nodes as a first step and, depending on the application and technology, expanding effector cells in a specific or nonspecific fashion for adoptive transfer. This article describes the rationale for adoptive T-cell therapy, the developments that have led to the translational application of this strategy for the treatment of cancer, the challenges that have been addressed, and future approaches to the development of adoptive therapy as a treatment modality.

SCIENTIFIC BASIS FOR ADOPTIVE THERAPY

Suppression of tumor cells by the immune response was hypothesized more than 40 years ago and has recently been supported by a number of murine models and clinical observations. In 1957, Burnet [1] postulated that "small accumulations of tumor cells may develop … and provoke an effective immunological reaction with regression of the tumor and no clinical hint of its existence." Not until the 1990s, however, were tumors found to arise more frequently and with shorter latency periods in mice deficient in lymphocyte-specific recombinase (the enzyme responsible for antigen receptor rearrangement) than in wild-type mice. These recombinase-deficient mice (RAG 2−/−) were completely lacking in natural-killer (NK), T, and B cells [2]. In subsequent experiments, mice deficient in perforin expression, the effector lytic mechanism of lymphocytes responsible for tumor cell killing, exhibited several-fold greater incidence of sarcomas and lymphomas than wild-type control mice [3]. It was surmised and later was proven that mice with an intact immune response were

Dr. Yee is a Damon Runyon Clinical Investigator supported in part by the Damon Runyon Cancer Research Foundation. This work was also supported by a grant from the National Institutes of Health (R01 CA104711) and the General Clinical Research Center (M01 RR00037).

* Clinical Research Division, Fred Hutchinson Cancer Research Center, 1100 Fairview Avenue North, D3-100, Seattle, WA 98109. E-mail address: cyee@fhcrc.org

0889-8588/06/$ – see front matter
doi:10.1016/j.hoc.2006.02.008

capable of rejecting "immunogenic" or virally induced tumor. It has become increasingly apparent in human cancer, however, that many T-cell–defined antigens are represented by normal self-proteins. In melanoma, these are pigment-producing proteins, such as tyrosinase, melanoma antigen recognized by T cells 1 (MART-1)/MelanA, and gp100, which also are expressed by normal melanocytes [4]. Under normal conditions (ie, in the absence of an inflammatory milieu), such nonimmunogenic targets, which often are self-proteins, do not induce a robust antigen-specific T-cell response. As a matter of self-preservation, thymic and extrathymic processes delete most autoreactive high-affinity T cells during development or render them anergic [5,6]. In a transgenic mouse model where a prototypic tumor-associated viral antigen is expressed in normal tissues during development, the T-cell response to the target antigen is anergic, and tumor cells are not rejected; however, T-cell function can be recovered after appropriate ex vivo manipulation [7–9]. Similarly the B16 melanoma cells expressing many of the dominant T-cell antigens shared by normal melanocytes are not rejected, unless a means of breaking the tolerance of the immune repertoire to an otherwise normal self-protein is used also. In this case, co-expression of B7, a costimulatory molecule, or co-administration of antibody (anti–cytotoxic T-lymphocyte antigen 4 [CTLA-4]) to counter autoregulatory mechanisms is sufficient to break the tolerance to self-proteins and mediate tumor rejection (in addition to some degree of autoimmunity) [10,11].

That tumor-specific T cells circulate in patients who have cancer but fail to reject tumor was demonstrated in a series of patients who had metastatic melanoma: CD8+ T cells were found to be selectively unresponsive to melanosomal antigens expressed by the tumor [12]. Ex vivo manipulation and expansion of tumor antigen–specific T cells represents one strategy to overcome tolerizing mechanisms and the influence of an immunosuppressive tumor microenvironment to augment a functional antitumor T-cell response [13–15]. Although it has been possible to perform this manipulation and expansion in vivo (ie, with vaccination strategies when an appropriate "danger" signal is provided to initiate a productive inflammatory response [16]), the ex vivo manipulation of effector cells provides a more rigorous means of controlling the intended immune response, free from the in vivo constraints of a potentially immunosuppressive environment in which the magnitude and function of the induced T-cell response may be limited.

EFFECTORS CELLS IN ADOPTIVE THERAPY

Effector cells operative in adoptive cellular therapy have been largely T cells, although a role for NK cells and other cytokine-induced lymphocytes is believed to exist. These cells are discussed individually here.

Cytokine-Induced Lymphocytes

NK cells, lymphokine-activated killer (LAK) cells, and (cytokine-induced killer cells (CIK) in are cytokine activated effectors that have been used for adoptive therapy. LAK cells are generated by in vitro exposure of peripheral blood mononuclear cells to high-dose interleukin (IL)-2 and are comprised predominantly of NK cells with a CD3−/CD56+ phenotype. NK cells do not display a T-cell receptor (TCR) and kill tumor cells after engagement of killer-activating receptors expressed on their surface [17] with nonpolymorphic ligands (eg, major histocompatability class I chain-related gene [MIC] A and MIC B) whose expression is increased in infected or "stressed" cells, such as tumor cells [18]. NK cells also engage self–major histocompatibility (MHC) class I molecules on target cells through inhibitory receptors (killer-inhibitory receptors), perhaps as a means of preventing autoreactivity. A role for NK cells in suppressing tumors that have lost MHC class I expression as a means of immune escape from antigen-specific T cells has been suggested. The clinical use of LAK often is coupled with co-administered IL-2 at high doses required to maintain LAK cell survival in vivo; although initially promising, responses were modest and often were accompanied by serious toxicities [19].

CIK cells are a unique population of lymphocytes that share phenotypic and functional properties of both T cells and NK cells. They are generated from peripheral blood mononuclear cells exposed in vitro to interferon-γ, anti-CD3, and IL-2, resulting in a population of CD3+/CD56+ lymphocytes [20]. These cells can be triggered through CD3/TCR but mediate killing of tumor cells in a non–MHC-restricted fashion [21]. Unlike LAK cells, co-administration of IL-2 is not required for adoptive therapy. In a recent clinical study, treatment with CIK resulted in partial responses or disease stabilization in four of nine patients who had refractory or relapsed non-Hodgkin's lymphoma or Hodgkin's disease [22]. In perhaps one of the largest phase III studies of adoptive cellular therapy, in which 150 patients who had hepatocellular carcinoma were assigned randomly to either surgery alone or surgery followed by infusions of cytokine-induced CD3+ lymphocytes, a 41% reduction in risk of recurrence and time to progression was observed in the adoptive therapy arm [23].

T Cells

T cells and their targets

T cells achieve specificity for cells expressing the target antigen through the surface TCR. The TCR recognizes fragments of antigen (peptide epitopes) presented by the MHC, which is encoded by highly polymorphic genes. Because T cells recognize tumor-derived peptides only when presented by the MHC complex, any disruption in the antigen-presentation machinery can lead to an absent or muted T-cell response [24,25]. The class I MHC complex, which restricts antigen presentation to CD8 T cells, is comprised of three parts: the MHC-encoded heavy α chain, a non–MHC-encoded β2-microglobulin chain, and an 8- to 11-mer peptide sitting in a groove formed by the polymorphic region of the α chain. Class I presentation to CD8 T cells classically is confined to endogenous proteins, although tumor fragments collected by specialized antigen-presenting cells, such as dendritic cells, can also cross-present tumor antigens. The class II MHC complex, which restricts antigen presentation to

CD4 T cells, is comprised of three parts, the polymorphic α and β chains and a 10- to 30(+)-mer peptide sitting in a groove formed by the two chains. Exogenous antigens are usually processed by the class II presenting pathway.

In addition to the TCR-triggered signal, it is believed that the activation of T cells can be modulated by the engagement of surface costimulatory or accessory molecules by their corresponding ligands on antigen-presenting cells. The most prominent are the signals provided by CD28 upon binding to B7-1 (CD80) or B7-2 (CD86) on antigen-presenting cells, which lead to full activation of an antigen-driven T-cell response during priming of naive T cells; however, CD28 has a far lesser role in the effector or killing phase of the T-cell response [26]. Other costimulatory molecules that deliver a positive signal to T cells include inducible costimulator, OX40, 4-1BB, and other B7 family members (eg, B7-H3); intracellular adhesion molecule-1 (ICAM-1) and leukocyte factor antigen-1 also are critical to T-cell recognition [27].

By contrast, CTLA-4 delivers a negative regulatory signal to activated T cells and competes with CD28 for binding to B7 on target cells [28]. Because many tumor target antigens are normal self-proteins, eliminating CTLA-4 inhibition may provide a means of breaking tolerance to self-antigens and augmenting an otherwise muted T-cell response to tumor. Administration of anti–CTLA-4 antibody in some murine models results in organ autoimmunity but also can lead to rejection of previously nonimmunogenic tumors [10]. The role of CTLA4 in the effector component is less well defined.

T cells and T-cell subsets

In animal studies using ex vivo expanded splenocytes for the treatment of tumor-bearing mice, CD8+ cytotoxic T lymphocytes (CTL) were identified as the predominant immune effector responsible for tumor eradication. Although most studies have assigned a role in tumor eradication to the CD8+ CTL, the helper CD4 T lymphocyte has also been shown to be a vital component in the induction and maintenance of a competent antitumor immune response [29]. Tumor antigen–specific responses been identified for CD4 T cells, and the presence of CD4 T cells may be required for CD8+ CTL responsiveness. Acting in concert, CD4 and CD8 T cells provide synergistic mechanisms of tumor killing. CD8 T cells kill tumor cells through the release of perforin and granzymes A and B or through engagement of the death receptor, Fas, through Fas ligand (FasL) expressed on activated T cells. FasL–Fas interaction leads to a form of cell death known as apoptosis. CD4 T cells can kill tumor cells directly by FasL–Fas engagement, as well as through indirect mechanisms that involve the recruitment of nonspecific effectors such as macrophages and eosinophils that can act even on MHC-negative tumors. One other type of T cell that has received renewed attention in the last few years is the regulatory T cell (Treg), which currently is characterized as a CD4+/CD25+ T cell, either naturally occurring (in 5%–10% of peripheral T cells) or induced from conventional CD4+/CD25− T cells [30–32]. Naturally occurring Tregs mediate their suppressive properties through cell-to-cell contact by an unknown mechanism. Induced or adaptive Tregs can be generated from conventional CD4+/CD25— T cells after in vitro exposure to antigen and IL-10; the induced Treg cells seem to mediate their inhibitory properties through the production of IL-10 and transforming growth factor-beta (TGF-β). Elimination of these regulatory components is believed to support the role of endogenous, vaccine-induced, or adoptively transferred T cells in tumor eradication.

Murine Models of Adoptive T-Cell Therapy

Adoptive T-cell therapy was established in murine models using ex vivo–expanded splenocytes as an effective antitumor strategy against syngeneic tumors. The antigen-specific CD8+ CTL was identified as an essential immune effector in several studies [33–35], although in some models CD4 T cells also were found to play an important helper role in both the transferred and endogenous CTL response [36,37]. In some cases, CD4 T cells alone were sufficient to mediate an antitumor effect [38,39]. The outcome of these and other murine studies led to the conclusions that the dose [40] and avidity [41,42] of adoptively transferred T cells are critical to tumor eradication and that preinfusion treatment with cytoxan to eliminate suppressor components [40,43,44] and a postinfusion source of helper function (ie, CD4 T cells or IL-2 [45–47]) are required. For larger, established tumors, a recent study demonstrated that, in addition to a combination of adoptive transfer and IL-2, postinfusion vaccination with a super-agonist peptide ligand may also be required [9]. Future studies to delineate requirements for effective therapy in mouse models and clinical trials are warranted.

CLINICAL TRIALS OF ADOPTIVE THERAPY

The implementation of clinical trials using adoptively transferred lymphocytes has progressed markedly during the last 2 decades as methods have been developed to harvest effector cells from the peripheral blood and tumor sites, to expand cells ex vivo using recombinant cytokines and novel TCR ligands, and then to enrich them selectively for a population of effectors targeting tumor-associated antigens. This section first describes the use of relatively nonspecific strategies, such as donor lymphocyte infusions, and then discusses more sophisticated strategies, made possible by scientific and technologic advances, that allow a broader and potentially less toxic application of adoptive therapy strategies to the treatment of Epstein-Barr virus (EBV)-associated diseases and solid tumors, using melanoma as a model human tumor.

Donor Lymphocyte Infusions

Allogeneic stem cell transplantation and donor lymphocyte infusions established proof of principle for adoptive therapy in the clinical setting and represent perhaps the most dramatic demonstration of its potential effectiveness. The observations that patients developing graft-versus-host disease (GVHD) after an allogeneic stem cell transplantation were less likely to relapse than those who did not develop GVHD [48,49] and that patients receiving unmanipulated stem cell infusions experienced a far lower incidence of relapse than seen in those receiving a T-cell–depleted infusion [50] suggested that donor lymphocytes play a significant role in host tumor eradication. Donor lymphocyte infusions (DLI) induced durable complete remissions in the majority of patients (60%–75%) who had chronic myeloid leukemia and who had relapsed after allogeneic stem cell transplantation [51–53]. Dose-limiting toxicities of myelosuppression and severe GVHD in these patients could be mitigated by a low initial dose (0.1 to 0.2 $\times$ 10^8 mononuclear cells/kg) and, in some cases, by selective T-cell depletion [54]. For patients who had acute myeloid leukemia, response rates with DLI were less favorable (<30%) [53], but DLI may be more effective when combined with chemotherapy (response rate >40%) [55] or used prophylactically for patients who have high-risk disease [56]. Response rates using DLI in the treatment of patients relapsing with acute lymphoblastic leukemia, lymphoma, and myeloma after allogeneic stem cell transplantation are somewhat less encouraging [53]. In acute lymphoblastic leukemia, the poor response to DLI may be attributed to weak immunogenicity of leukemic cells and other factors, including more rapid disease progression and complications of GVHD. Graft-versus-lymphoma and graft-versus-myeloma effects have been described occasionally but not consistently [57,58]. For myeloma, enhancing the antitumor potency of the donor-derived lymphocytes by preimmunizing the donor against patient-specific myeloma idiotype has shown promising results in early clinical trials [59,60].

Future uses of DLI will focus on prophylactic indications in the case of high-risk leukemias or at the earliest identification of relapse. Efforts to minimize toxicities associated with DLI, such as GVHD, have incorporated genetic safeguards (eg, an inducible suicide gene) to eliminate potential GVHD effects in vivo once a graft-versus-tumor response has been achieved [61]. Although it is believed that the T-cell component of a donor allograft or DLI is critical for the antitumor response, for patients receiving a haploidentical transplant, NK cells have a regulatory role (in suppressing GVHD and rejection) and also eradicate measurable disease, leading to successful engraftment and long-term remission across major MHC barriers [62]. For patients receiving reduced-intensity conditioning or a nonmyeloablative transplant, in which full donor hematopoietic chimerism is achieved largely through the donor lymphocyte antihost response, DLI has successfully augmented response rates, especially among patients who have relapsing disease who do not achieve full donor chimerism after stem cell transplantation [63].

Malignancies Associated with Epstein-Barr Virus

Targeting viral antigens associated with a tumorigenic phenotype is a potentially powerful strategy using adoptive therapy. EBV-reactive T cells have been used to treat patients who have posttransplant lymphoproliferative diseases (EBV-LPD) [64] and, to a lesser extent, nasopharyngeal cancer and Hodgkin's disease. In all these cases, the EBV antigens represent targets for T-cell therapy, although some antigen-specific responses are more elusive than others. For patients who have EBV-associated LPD occurring during the T-cell–deficient state after hematopoietic stem cell or solid-organ transplantation, the malignant lymphoproliferative cells express most of the EBV latent antigens against which robust T-cell responses exist in the peripheral blood of seropositive adults (>95% of population) [64,65]. A causative role for immune suppression in the etiology of EBV-LPD is borne out by studies demonstrating that an elevated EBV-DNA level and viral load is necessary [66] and that a concurrent deficiency in the EBV-specific immune response can be highly predictive for the development of EBV-LPD in allogeneic stem cell transplant recipients [67]. Relatively high T-cell responses to the EBV latent antigens—EBNA3, A, B, and C—are present endogenously in donor peripheral blood and can be transferred to stem cell recipients through DLI [68,69]. Response rates are as high as 90% in some studies [66,70]. To prevent potentially life-threatening complications such as the development of severe GVHD [66,68], inducible suicide genes (such as Herpes simplex virus-thymidine kinase, HSV-TK) have been introduced into donor T cells so that any untoward effects following treatment of EBV-LPD can be abrogated by in vivo elimination of infused donor lymphocytes [61,71]. Because HSV-TK, containing foreign epitopes, can itself induce immune-mediated rejection of transduced T cells, other suicide genes composed of less immunogenic sequences such as Fas/FK50 chimeric proteins are being evaluated [72,73].

Selective expansion of EBV-specific CTLs ex vivo provides a means of decreasing toxicity caused by alloreactive responses and of improving efficacy. Studies in patients at high risk for developing EBV-LPD (T-cell–depleted stem cell recipients or those with a diagnosis of EBV-associated lymphoma) who received donor-derived EBV-specific T-cell lines generated ex vivo using EBV-transformed B-lymphoblastoid cell lines demonstrated this prophylactic strategy to be highly effective, capable of reconstituting the EBV-specific response in these patients with minimal toxicity [74,75] As a therapeutic strategy for patients developing EBV-LPD after hematopoietic stem cell or solid-organ transplantation (although the number of patients in individual trials were fewer), the total experience demonstrated significant tumor regression or complete responses in the majority of patients treated, for whom disease otherwise would have been fatal [75–77].

In contrast to EBV-associated lymphoproliferative diseases, Hodgkin's disease and nasopharyngeal carcinomas arising in an immunocompetent host express only a handful of largely subdominant antigens (eg, Epstein-Barr nuclear antigen, EBNA-1, latent membrane protein-1 and -2) against which T-cell responses are more infrequent and more difficult to elicit ex vivo [78]. Adoptive transfer of polyclonal T cells generated in vitro using lymphoblastoid cell lines, which are comprised of only a minor population (<10%) of latent membrane protein-2–specific CTL, is capable of mediating antitumor responses, however. These CTL persist in vivo, traffic to tumor sites, and expand several-fold in vivo. Among six patients who had refractory nasopharyngeal carcinomas, two achieved complete responses and remained in remission for 11 and 23 months, respectively, after adoptive therapy with EBV-specific CTL [79]. Among 14 patients treated for relapsed EBV-positive Hodgkin's disease, 5 patients achieved a complete remission, 1 had a partial response, and 5 had stabilization of disease [80].

Adoptive Therapy of Melanoma

Studies targeting EBV antigens expressed by malignant cells have led to significant and occasionally durable objective responses. These responses have not yet been achieved with any consistency in solid tumors but are instructive for solid tumor immunotherapies because they demonstrate the feasibility of targeting tumor-associated antigens to eradicate life-threatening diseases. Because solid tumors, such as melanoma, exhibit physical and immunologic barriers distinct from EBV-associated tumors (eg, the lower affinity and frequency of the T-cell repertoire for non–viral tumor–associated antigens), the obstacles to success are likely to be more formidable. Initial attempts, before the identification of T-cell–defined tumor antigens, used nonspecific ex vivo expansion strategies. Once tumor-associated T-cell–defined antigens were identified, adoptive therapy evolved to include more precise targeting. As ex vivo selection and expansion methods developed, efforts were made to translate the design and potential success observed in murine studies into the clinical arena.

Adoptive therapy using lymphokine-activated killer cells and tumor-infiltrating lymphocytes
Before tumor-associated antigens had been identified, in vitro studies had demonstrated that exposure of peripheral blood mononuclear cells to high doses of IL-2 produced activated lymphocytes with antitumor potential. It was hoped that nonspecific expansion of NK cells and LAK cells would lead to tumor eradication after adoptive transfer. Responses were modest, however, and a prospective, randomized trial comparing high-dose IL-2 given with and without LAK failed to demonstrate an enhanced outcome in patients who had melanoma or renal cell cancer. Alternative approaches to expanding polyclonal T cells in vitro by triggering the TCR and costimulatory molecules have recently become available in the form of agonist monoclonal antibodies to CD3 and CD28 [81–83]. Early studies demonstrate that expansion using anti-CD3 and CD28 antibodies is safe, efficient, and may have a role in reconstituting immunity in immunodeficient states. The role of these cells for the treatment of cancer is currently being defined in clinical trials.

Murine models demonstrated that tumor-infiltrating lymphocytes (TIL cells), a population of T cells enriched for tumor reactivity, confer improved efficacy over activated peripheral lymphocytes [84]. TILs harvested from tumor sites (in some cases after vaccination [85]) could be expanded ex vivo and adoptively transferred [86–89]. A series of clinical trials using TIL for the treatment of renal cell cancer and melanoma demonstrated measurable clinical responses, but in general such responses were transient, and confounding effects of concomitantly administered high-dose IL-2 (needed to sustain the survival of the transferred TIL cells) could not be excluded as a reason for the observed responses.

The limited efficacy of these cellular therapies potentially resulted from inadequate numbers of the requisite effector cells in the heterogeneous TIL or LAK population, failure of the cells to recognize antigens expressed in all cells, or suboptimal in vivo survival of transferred cells. Recent advances in tumor immunology, heralded by the identification of tumor antigens recognized by autologous T cells, have enabled the design of more specific and improved therapeutic strategies.

Identification of tumor-associated antigens
The identification of tumor-associated antigens for T-cell therapy (either adoptive therapy or vaccine therapy) has been aided by technologic advances in the last decade. Although it had been possible to isolate tumor antigen-specific T cells from patients who had cancer, it was not until 1991, that P. van der Bruggen and colleagues [90] at the Ludwig Institute (Brussels) first described a human T-cell–defined antigen. Using target cells engineered to express the restricting allele and transfected with the tumor cDNA library, they were able to screen for the target gene using autologous tumor-reactive CTL clones. The cDNA of cells lysed by tumor-specific CTL was sequenced and compared with a gene database to identify the target gene. Based on this strategy, others have identified tumor-associated antigens, including several MHC class II–restricted antigens [91–94].

An alternative strategy known as serologic recombinant expression cloning (SEREX) has also provided a rich source of potentially immunogenic tumor antigens for a broad spectrum of human cancers [95]. In this method, autoantibodies circulating in patient serum are used to screen for tumor proteins expressed by tumor-derived cDNA expression libraries. Because SEREX immunoscreening identifies tumor antigens on the basis of a T-cell–dependent IgG antibody response, it is possible that such antigens might elicit a T-cell response as well. Indeed, both antibody and T-cell responses to several human tumor antigens, such as NY-ESO-1, prostate-specific antigen, and Her2/neu have been detected. More than 2000 SEREX clones have been identified using this approach, most notably, the group of cancer-testis antigens, which are expressed in a variety of tumors and germinal tissues [96].

Finally, gene-expression profiling, such as serial analysis of gene expression, has been used to identify genes that are overexpressed in tumor cells compared with normal tissues and to provide a starting point for increasingly sophisticated algorithms that predict potential immunogenic epitopes [97]. These putative epitopes are validated empirically using in vitro T-cell assays before being confirmed as tumor-associated antigens.

In general the tumor-associated antigens can be divided into five major categories: self-antigens associated with normal differentiation (pigmented genes such as tyrosinase, MART-1 in melanoma [98,99], or Her2 neu in breast or ovarian cancer [100]); self-antigens associated with a tumorigenic phenotype, such as survivin [101] or telomerase [102], which are expressed in some normal tissues but are overexpressed in tumor cells; cancer-testis antigens, such as melanoma-associated antigen 1 (MAGE-1) [90] and NY-ESO-1 [103], which are expressed in a variety of solid tumors and confined to tumor and germinal tissues (eg, testis); mutated antigens that represent truly tumor-specific proteins, such as the CDK4-kinase mutations [104] or beta-catenin [105]; and finally viral antigens such as EBV and human papilloma virus for cervical cancer [106].

Antigen-Specific Adoptive T-Cell Therapy

The arrival of antigen-specific adoptive T-cell therapy into the clinical arena was made possible by at least three major developments: (1) the identification of T-cell–defined tumor antigens and associated immunogenic peptide epitopes, (2) the availability of clinical-grade peptides corresponding to such epitopes for clinical use, and (3) methods of isolating and expanding antigen-specific T cells in vitro to doses sufficient for adoptive transfer (Fig. 1).

The ability to manipulate immune effectors ex vivo for adoptive transfer allows control of the effector component to an extent not possible with other immunotherapeutic means. In general, these parameters include the magnitude or cell dose, the structural and functional phenotype of the effector cells, and the specificity of the targeted response. In murine models, the cell dose has been shown to be critical to tumor eradication and long-term survival in tumor-bearing mice [40]. Although an optimal dose in patients cannot be defined readily, especially when tumor burden is substantial, it is likely that there is a threshold below which a response is unlikely. Experience in tumor-bearing murine models suggests that effective therapy requires antigen-specific T cells represent at least 1% to 10% of all CD8 T cells, a level that translates to a dose of 2 to 20×10^9 antigen-specific T cells in humans. Equally important is the in vivo persistence of the transferred T cells. It is conceivable that among the population of transferred T cells, there may exist a small subset of tumor-eradicating T cells that have greater replicative potential and that the effectiveness of a larger cell dose, which is more likely to harbor such a subset, merely reflects these probabilities. It then would follow that lower doses might be adequate if the "right" effector cell or cell types are present in sufficient numbers [107].

The question of what is the "right" effector cell is an open one, but it can be answered by exploiting one major advantage that adoptive T-cell therapy has over other immunotherapeutic strategies. It might be possible to define the requirements for successful T-cell–based therapy by selectively enriching for effector cells of a specific phenotype (eg, helper CD4 T cells, which provide critical signals for CD8 T cell survival and function, or T cells with enhanced TCR affinity so that endogenously expressed tumor antigens are more efficiently recognized [108]).

In recent years, six trials of T-cell therapy using adoptively transferred antigen-specific T cells have been reported, in all cases for the treatment of patients who had metastatic melanoma. The methods of generating antigen-specific T cells, the cell doses used, and incorporation of adjuvant measures such as lymphodepletion or co-administered cytokine into the clinical trials varied among the individual trials. Doses from as few as 10^8 to as high as more than

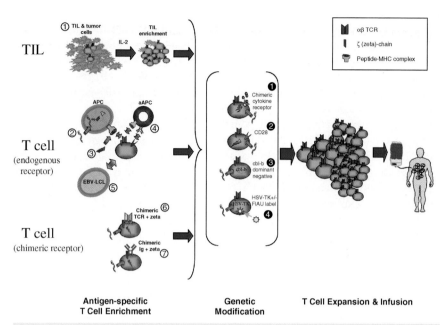

Fig. 1. Adoptive therapy using antigen-specific T cells—state of the art. Antigen-specific T cells can be enriched from tumor-infiltrating lymphocyte (TIL) cultures exposed to IL-2 (①), peripheral blood lymhocytes following in vitro stimulation with antigen-presenting cells (②③④⑤⑥⑦), or by genetically modifying T cells to express a chimeric TCR or Ig receptor. TIL cells harvested from tumor sites and exposed to IL-2 in vitro provide a reactive population of T cells that can be further expanded for T cell therapy①. ②③④⑤: Autologous APC (eg, dendritic cells) can be engineered to express the target antigens of interest following recombinant viral transduction ②, RNA transfection ② or peptide loading ③. Artificial APCs (bead-based, insect cells or xenogeneic cell lines, or liposomes) expressing the TCR ligand and costimulatory counter-receptor (B7 for CD28, 4-1BBL for 4-1BB)④. EBV-transformed B-LCL (lymphoblastoid cell lines) can be used as APC to elicit T cell responses for treatment of EBV-associated malignancies ⑤. T cells can be endowed with desired antigen specificity following introduction of a chimeric receptor comprised of the αβ chains of a high-affinity TCR ⑥ or the Ig domains of an antibody binding a tumor surface receptor ⑦, fused to the TCR ζ (zeta) chain that mediates T cell signaling upon receptor engagement. ❶❷❸❹: Antigen-specific T cells can be genetically modified to enhance function. A chimeric cytokine receptor comprised of the extracellular domain of a cytokine such as GM-CSF produced upon TCR engagement and the intracellular domain of TCR-zeta chain or CD28 signaling domain provides an antigen-driven autocrine source of helper function ❶. Direct transduction of CD28 into memory effector CD8 T cells can enhance T cell survival ❷. Introducing a dominant-negative transgene, such as cbl-b or TGF-β receptor will counteract negative regulatory or suppressive signals ❸. Transduction of a thymidine kinase gene (HSV-TK) provides a genetic safeguard as an inducible suicide gene and as a means of activating reporter molecules to permit non-invasive PET imaging ❹.

100×10^9 T cells have been infused without a demonstrable linear relationship between cell dose and in vivo persistence or clinical outcome. In part this finding results from some of the reasons stated previously and reflects the method of T-cell generation and source of T cells used. For example, T cells generated from previously vaccinated patients who did not respond to peptide vaccine therapy, using the identical epitope and exposed to high-dose IL-2 in vitro [109,110] are likely to have properties different from those of T cells obtained from previously untreated patients and stimulated in vitro under more physiologic conditions of cyclical antigen exposure with low-dose IL-2 [15,111]. These latter T cells, even after undergoing multiple cycles of in vitro replication, may experience longer periods of in vivo persistence than T cells generated from previously vaccinated patients and exposed to high-dose IL-2 in vivo. One of the first studies of antigen-specific adoptive T-cell therapy used insect cells engineered to present the antigenic epitope [112]; however, T-cell survival in vivo was short-lived, possibly because of the absence of requisite costimulatory signals not provided by the gene-modified antigen-presenting cells during in vitro stimulation and expansion. Recent developments in the production of artificial antigen-presenting cells, which express the MHC restriction molecule and cognate peptide along with costimulators such as anti-CD28 or B7, 4-1BBL, and ICAM-1, have led to a number of studies that include the use of genetically modified insect cells [113–115], bead-based technologies [116–118], liposomes [119], exosomes [120], K562 [117], and mouse fibroblast cell lines [121–123]. These reagents have been used successfully in vitro to elicit high frequencies of tumor-reactive T cells in a reproducible manner and may represent a more efficient strategy than the use of autologous antigen-presenting cells in the ex vivo expansion of antigen-specific CD4 and CD8 T cells for adoptive therapy. Several of these reagents are now in clinical use.

Of the published reports involving adoptive therapy using antigen-specific T cells, clinical responses were noted in three of the six studies [13,15,111]. Where clinical responses were observed, infusions were comprised of T cells with relatively uniform specificity against a melanosomal antigen (MART-1 or gp100) with a measurable period of in vivo persistence from 2 to more than 60 days. In one study involving patients who had disease refractory to conventional therapy, who historically have a median survival of less than 6 months, T cells generated from the peripheral blood of previously untreated patients were administered with low-dose exogenous IL-2. There was one near-complete response (by positron emission tomographic [PET] scanning) and one partial response; disease was stabilized in five other patients for up to 36 months [15]. In patients who had persistent or recurrent disease, examination of tumor nodules revealed selective loss of expression of the targeted antigen, suggesting a potent antigen-specific immune response that was subverted by the outgrowth of antigen-loss variants [15]. In a study conducted at the National Cancer Institute using ex vivo–expanded tumor-infiltrating T cells after lymphodepletion with cyclophosphamide (60 mg/kg for 2 days) and fludarabine (25 mg/m^2 for 5 days) and followed by high dose IL-2 (720,000 U/kg three times/d), significant objective clinical responses were observed in patients who had refractory metastatic melanoma [13]. Six of the first 13 patients in this study demonstrated objective responses, and a follow-up study of 35 patients reported that 18 achieved a partial or complete response. Clonotypic analysis of the transferred T cells demonstrated a positive correlation between the duration of in vivo persistence and clinical response [124]. The success of this approach is mitigated by auto-immune and other complications (vision- and life-threatening side effects such as uveitis and lymphoproliferative disease), probably resulting from severe immune depletion and replacement with an oligoclonal repertoire of T cells. Although this study underlines the potential effectiveness of adoptive therapy as a treatment modality, it is limited to patients who have accessible TIL and does not clearly define the requirements for successful therapy. Future studies will be needed to answer questions related to the nature and phenotype of long-term proliferating T cells, whether such cells can be propagated, the requirement for lymphodepletion and degree of lymphodepletion necessary, and the individual contribution of high-dose IL-2 and of CD4+ T cells in adoptive therapy.

TRACKING ANTIGEN-SPECIFIC T CELLS

Precise and comprehensive immunologic monitoring is required to understand why and how a given adoptive therapy strategy succeeds or fails and to answer many of the questions raised in existing studies. Although the reagent (in this case, the effector cells) can be "dosed" and manipulated ex vivo, a set of tools analogous to those pharmacologists use when studying a drug reagent in vivo has only recently allowed tracking of infused cells in a meaningful and reliable fashion. Tetramer-based and other antigen-specific technologies, such as ELISPOT assays, have added new and important dimensions to T-cell analysis. They are presented briefly here and are reviewed more extensively elsewhere [125].

In general, antigen-specific immunologic monitoring can be described as structure-based or function-based strategies. The classic chromium release and proliferation assays that lead to estimates of T cell frequency by limiting dilution analysis are unidimensional function-based assays that are subject to confounding variables of prolonged in vitro culture and iterative stimulations [126,127]. Current function-based assays representing cytokine production at the single-cell level after a brief period of in vitro stimulation (eg, ELISPOT analysis [128] or flow cytometry analysis of intracellular cytokines [129]) provide a more proximal assessment of T-cell frequency. By contrast, peptide-MHC multimers can identify and enumerate T cells on the basis of a structural feature, (the antigen-specific TCR), in a nondestructive fashion [130,131]. Coupled with assays describing the T-cell surface or functional phenotype in the type of multiparametric analysis afforded by flow cytometry, multimer- or tetramer-based technologies revolutionized the capabilities of investigators studying the antigen-specific response. For example, it became possible to ascribe a denominator representing the total number of antigen-specific effectors from which the fraction of functional (or nonfunctional) T cells could be calculated, leading to novel insights into the endogenous and manipulated antitumor response [12,132,133]. Peptide-MHC multimers also led to more direct methods of assessing T-cell affinity, an important but often elusive measurement that can influence the ability of T cells to recognize and eradicate tumor [14,134,135].

Ex vivo–manipulated T cells also can be genetically marked, and often such modifications are coincident with a transgene function, such as an inducible suicide gene or ex vivo selection marker [73,136,137]. When T-cell clones are used for adoptive transfer, genetic marking may not be required, because T-cell clones can be tracked by probing with clone-specific sequences flanking the hypervariable complimentary determining region-3 (CDR3) of the T-cell receptor [138,139]. For these structure-based methods of evaluating T-cell frequency, the development of real-time polymerase chain reaction analysis for the transgene or CDR3 region has led to highly sensitive and reliable quantitative assays, especially when cell viability of collected specimens is not a prerequisite.

Assessments of T-cell frequency and function currently are limited to accessible sites (ie, peripheral blood, excised tumor). In situ assessments of the geographic localization of infused T cells within tumor nodules or draining lymph nodes can provide critical information (eg, using tetramers for immunohistochremistry staining) [140]. A more dynamic evaluation of T-cell persistence and trafficking in patients would be desirable. In part, this need has been addressed by the use of serial fine-needle aspirates together with molecular immunologic profiling, which provide a more comprehensive understanding of other fundamental T-cell properties after T-cell transfer [141,142]. Several groups are evaluating the use of imaging techniques in animals and humans to track infused T cells noninvasively over time. Optical (bioluminescent) imaging using T cells endowed with a luciferase gene has been a powerful technique in rodent models, especially when combined with differentially luminescent tumor [143], but signal attenuation through tissues and lack of tomographic information make this technology difficult to translate into human studies. The use of Indium to label T cells before adoptive transfer has provided a short-term method for assessing initial trafficking patterns (generally to lung and spleen but eventually to tumor sites) but often yields a noisy image with low sensitivity. Recently, the use of a reporter gene coupled with PET imaging has led to an innovative approach to noninvasive serial monitoring. T cells transduced with the HSV-TK enzyme selectively phosphorylate radiolabeled thymidine analogues ($[^{124}I]$ fialuridine or $[^{18}F]$ [fluoro-3-(hydroxymethyl)butyl]guanine) that accumulate intracellularly and can be detected by PET imaging [144,145]. In addition to providing a means of assessing T-cell kinetics, the thymidine kinase gene also would allow in vivo ablation of infused T cells using low-dose ganciclovir should toxicity occur.

GENETIC MODIFICATION OF T CELLS FOR ADOPTIVE THERAPY

One advantage of adoptive T-cell therapy over vaccination strategies is the ability to modify antigen-specific T-cell clones genetically ex vivo to enhance safety or function. Introduction of a chimeric antigen receptor comprised of immunoglobulin-binding domains for a surface protein and the intracellular domains for T-cell signaling (eg, the CD3-zeta chain) provide an efficient means of redirecting T-cell responses to surface tumor antigens that are prevalent for a given tumor type, such as CD20 or CD19 in B-cell malignancies [146,147]. Uniform specificity for T-cell target antigens, for example when high-affinity T-cell responses are difficult to elicit in vitro, may be achieved by peripheral blood lymphocytes with cloned TCR of high target affinity leading to the generation of tumor-reactive CD4 and CD8 T cells [148–150]. Methods to enhance survival of adoptively transferred T cells (eg, CD8+ CTL) include the introduction of costimulatory molecules (eg, CD28 [151]) or chimeric cytokine receptors comprised of an extracellular domain (eg, GM-CSF receptor) and the intracellular signaling molecule for the IL-2 receptor to allow antigen-driven helper-independent proliferation [152]. Strategies to improve effector function may be achieved by countering inhibitory proteins expressed by T cells, such as CTLA-4, src homology phosphatase-1, suppressor of cytokine signaling, or cbl-b [153]. Decreased expression of cbl-b, for example, can lead to a decreased threshold for TCR activation and enhanced effector function and may be achieved by introducing a dominant-negative transgene into T cells [153]. Inhibitory signals in the tumor microenvironment may also be countered by genetically modifying adoptively transferred T cells. TGF-β, an immunosuppressive cytokine found in many tumor sites, can lead to immune evasion by directly engaging T cells. T cells modified to express the dominant negative TGF-β receptor type II have been rendered unresponsive to TGF-β [154], resulting in a more potent tumor-specific T-cell response and tumor eradication [155]. In the current regulatory climate, the means to transduce T cells efficiently and to maintain transgene function in T cells for adoptive transfer represent surmountable challenges, and several promising clinical studies are already under way to evaluate the use of genetically modified T cells in cancer.

SUMMARY

Adoptive T-cell therapy provides a rigorous means of dissecting the requirements for successful immunotherapy and is an increasingly feasible treatment modality for patients who have cancer. With recent scientific and technologic advances, lessons learned from murine models gradually are being translated into clinical trials. One limitation continues to be the identification of immunogenic targets for solid tumors other than melanoma, although this limitation has been addressed partially by the identification of "universal" antigens such as survivin, p53, and telomerase and the family of cancer-testis antigens that are more broadly expressed among tumor types. Although the majority of studies have been performed in patients who have advanced disease, immunotherapy is particularly well suited for prevention and for treatment of patients who have low tumor burden. The convergence of early disease detection and antigen-specific immunotherapy may lead to safe and effective strategies for long-term tumor immunoprotection. For the treatment of established tumors, the development of strategies to undermine tumor immune escape mechanisms and the integration of adoptively transferred antigen-specific T cells in combination with chemotherapy, anti-angiogenesis agents, or other targeted molecules will enhance the prospect of achieving and maintaining clinical responses in patients who have otherwise refractory disease.

References

[1] Burnet FM. Cancer—a biological approach. BMJ 1957;1:841–7.
[2] Shankaran V. IFNgamma and lymphocytes prevent primary tumour development and shape tumour immunogenicity. Nature 2001;410:1107–11.
[3] Street SE, Cretney E, Smyth MJ. Perforin and interferon-gamma activities independently control tumor initiation, growth, and metastasis. Blood 2001;97:192–7.
[4] Houghton AN, Vijayasaradhi S, Bouchard B, et al. Recognition of autoantigens by patients with melanoma. Ann N Y Acad Sci 1993;690:59–68.
[5] Blackman M, Kappler J, Marrack P. The role of the T cell receptor in positive and negative selection of developing T cells. Science 1990;248:1335–41.
[6] Morahan G, Allison J, Miller JF. Tolerance of class I histocompatibility antigens expressed extrathymically. Nature 1989;339:622–4.
[7] Ohlen C, Kalos M, Cheng LE, et al. CD8(+) T cell tolerance to a tumor-associated antigen is maintained at the level of expansion rather than effector function. J Exp Med 2002; 195:1407–18.
[8] Ohlen C, Kalos M, Hong DJ, et al. Expression of a tolerizing tumor antigen in peripheral tissue does not preclude recovery of high-affinity CD8 + T cells or CTL immunotherapy of tumors expressing the antigen. J Immunol 2001;166:2863–70.
[9] Overwijk WW, Theoret MR, Finkelstein SE, et al. Tumor regression and autoimmunity after reversal of a functionally tolerant state of self-reactive CD8 + T cells. J Exp Med 2003; 198:569–80.
[10] Leach DR, Krummel MF, Allison JP. Enhancement of antitumor immunity by CTLA-4 blockade [see comments]. Science 1996;271:1734–6.
[11] Townsend SE, Allison JP. Tumor rejection after direct costimulation of CD8 + T cells by B7-transfected melanoma cells [see comments]. Science 1993;259:368–70.
[12] Lee PP, Yee C, Savage PA, et al. Characterization of circulating T cells specific for tumor-associated antigens in melanoma patients. Nat Med 1999;5:677–85.
[13] Dudley ME, Wunderlich JR, Robbins PF, et al. Cancer regression and autoimmunity in patients after clonal repopulation with antitumor lymphocytes. Science 2002;298: 850–4.
[14] Yee C, Savage PA, Lee PP, et al. Isolation of high avidity melanoma-reactive CTL from heterogeneous populations using peptide-MHC tetramers. J Immunol 1999;162: 2227–34.
[15] Yee C, Thompson JA, Byrd D, et al. Adoptive T cell therapy using antigen-specific CD8 + T cell clones for the treatment of patients with metastatic melanoma: In vivo persistence, migration, and antitumor effect of transferred T cells. Proc Natl Acad Sci U S A 2002; 99:16168–73.
[16] Gallucci S, Matzinger P. Danger signals: SOS to the immune system. Curr Opin Immunol 2001;13:114–9.
[17] Lanier LL. Natural killer cell receptor signaling. Curr Opin Immunol 2003;15:308–14.
[18] Bauer S, Groh V, Wu J, et al. Activation of NK cells and T cells by NKG2D, a receptor for stress-inducible MICA. Science 1999;285:727–9.
[19] Rosenberg SA, Lotze MT, Muul LM, et al. Observations on the systemic administration of autologous lymphokine-activated killer cells and recombinant interleukin-2 to patients with metastatic cancer. N Engl J Med 1985;313:1485–92.

[20] Schmidt-Wolf IG, Lefterova P, Mehta BA, et al. Phenotypic characterization and identification of effector cells involved in tumor cell recognition of cytokine-induced killer cells. Exp Hematol 1993;21:1673–9.

[21] Lu PH, Negrin RS. A novel population of expanded human CD3 + CD56 + cells derived from T cells with potent in vivo antitumor activity in mice with severe combined immuno-deficiency. J Immunol 1994;153:1687–96.

[22] Leemhuis T, Wells S, Scheffold C, et al. A phase I trial of autologous cytokine-induced killer cells for the treatment of relapsed Hodgkin disease and non-Hodgkin lymphoma. Biol Blood Marrow Transplant 2005;11:181–7.

[23] Takayama T, Sekine T, Makuuchi M, et al. Adoptive immunotherapy to lower postsurgical recurrence rates of hepatocellular carcinoma: a randomised trial. Lancet 2000;356: 802–7.

[24] Kageshita T, Hirai S, Ono T, et al. Down-regulation of HLA class I antigen-processing molecules in malignant melanoma: association with disease progression. Am J Pathol 1999;154:745–54.

[25] Whiteside TL, Stanson J, Shurin MR, et al. Antigen-processing machinery in human dendritic cells: up-regulation by maturation and down-regulation by tumor cells. J Immunol 2004;173:1526–34.

[26] Boise LH, Noel PJ, Thompson CB. CD28 and apoptosis. Curr Opin Immunol 1995;7: 620–5.

[27] Bromley SK, Burack WR, Johnson KG, et al. The immunological synapse. Annu Rev Immunol 2001;19:375–96.

[28] Krummel MF, Allison JP. CD28 and CTLA-4 have opposing effects on the response of T cells to stimulation. J Exp Med 1995;182:459–65.

[29] Hung K, Hayashi R, Lafond-Walker A, et al. The central role of CD4(+) T cells in the antitumor immune response. J Exp Med 1998;188:2357–68.

[30] Bluestone JA, Abbas AK. Natural versus adaptive regulatory T cells. Nat Rev Immunol 2003;3:253–7.

[31] Sakaguchi S. Naturally arising CD4 + regulatory t cells for immunologic self-tolerance and negative control of immune responses. Annu Rev Immunol 2004;22:531–62.

[32] Suri-Payer E. CD4 + CD25 + T cells inhibit both the induction and effector function of autoreactive T cells and represent a unique lineage of immunoregulatory cells. J Immunol 1998;160:1212–8.

[33] Greenberg PD. Therapy of murine leukemia with cyclophosphamide and immune Lyt-2 + cells: cytolytic T cells can mediate eradication of disseminated leukemia. J Immunol 1986;136:1917–22.

[34] Overwijk WW, Tsung A, Irvine KR, et al. gp100/pmel 17 is a murine tumor rejection antigen: induction of "self"-reactive, tumoricidal T cells using high-affinity, altered peptide ligand. J Exp Med 1998;188:277–86.

[35] Sakai K, Chang AE, Shu SY. Phenotype analyses and cellular mechanisms of the pre-effector T-lymphocyte response to a progressive syngeneic murine sarcoma. Cancer Res 1990;50:4371–6.

[36] Ossendorp F, Mengede E, Camps M, et al. Specific T helper cell requirement for optimal induction of cytotoxic T lymphocytes against major histocompatibility complex class II negative tumors. J Exp Med 1998;187:693–702.

[37] Surman DR, Dudley ME, Overwijk WW, et al. Cutting edge: CD4 + T cell control of CD8 + T cell reactivity to a model tumor antigen. J Immunol 2000;164:562–5.

[38] Frey AB, Cestari S. Killing of rat adenocarcinoma 13762 in situ by adoptive transfer of CD4 + anti-tumor T cells requires tumor expression of cell surface MHC class II molecules. Cell Immunol 1997;178:79–90.

[39] Greenberg PD, Kern DE, Cheever MA. Therapy of disseminated murine leukemia with cyclophosphamide and immune Lyt-1 +, 2- T cells. Tumor eradication does not require participation of cytotoxic T cells. J Exp Med 1985;161:1122–34.

[40] Greenberg PD. Adoptive T cell therapy of tumors: mechanisms operative in the recognition and elimination of tumor cells. Adv Immunol 1991;49:281–355.

[41] Alexander-Miller MA, Leggatt GR, Berzofsky JA. Selective expansion of high- or low-avidity cytotoxic T lymphocytes and efficacy for adoptive immunotherapy. Proc Natl Acad Sci U S A 1996;93:4102–7.

[42] Zeh HJ, Perry-Lalley D, Dudley ME, et al. High avidity CTLs for two self-antigens demonstrate superior in vitro and in vivo antitumor efficacy. J Immunol 1999;162:989–94.

[43] Awwad M, North RJ. Cyclophosphamide-induced immunologically mediated regression of a cyclophosphamide-resistant murine tumor: a consequence of eliminating precursor L3T4 + suppressor T-cells. Cancer Res 1989;49:1649–54.

[44] North RJ, Awwad M. T cell suppression as an obstacle to immunologically-mediated tumor regression: elimination of suppression results in regression. Prog Clin Biol Res 1987;244:345–58.

[45] Cameron RB, Spiess PJ, Rosenberg SA. Synergistic antitumor activity of tumor-infiltrating lymphocytes, interleukin 2, and local tumor irradiation. Studies on the mechanism of action. J Exp Med 1990;171:249–63.

[46] Cheever MA, Greenberg PD, Fefer A, et al. Augmentation of the anti-tumor therapeutic efficacy of long-term cultured T lymphocytes by in vivo administration of purified interleukin 2. J Exp Med 1982;155:968–80.

[47] Cheever MA, Thompson JA, Kern DE, et al. Interleukin 2 (IL 2) administered in vivo: influence of IL 2 route and timing on T cell growth. J Immunol 1985;134:3895–900.

[48] Porter DL, Roth MS, McGarigle C, et al. Induction of graft-versus-host disease as immunotherapy for relapsed chronic myeloid leukemia. N Engl J Med 1994;330:100–6.

[49] Weiden PL, Sullivan KM, Flournoy N, et al. Antileukemic effect of chronic graft-versus-host disease: contribution to improved survival after allogeneic marrow transplantation. N Engl J Med 1981;304:1529–33.

[50] Goldman JM, Gale RP, Horowitz MM, et al. Bone marrow transplantation for chronic myelogenous leukemia in chronic phase. Increased risk for relapse associated with T-cell depletion. Ann Intern Med 1988;108:806–14.

[51] Dazzi F, Szydlo RM, Cross NC, et al. Durability of responses following donor lymphocyte infusions for patients who relapse after allogeneic stem cell transplantation for chronic myeloid leukemia. Blood 2000;96:2712–6.

[52] Kolb HJ, Mittermuller J, Clemm C, et al. Donor leukocyte transfusions for treatment of recurrent chronic myelogenous leukemia in marrow transplant patients. Blood 1990;76:2462–5.

[53] Kolb HJ, Schattenberg A, Goldman JM, et al. Graft-versus-leukemia effect of donor lymphocyte transfusions in marrow grafted patients. Blood 1995;86:2041–50.

[54] Soiffer RJ, Alyea EP, Hochberg E, et al. Randomized trial of CD8 + T-cell depletion in the prevention of graft-versus-host disease associated with donor lymphocyte infusion. Biol Blood Marrow Transplant 2002;8:625–32.

[55] Levine JE, Braun T, Penza SL, et al. Prospective trial of chemotherapy and donor leukocyte infusions for relapse of advanced myeloid malignancies after allogeneic stem-cell transplantation. J Clin Oncol 2002;20:405–12.

[56] Schmid C, Schleuning M, Ledderose G, et al. Sequential regimen of chemotherapy, reduced-intensity conditioning for allogeneic stem-cell transplantation, and prophylactic donor lymphocyte transfusion in high-risk acute myeloid leukemia and myelodysplastic syndrome. J Clin Oncol 2005;23:5675–87.

[57] Seropian S, Bahceci E, Cooper DL. Allogeneic peripheral blood stem cell transplantation for high-risk non-Hodgkin's lymphoma. Bone Marrow Transplant 2003;32:763–9.

[58] Verdonck LF, Lokhorst HM, Dekker AW, et al. Graft-versus-myeloma effect in two cases. Lancet 1996;347:800–1.

[59] Kwak LW, Neelapu SS, Bishop MR. Adoptive immunotherapy with antigen-specific T cells in myeloma: a model of tumor-specific donor lymphocyte infusion. Semin Oncol 2004;31:37–46.

[60] Neelapu SS, Munshi NC, Jagannath S, et al. Tumor antigen immunization of sibling stem cell transplant donors in multiple myeloma. Bone Marrow Transplant 2005;36:315–23.

[61] Bonini C, Ferrari G, Verzeletti S, et al. HSV-TK gene transfer into donor lymphocytes for control of allogeneic graft-versus-leukemia [see comments]. Science 1997;276:1719–24.

[62] Ruggeri L, Capanni M, Urbani E, et al. Effectiveness of donor natural killer cell alloreactivity in mismatched hematopoietic transplants. Science 2002;295:2097–100.

[63] Bethge WA, Hegenbart U, Stuart MJ, et al. Adoptive immunotherapy with donor lymphocyte infusions after allogeneic hematopoietic cell transplantation following nonmyeloablative conditioning. Blood 2004;103:790–5.

[64] Babcock GJ, Decker LL, Freeman RB, et al. Epstein-Barr virus-infected resting memory B cells, not proliferating lymphoblasts, accumulate in the peripheral blood of immunosuppressed patients. J Exp Med 1999;190:567–76.

[65] Callan MFC, Tan L, Annels N, et al. Direct visualization of antigen-specific Cd8(+) T cells during the primary immune response to Epstein-Barr virus in vivo. J Exp Med 1998;187: 1395–402.

[66] Lucas KG, Burton RL, Zimmerman SE, et al. Semiquantitative Epstein-Barr virus (EBV) polymerase chain reaction for the determination of patients at risk for EBV-induced lymphoproliferative disease after stem cell transplantation. Blood 1998;91:3654–61.

[67] Clave E, Agbalika F, Bajzik V, et al. Epstein-Barr virus (EBV) reactivation in allogeneic stem-cell transplantation: relationship between viral load, EBV-specific T-cell reconstitution and rituximab therapy. Transplantation 2004;77:76–84.

[68] Heslop HE, Brenner MK, Rooney CM. Donor T cells to treat EBV-associated lymphoma. N Engl J Med 1994;331:679–80.

[69] Papadopoulos EB, Ladanyi M, Emanuel D, et al. Infusions of donor leukocytes to treat Epstein-Barr virus-associated lymphoproliferative disorders after allogeneic bone marrow transplantation [see comments]. N Engl J Med 1994;330:1185–91.

[70] O'Reilly RJ, Small TN, Papadopoulos E, et al. Adoptive immunotherapy for Epstein-Barr virus-associated lymphoproliferative disorders complicating marrow allografts. Springer Semin Immunopathol 1998;20:455–91.

[71] Tiberghien P, Ferrand C, Lioure B, et al. Administration of herpes simplex-thymidine kinase-expressing donor T cells with a T-cell-depleted allogeneic marrow graft. Blood 2001;97:63–72.

[72] Berger C, Blau CA, Huang ML, et al. Pharmacologically regulated Fas-mediated death of adoptively transferred T cells in a nonhuman primate model. Blood 2004;103: 1261–9.

[73] Thomis DC, Marktel S, Bonini C, et al. A Fas-based suicide switch in human T cells for the treatment of graft-versus-host disease. Blood 2001;97:1249–57.

[74] Heslop HE, Ng CY, Li C, et al. Long-term restoration of immunity against Epstein-Barr virus infection by adoptive transfer of gene-modified virus-specific T lymphocytes. Nat Med 1996;2:551–5.

[75] Rooney CM, Smith CA, Ng CY, et al. Infusion of cytotoxic T cells for the prevention and treatment of Epstein-Barr virus-induced lymphoma in allogeneic transplant recipients. Blood 1998;92:1549–55.

[76] Haque T, Wilkie GM, Taylor C, et al. Treatment of Epstein-Barr-virus-positive posttransplantation lymphoproliferative disease with partly HLA-matched allogeneic cytotoxic T cells. Lancet 2002;360:436–42.

[77] Khanna R, Bell S, Sherritt M, et al. Activation and adoptive transfer of Epstein-Barr virus-specific cytotoxic T cells in solid organ transplant patients with posttransplant lymphoproliferative disease. Proc Natl Acad Sci U S A 1999;96:10391–6.

[78] Bollard CM, Straathof KC, Huls MH, et al. The generation and characterization of LMP2-specific CTLs for use as adoptive transfer from patients with relapsed EBV-positive Hodgkin disease. J Immunother 2004;27:317–27.

[79] Straathof KC, Bollard CM, Popat U, et al. Treatment of nasopharyngeal carcinoma with Epstein-Barr virus–specific T lymphocytes. Blood 2005;105:1898–904.

[80] Bollard CM, Aguilar L, Straathof KC, et al. Cytotoxic T lymphocyte therapy for Epstein-Barr virus + Hodgkin's disease. J Exp Med 2004;200:1623–33.

[81] Garlie NK, LeFever AV, Siebenlist RE, et al. T cells coactivated with immobilized anti-CD3 and anti-CD28 as potential immunotherapy for cancer. J Immunother 1999;22: 336–45.

[82] Curti BD, Ochoa AC, Powers GC, et al. Phase I trial of anti-CD3-stimulated CD4 + T cells, infusional interleukin-2, and cyclophosphamide in patients with advanced cancer. J Clin Oncol 1998;16:2752–60.

[83] Ito F, Carr A, Svensson H, et al. Antitumor reactivity of anti-CD3/anti-CD28 bead-activated lymphoid cells: implications for cell therapy in a murine model. J Immunother 2003;26:222–33.

[84] Spiess PJ, Yang JC, Rosenberg SA. In vivo antitumor activity of tumor-infiltrating lymphocytes expanded in recombinant interleukin-2. J Natl Cancer Inst 1987;79:1067–75.

[85] Meijer SL, Dols A, Urba WJ, et al. Adoptive cellular therapy with tumor vaccine draining lymph node lymphocytes after vaccination with HLA-B7/beta2-microglobulin gene-modified autologous tumor cells. J Immunother 2002;25:359–72.

[86] Arienti F, Belli F, Rivoltini L, et al. Adoptive immunotherapy of advanced melanoma patients with interleukin-2 (IL-2) and tumor-infiltrating lymphocytes selected in vitro with low doses of IL-2. Cancer Immunol Immunother 1993;36:315–22.

[87] Dillman RO, Oldham RK, Barth NM, et al. Continuous interleukin-2 and tumor-infiltrating lymphocytes as treatment of advanced melanoma. A national biotherapy study group trial. Cancer 1991;68:1–8.

[88] Rosenberg SA, Yannelli JR, Yang JC, et al. Treatment of patients with metastatic melanoma with autologous tumor-infiltrating lymphocytes and interleukin 2. J Natl Cancer Inst 1994; 86:1159–66.

[89] Topalian SL, Solomon D, Avis FP, et al. Immunotherapy of patients with advanced cancer using tumor-infiltrating lymphocytes and recombinant interleukin-2: a pilot study. J Clin Oncol 1988;6:839–53.

[90] van der Bruggen P, Traversari C, Chomez P, Lurquin C, De Plaen E, Van den Eynde B, Knuth A, Boon T. A gene encoding an antigen recognized by cytolytic T lymphocytes on a human melanoma. Science 1991;254:1643–7.

[91] Chaux P, Vantomme V, Stroobant V, et al. Identification of MAGE-3 epitopes presented by HLA-DR molecules to CD4(+) T lymphocytes. J Exp Med 1999;189:767–77.

[92] Kawakami Y, Eliyahu S, Delgado CH, et al. Identification of a human melanoma antigen recognized by tumor-infiltrating lymphocytes associated with in vivo tumor rejection. Proc Natl Acad Sci U S A 1994;91:6458–62.

[93] Kawakami Y, Eliyahu S, Sakaguchi K, et al. Identification of the immunodominant peptides of the MART-1 human melanoma antigen recognized by the majority of HLA-A2-restricted tumor infiltrating lymphocytes. J Exp Med 1994;180:347–52.

[94] Robbins PF, el-Gamil M, Kawakami Y, et al. Recognition of tyrosinase by tumor-infiltrating lymphocytes from a patient responding to immunotherapy [erratum published in Cancer Res 1994;54(14):3952]. Cancer Res 1994;54:3124–6.

[95] Sahin U, Tureci O, Pfreundschuh M. Serological identification of human tumor antigens. Curr Opin Immunol 1997;9:709–16.

[96] Scanlan MJ, Gure AO, Jungbluth AA, et al. Cancer/testis antigens: an expanding family of targets for cancer immunotherapy. Immunol Rev 2002;188:22–32.

[97] Hermeking H. Serial analysis of gene expression and cancer. Curr Opin Oncol 2003; 15:44–9.

[98] Brichard V, Van Pel A, Wolfel T, et al. The tyrosinase gene codes for an antigen recognized by autologous cytolytic T lymphocytes on HLA-A2 melanomas. J Exp Med 1993;178:489–95.

[99] Coulie PG, Brichard V, Van Pel A, et al. A new gene coding for a differentiation antigen recognized by autologous cytolytic T lymphocytes on HLA-A2 melanomas [see comments]. J Exp Med 1994;180:35–42.

[100] Disis ML, Smith JW, Murphy AE, et al. In vitro generation of human cytolytic T-cells specific for peptides derived from the HER-2/neu protooncogene protein. Cancer Res 1994;54:1071–6.

[101] Ambrosini G. A novel anti-apoptosis gene, survivin, expressed in cancer and lymphoma. Nat Med 1997;3:917–21.

[102] Kim NW, Piatyszek MA, Prowse KR, et al. Specific association of human telomerase activity with immortal cells and cancer. Science 1994;266:2011–5.

[103] Chen YT, Scanlan MJ, Sahin U, et al. A testicular antigen aberrantly expressed in human cancers detected by autologous antibody screening. Proc Natl Acad Sci U S A 1997; 94:1914–8.

[104] Wolfel T, Hauer M, Schneider J, et al. A p16INK4a-insensitive CDK4 mutant targeted by cytolytic T lymphocytes in a human melanoma. Science 1995;269:1281–4.

[105] Robbins PF, El-Gamil M, Li YF, et al. A mutated beta-catenin gene encodes a melanoma-specific antigen recognized by tumor infiltrating lymphocytes. J Exp Med 1996;183: 1185–92.

[106] Ressing ME, Sette A, Brandt RM, et al. Human CTL epitopes encoded by human papillomavirus type 16 E6 and E7 identified through in vivo and in vitro immunogenicity studies of HLA-A*0201-binding peptides. J Immunol 1995;154:5934–43.

[107] Gattinoni L, Klebanoff CA, Palmer DC, et al. Acquisition of full effector function in vitro paradoxically impairs the in vivo antitumor efficacy of adoptively transferred CD8 + T cells. J Clin Invest 2005;115:1616–26.

[108] Stuge TB, Holmes SP, Saharan S, et al. Diversity and recognition efficiency of T cell responses to cancer. PLoS Med 2004;1:149–60.

[109] Dudley ME. Adoptive transfer of cloned melanoma-reactive T lymphocytes for the treatment of patients with metastatic melanoma. J Immunother 2001;24:363–73.

[110] Dudley ME, Wunderlich JR, Yang JC, et al. A phase I study of nonmyeloablative chemotherapy and adoptive transfer of autologous tumor antigen-specific T lymphocytes in patients with metastatic melanoma. J Immunother 2002;25:243–51.

[111] Meidenbauer N, Marienhagen J, Laumer M, et al. Survival and tumor localization of adoptively transferred Melan-A-specific T cells in melanoma patients. J Immunol 2003; 170:2161–9.

[112] Mitchell MS. Phase I trial of adoptive immunotherapy with cytolytic T lymphocytes immunized against a tyrosinase epitope. J Clin Oncol 2002;20:1075–86.

[113] Cai Z, Brunmark A, Jackson MR, et al. Transfected Drosophila cells as a probe for defining the minimal requirements for stimulating unprimed CD8 + T cells. Proc Natl Acad Sci U S A 1996;93:14736–41.

[114] Jackson MR, Song ES, Yang Y, et al. Empty and peptide-containing conformers of class I major histocompatibility complex molecules expressed in Drosophila melanogaster cells. Proc Natl Acad Sci U S A 1992;89:12117–21.

[115] Sun S, Cai Z, Langlade-Demoyen P, et al. Dual function of Drosophila cells as APCs for naive CD8 + T cells: implications for tumor immunotherapy. Immunity 1996;4: 555–64.

[116] Maus MV, Riley JL, Kwok WW, et al. HLA tetramer-based artificial antigen-presenting cells for stimulation of CD4 + T cells. Clin Immunol 2003;106:16–22.

[117] Maus MV, Thomas AK, Leonard DG, et al. Ex vivo expansion of polyclonal and antigen-specific cytotoxic T lymphocytes by artificial APCs expressing ligands for the T-cell receptor, CD28 and 4–1BB. Nat Biotechnol 2002;20:143–8.

[118] Oelke M, Maus MV, Didiano D, et al. Ex vivo induction and expansion of antigen-specific cytotoxic T cells by HLA-Ig-coated artificial antigen-presenting cells. Nat Med 2003;9: 619–24.

[119] Prakken B, Wauben M, Genini D, et al. Artificial antigen-presenting cells as a tool to exploit the immune 'synapse'. Nat Med 2000;6:1406–10.

[120] Zitvogel L, Regnault A, Lozier A, et al. Eradication of established murine tumors using a novel cell-free vaccine: dendritic cell-derived exosomes. Nat Med 1998;4:594–600.

[121] Dupont J, Latouche JB, Ma C, et al. Artificial antigen-presenting cells transduced with telomerase efficiently expand epitope-specific, human leukocyte antigen-restricted cytotoxic T cells. Cancer Res 2005;65:5417–27.

[122] Latouche JB, Sadelain M. Induction of human cytotoxic T lymphocytes by artificial antigen-presenting cells. Nat Biotechnol 2000;18:405–9.

[123] Schoenberger SP, Jonges LE, Mooijaart RJ, et al. Efficient direct priming of tumor-specific cytotoxic T lymphocyte in vivo by an engineered APC. Cancer Res 1998;58: 3094–100.

[124] Robbins PF, Dudley ME, Wunderlich J, et al. Cutting edge: persistence of transferred lymphocyte clonotypes correlates with cancer regression in patients receiving cell transfer therapy. J Immunol 2004;173:7125–30.

[125] Yee C, Greenberg P. Modulating T-cell immunity to tumours: new strategies for monitoring T-cell responses. Nat Rev Cancer 2002;2:409–19.

[126] Cerottini JC, Nordin AA, Brunner KT. Specific in vitro cytotoxicity of thymus-derived lymphocytes sensitized to alloantigens. Nature 1970;228:1308–9.

[127] Taswell C. Limiting dilution assays for the determination of immunocompetent cell frequencies. I. Data analysis. J Immunol 1981;126:1614–9.

[128] Herr W, Schneider J, Lohse AW, et al. Detection and quantification of blood-derived CD8 + T lymphocytes secreting tumor necrosis factor alpha in response to HLA-A2.1-binding melanoma and viral peptide antigens. J Immunol Methods 1996;191:131–42.

[129] Pala P, Hussell T, Openshaw PJM. Flow cytometric measurement of intracellular cytokines. J Immunol Methods 2000;243:107–24.

[130] Altman JD, Moss PAH, Goulder PJR, et al. Phenotypic analysis of antigen-specific T lymphocytes [erratum published in Science 1998;280(5371):1821]. Science 1996;274: 94–6.

[131] Schneck JP. Monitoring antigen-specific T cells using MHC-Ig dimers. Immunol Invest 2000;29:163–9.

[132] Murali-Krishna K, Altman JD, Suresh M, et al. Counting antigen-specific CD8 T cells: a reevaluation of bystander activation during viral infection. Immunity 1998;8:177–87.

[133] Zajac AJ, Blattman JN, Murali-Krishna K, et al. Viral immune evasion due to persistence of activated T cells without effector function. J Exp Med 1998;188:2205–13.

[134] Dutoit V, Rubio-Godoy V, Doucey MA, et al. Functional avidity of tumor antigen-specific CTL recognition directly correlates with the stability of MHC/peptide multimer binding to TCR. J Immunol 2002;168:1167–71.

[135] Savage PA. A kinetic basis for T cell receptor repertoire selection during an immune response. Immunity 1999;10:485–92.

[136] Riddell SR, Elliott M, Lewinsohn DA, et al. T-cell mediated rejection of gene-modified HIV-specific cytotoxic T lymphocytes in HIV-infected patients [see comments]. Nat Med 1996;2:216–23.

[137] Rosenberg SA, Aebersold P, Cornetta K, et al. Gene transfer into humans—immunotherapy of patients with advanced melanoma, using tumor-infiltrating lymphocytes modified by retroviral gene transduction [see comments]. N Engl J Med 1990;323: 570–8.

[138] Gallard A, Foucras G, Coureau C, et al. Tracking T cell clonotypes in complex T lymphocyte populations by real-time quantitative PCR using fluorogenic complementarity-determining region-3-specific probes. J Immunol Methods 2002;270:269–80.

[139] Walter EA, Greenberg PD, Gilbert MJ, et al. Reconstitution of cellular immunity against cytomegalovirus in recipients of allogeneic bone marrow by transfer of T-cell clones from the donor [see comments]. N Engl J Med 1995;333:1038–44.

[140] Haanen J, Van Oijen M, Tirion F, et al. In situ detection of virus- and tumor-specific T-cell immunity. Nat Med 2000;6:1056–60.

[141] Mocellin S, Ohnmacht GA, Wang E, et al. Kinetics of cytokine expression in melanoma metastases classifies immune responsiveness. Int J Cancer 2001;93:236–42.

[142] Panelli MC, Riker A, Kammula U, et al. Expansion of tumor-T cell pairs from fine needle aspirates of melanoma metastases. J Immunol 2000;164:495–504.

[143] Hardy J, Edinger M, Bachmann MH, et al. Bioluminescence imaging of lymphocyte trafficking in vivo. Exp Hematol 2001;29:1353–60.

[144] Hildebrandt IJ, Gambhir SS. Molecular imaging applications for immunology. Clin Immunol 2004;111:210–24.
[145] Koehne G, Doubrovin M, Doubrovina E, et al. Serial in vivo imaging of the targeted migration of human HSV-TK-transduced antigen-specific lymphocytes. Nat Biotechnol 2003;21:405–13.
[146] Brentjens RJ, Latouche JB, Santos E, et al. Eradication of systemic B-cell tumors by genetically targeted human T lymphocytes co-stimulated by CD80 and interleukin-15. Nat Med 2003;9:279–86.
[147] Wang J, Press OW, Lindgren CG, et al. Cellular immunotherapy for follicular lymphoma using genetically modified CD20-specific CD8 + cytotoxic T lymphocytes. Mol Ther 2004;9:577–86.
[148] Kessels HW, van Den Boom MD, Spits H, et al. Changing T cell specificity by retroviral T cell receptor display. Proc Natl Acad Sci U S A 2000;97:14578–83.
[149] Roszkowski JJ, Lyons GE, Kast WM, et al. Simultaneous generation of CD8 + and CD4 + melanoma-reactive T cells by retroviral-mediated transfer of a single T-cell receptor. Cancer Res 2005;65:1570–6.
[150] Zhao Y, Zheng Z, Cohen CJ, et al. High-efficiency transfection of primary human and mouse T lymphocytes using RNA electroporation. Mol Ther 2005;13:151–9.
[151] Topp MS, Riddell SR, Akatsuka Y, et al. Restoration of CD28 expression in CD28- CD8 + memory effector T cells reconstitutes antigen-induced IL-2 production. J Exp Med 2003;198:947–55.
[152] Cheng LE, Ohlen C, Nelson BH, et al. Enhanced signaling through the IL-2 receptor in CD8 + T cells regulated by antigen recognition results in preferential proliferation and expansion of responding CD8 + T cells rather than promotion of cell death. Proc Natl Acad Sci U S A 2002;99:3001–6.
[153] Chiang YJ, Kole HK, Brown K, et al. Cbl-b regulates the CD28 dependence of T-cell activation. Nature 2000;403:216–20.
[154] Bollard CM, Rossig C, Calonge MJ, et al. Adapting a transforming growth factor beta-related tumor protection strategy to enhance antitumor immunity. Blood 2002;99:3179–87.
[155] Gorelik L, Flavell RA. Immune-mediated eradication of tumors through the blockade of transforming growth factor-beta signaling in T cells. Nat Med 2001;7:1118–22.

HEMATOLOGY/ONCOLOGY CLINICS
OF NORTH AMERICA

ELSEVIER
SAUNDERS

Immunoprevention of Cancer

Radek Spisek, MD, PhD[a], Madhav V. Dhodapkar, MD[a,b,*]

[a]Laboratory of Tumor Immunology and Immunotherapy, The Rockefeller University, New York, NY, USA
[b]Hematology Service, Memorial Sloan-Kettering Cancer Center, New York, NY, USA

The eradication of smallpox by preventive vaccination represents one of the most impressive triumphs of modern medicine and immunology [1]. The primary function of the immune system is to protect the host against pathogens. The success of vaccination in the context of infectious diseases has inspired efforts to harness the immune system to protect against cancer. The remarkable specificity of the immune system, if harnessed, holds much promise for improving cancer therapy. But can the immune system be harnessed to prevent cancer? There is one fundamental difference between vaccines against cancer and vaccines against pathogens. Vaccines against pathogens have been largely tried and proven effective in the preventive setting, in otherwise healthy individuals [2]. In contrast, vaccination against cancer generally has been attempted in the context of therapy, in patients who already have tumors [3]. This strategy itself may be at the heart of why cancer vaccines have proved disappointing in the clinic. This article discusses the emerging body of evidence in animal and human studies that points to the need to consider an alternate approach, harnessing the immune system to prevent, rather than treat, cancer (Table 1).

ROLE OF IMMUNE SYSTEM IN PROTECTION FROM CANCER
Immunosurveillance and Immune Editing
The essential prerequisite for the rational use of immunoprevention of cancer is the assumption that the immune system can recognize transformed cells and destroy them before the onset of clinically apparent disease. The idea that the immune system can recognize and respond to tumors was initially suggested in the late nineteenth century, when Coley noted that rare events of spontaneous tumor regression sometimes were preceded by severe infections. In the 1950s, it

M.V. Dhodapkar is supported in part by funds from the National Institutes of Health (CA84512, CA106802, and CA109465), Damon Runyon Cancer Research Fund, Irene Diamond Foundation, Fund to Cure Myeloma, Dana Foundation, and Irma T. Hirschl Foundation.
* Corresponding author. Laboratory of Tumor Immunology and Immunotherapy, The Rockefeller University, 1230 York Avenue, New York, NY, 10021. *E-mail address:* dhodapm@rockefeller.edu (M.V. Dhodapkar).

0889-8588/06/$ – see front matter
doi:10.1016/j.hoc.2006.02.009

Table 1
Immunoprevention versus immunotherapy of cancer

	Immunoprevention	Immunotherapy
Patients	Patients at increased risk of cancer and preneoplastic diseases	Patients with clinical diagnosis of cancer
Patient immune status	Mostly immunocompetent	Tumor-induced or therapy-induced immunosuppression
Requirements for induced immune response	Broad immune response consisting of the activation of innate and adaptive immune mechanisms, generation of memory T and B cells population	Rapid effector immune response capable of eliminating tumor cell population
Tumor cell population	None (in the case of primary prevention), small population of preneoplastic cells at early stages of transformation (secondary prevention). Absence of tumor escape variants, absence of reactive tumor stroma	Large and heterogeneous population of tumor cells, high genetic instability, and existence of tumor escape variants
Criteria for efficacy	Induction of broad immune response, presence of memory cells	Induction of detectable immune response, induction of objective clinical response
Goals	Prevention of tumor onset, delay in progression of preneoplastic lesions	Tumor elimination, stabilization of tumor growth, prolonged survival

was shown that inbred mice could be immunized against carcinogen-induced transplantable tumors, and that the tumor rejection antigens were tumor specific. These discoveries led, in 1957, to the formulation of the cancer immunosurveillance hypothesis proposed by Thomas and Burnet, which stated that "sentinel thymus dependent cells of the body constantly surveyed host tissues for nascent transformed cells" [4]. The logical prediction of cancer immunosurveillance is that immunodeficient individuals would exhibit an increased incidence of tumors [5]. Early studies in mice with experimentally induced immunosuppression showed a higher incidence of virally induced tumors [6]. These experiments and experiments performed in athymic nude mice failed to show an increase in the incidence of spontaneous tumors, however, and the immunosurveillance concept was nearly abandoned in the late 1970s. Resurrection of this hypothesis in the last 5 years has been enabled by new experiments in truly immunodeficient mice, which provide evidence for the existence of immunosurveillance.

Effector Cells in Immunoprotection
Nude athymic mice are not completely immunodeficient because they have detectable levels of circulating $\alpha\beta$ T cells [6]. One of the most definitive stud-

ies employed gene-targeted mice lacking recombinase-activating genes (RAG) RAG-1 or RAG-2. These mice fail to rearrange lymphocyte antigen-specific receptors and lack T and B lymphocytes and natural killer T (NKT) cells [7]. RAG$^{-/-}$ mice not only developed chemically induced tumors more rapidly and with greater frequency than immunocompetent controls, but also they formed much more spontaneous tumors [8].

Studies in other mice models identified the role of other cellular components of the immune system in cancer prevention. Selective depletion of natural killer (NK) cells by anti-asialo-GM$_1$ rendered mice three times more susceptible to chemically induced tumors [9]. Similarly, Jα281$^{-/-}$ mice lacking NKT cells had a higher incidence of chemically induced tumors [9–11]. Administration of NKT cell–activating ligand α-galactosylceramide in models of chemically induced tumorigenesis decreased the incidence of tumors and prolonged the latency period to tumor formation compared with control mice. These studies not only provide support for a role of the immune system in the control of tumor formation, but also reveal the involvement of innate and adaptive immunity in this process.

Pioneering studies in Schreiber's laboratory at Washington University showed a crucial role of interferon (IFN)-γ in immunosurveillance [12]. Abrogation of IFN-γ function by neutralization with monoclonal antibodies or by genetic manipulation of its expression or signaling pathways enhanced susceptibility to chemically induced and spontaneous tumors [13]. IFN-γ is likely to act at the level of the host and the tumor. It promotes the generation of antigen-specific CD4 Th1 T cells and cytotoxic T lymphocytes (CTL), enhances activation of dendritic cells and macrophages, and inhibits angiogenesis [14,15]. The tumor cells themselves also have been shown to represent a crucial cellular target of IFN-γ. IFN-γ induces increased expression of several components of MHC class I, antigen processing, and presentation pathway [16]. Another key finding was the observation that mice lacking perforin (perforin$^{-/-}$), a crucial cytolytic molecule, developed significantly more chemically induced tumors compared with perforin-sufficient mice [17]. Untreated perforin$^{-/-}$ mice also showed an increased incidence of spontaneous disseminated lymphomas. In addition to perforin, a component of cytolytic granules of CTL and NK cells, subsequent studies also revealed an important role of tumor necrosis factor–related apoptosis-inducing ligand, an important mediator of the cytotoxic function of the innate immune system. Lymphocytes and IFN-γ seem to be crucial and independent components of the protection mechanisms against tumors.

Cancer Immune Editing

In discussing the theoretical and experimental basis for the advantages of cancer immunoprevention, it is important to mention the cancer immune editing hypothesis proposed by Dunn et al [18], which complements and extends the initial immunosurveillance postulate. The same RAG-2$^{-/-}$ mouse model that was used for the validation of the immunosurveillance concept was used in experiments that looked at the differences in the immunogenicity of tumors

originally generated in the presence or absence of the functional immune system
[8]. When tumors isolated from wild-type or RAG-2$^{-/-}$ mice were transplanted
into RAG-2$^{-/-}$ mice, they grew with similar kinetics. Transfer of tumors grown
in immunocompetent mice into the naive immunocompetent mice also led to the
rapid establishment and progression of all tumors. Almost 50% of tumors
generated in RAG-2$^{-/-}$ mice were rejected after the transfer into the immunocompetent host. Tumors formed in the absence of a functional immune system
are more immunogenic than tumors generated in immunocompetent hosts.
Similar findings, showing higher immunogenicity of tumors grown in immunodeficient hosts, also were reported for Jα281$^{-/-}$ [11] and perforin$^{-/-}$ mice [19].
   The aforementioned results suggest that an immune reaction initiated against
transforming tumor cells exerts a continuous evolutionary pressure and favors
the development and survival of cells that can escape the control of the immune
system. Dunn et al [20] proposed to distinguish three separate stages in the
process of cancer immune editing—elimination, equilibrium, and escape. The
occurrence of tumor cells in an organism does not mean that the cancer immune
editing process would follow all three phases. Most likely, a transformed tumor
cell would be recognized and destroyed, and the process would terminate in the
elimination phase. In the equilibrium phase, the host immune system and any
surviving tumor cell variants enter into the state of dynamic equilibrium. The
enormous plasticity of cancer cells arising from increasing genetic instability
eventually may give rise to new phenotypes that have reduced immunogenicity
and can progress to the escape phase. It is likely that equilibrium is the longest of
the three processes and clinically most likely corresponds to the preneoplastic
disease that most frequently remains undiagnosed. Three possible scenarios
could be envisaged for transformed cells in the equilibrium stage: (1) complete
elimination of tumor cell population; (2) long-term, possibly permanent maintenance of dynamic equilibrium between active immune response and restricted
population of tumor cells; and (3) escape from the control of the immune
reaction and progression to the clinically overt disease. The degree to which
immune editing occurs in the context of human cancer remains to be defined. If
such editing is really occurring in vivo, however, it would provide a strong
rationale for prevention-based approaches rather than therapy-based approaches
to human cancer.

Role of Antigen-Presenting Cells in Tumor Immunity Versus Tolerance

The cancer immune editing hypothesis may not be the only mechanism accounting for the escape of tumors from the control of the immune system. Induction of
tolerance to tumor cells, possibly by their recognition in the absence of appropriate costimulatory signals, also has been shown to result in the progressive
growth of previously immunogenic tumors [21]. Tumors by themselves are poor
antigen-presenting cells. The generation of protective immunity requires that
tumor antigens be processed and presented by professional antigen-presenting
cells, such as dendritic cells [22]. The context in which these antigens are
presented is a major determinant of immunity versus tolerance, however. Tu-

mors often take advantage of this mechanism and induce tolerance early in the course of tumorigenesis [23,24]. Overcoming this tumor-induced tolerance is a major goal in design of cancer immunotherapies.

Mechanisms of Immune Escape

Tumor cells have evolved several strategies to evade the immune system. Tumors often induce the expression or production of factors such as transforming growth factor-β and interleukin-10 that may suppress or attenuate the antitumor immune response. Tumors also may escape the immune system by mutations in the antigen-processing pathway, such as mutations in β_2-microglobulin, the transporter associated with antigen processing (TAP), or proteasome components [25]. These mutations are sufficient to confer a resistance to the CD8 T lymphocytes that is difficult to overcome despite the fact that downregulation of MHC class I expression can make tumor cells more susceptible to NK cell–mediated death. It is hoped that the induction of a broad immune response, including the activation of CD4 T cells and antibody production by B cells, could compensate for this defect as indicated by murine studies [26,27].

In addition to tumor cell–derived mechanisms of immune system evasion, tumor progression depends on the adjacent stroma [28]. Immunizing against products specific for stromal cells also could affect tumor growth. Stimulating immune responses against angiogenesis-associated products that are expressed in tumor vascular bed could interfere with the formation of new vessels and inhibit tumor growth. This problem was shown in studies in which immunization of mice with vascular endothelial growth factor receptor 2 (VEGFR2) protein loaded dendritic cells [29] or dendritic cells transfected with VEGFR2 mRNA [30].

IMMUNE SYSTEM AS A TWO-EDGED SWORD: IMMUNE STIMULATION OF CANCER

There is a growing body of multidisciplinary evidence that inflammation is strongly linked to cancer [31,32]. In some situations, this inflammatory response may drive the development of the tumor [33]. One example of such a process may be the stimulation of germinal center lymphomas in mice by T cells in response to retrovirus-derived superantigens [34]. These findings do not contradict the immunosurveillance hypothesis, however. Specific immune response targeted against tumor cells can lead to their elimination, whereas chronic inflammation maintained by persistent viral infection or chronic exposure to carcinogens leads to the production of cytokines, chemokines, and growth factors and to an increase in genetic instability [35]. It also is possible that chronic inflammation suppresses the specific immune response against cancer. Changes in the tumor microenvironment (as opposed to tumor cells themselves) may be among the major obstacles for immunotherapy of cancer and support the consideration of preventive approaches, wherein these microenvironmental changes would not be as robust.

RATIONALE FOR IMMUNOPREVENTION
Lessons from Animal Models
Difficulties in addressing some fundamental immunotherapeutic questions directly in humans urge for the development of suitable animal models. Technical advances over the past 2 decades have allowed researchers to introduce alterations in the mouse genome that constitutively or conditionally alter the expression of crucial genes, leading to the development of particular tumors. These genetically engineered mice help to elucidate molecular pathways involved in oncogenesis [36,37]. More recently, these models have been used to test targeted therapies, cancer vaccines, and other preventive or therapeutic approaches. Generation of animal models has become increasingly sophisticated and relevant for the preclinical testing of prevention strategies [36]. Elegant models of gradual development of preneoplastic lesions and cancer now exist for colon cancer [38–40], pancreatic cancer [41], and breast cancer [42]. Forni and others extensively investigated preclinical approaches for cancer prevention in transgenic mice overexpressing rat HER-2/neu proto-oncogene or its mutated form. The slow carcinogenesis of mammary cancer driven by Her2/neu proto-oncogene and the aggressive carcinogenesis caused by mutated Her2/neu are inhibited by vaccination with proteins, peptides, or DNA plasmids [43–48]. Inhibition of tumor growth depends mainly on IFN-γ and antibody directed against Her2/neu protein. For the complete inhibition of tumor growth in the case of mutated oncogenic protein, interleukin-12 needs to be administered together with the Her2/neu construct [49–51]. Another study extended tumor prevention to a model of spontaneous preneoplasia. Dendritic cells fused with preneoplastic cells were shown to protect against colon polyps in a mouse model of spontaneous cancer [52]. In accordance with above-discussed data, mechanisms other than just CTL activity likely are crucial to inhibit carcinogenesis. Simultaneous stimulation of innate and adaptive immunity and the induction of broad cellular and humoral immune response may be the key to the prevention of escape of preneoplastic cells from immune control.

A spontaneous pancreatic cancer model has been developed in which the potential of mucin-1 (MUC-1)–specific immunity to eliminate preneoplastic lesions and prevent tumor progression can be studied. Early in life, these mice exhibit dysplasia in the pancreas that progresses to microadenomas and then to fully transformed MUC-1-positive pancreatic adenocarcinomas [53]. The process of carcinogenesis is accompanied by the appearance of low-frequency MUC-1-specific CD8 T cells that disappear as the tumor progresses [54]. When expanded in vitro and adoptively transferred in large numbers, however, these T cells can prevent the growth of a transplanted tumor [55]. These results suggest that inducing a robust anti-MUC-1 response before tumor occurrence could serve to prevent the development and progression of pancreatic cancer. Although mouse models have proved useful in providing the rationale for immunoprevention, fundamental differences between human and mouse cells require that principles established in mouse models be complemented by appropriate human studies (Box 1).

BOX 1: PREREQUISITES FOR IMMUNOPREVENTION OF CANCER

- Development of protocols identifying individuals at increased risk for development of cancer (hereditary cancer syndromes, virally induced cancers, cancer-causing genetic mutations)—*primary prevention*
- Implementation of population-wide screening programs for major cancers for early detection of preneoplastic lesions (breast cancer, colon cancer, lung cancer, prostate cancer)—*secondary prevention*
- Identification of shared tumor rejection antigens expressed on premalignant cells and allowing for the production of large-scale tumor vaccines relevant for most of the target population
- Definition and design of vaccination protocols
- Need for clinical trials involving large numbers of patients and long-term follow-up to establish efficacy and safety of cancer immunoprevention
- Definition of relevant criteria for the evaluation of clinical efficacy and definition of surrogate end points

Immune Recognition of Human Preneoplastic States

As reviewed previously, experimental findings in mice have helped validate the concept of cancer immunosurveillance. If applied to the immunotherapy settings, these findings imply that immune intervention directed against tumor cells at the early stages of transformation that have not been shaped by long-term interaction with host immune system could lead to the more effective elimination of malignant cells (Fig. 1). Skepticism remains, however, regarding the relevance of animal data to human tumor immunology. The key question is whether cells in the early stages of their transformation provide signals that can alert various physiologic repair and control mechanisms (including the immune system) of the presence of danger and allow for its elimination. This section discusses evidence emerging from studies in humans that preneoplastic cells are readily recognized by the immune system and cellular repair mechanisms and eliminated or kept under control at their earliest manifestation.

If immunoprevention becomes a stated goal of cancer immunotherapy, it would be important to obtain evidence that preneoplastic cells can become targets of specific immune response [56]. In addition to evidence that human cells in the early stages of neoplastic transformation activate inducible barriers against tumor progression [57], there is evidence that these cells provide signals that make them visible to the immune system and activate immune response. To document the existence of cancer surveillance in humans, the authors focused on patients with monoclonal gammopathy of unknown significance (MGUS), who have a clonal expansion of plasma cells in the bone marrow that often remains clinically stable for years without the development of clinical malignancy [58]. In this system, preneoplastic and immune cells can be readily isolated from the bone marrow and used immediately for further studies without the need for further isolation by enzyme treatment. T cells isolated from the bone marrow of MGUS patients recognized autologous tumor cell–loaded

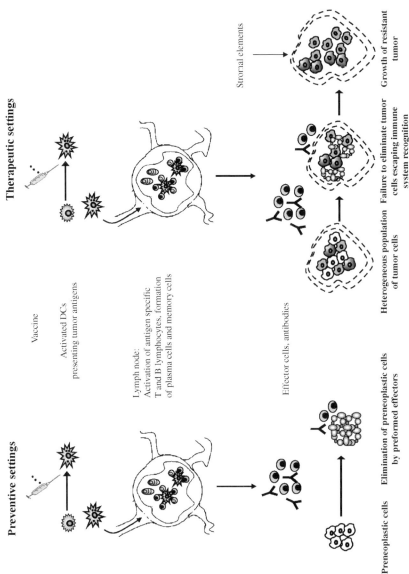

dendritic cells without the need for any ex vivo stimulation [59]. In contrast, in multiple myeloma, a malignant counterpart of preneoplastic monoclonal gammopathy, T cells must be expanded for 1 to 2 weeks in culture before tumor-specific T cells can be detected [60]. These data provide evidence that the human immune system is capable of recognizing and responding to preneoplastic lesions. Further studies are needed to assess if such responses occur in other preneoplastic states and to identify the nature of antigenic targets of these responses.

IMMUNOLOGIC CONSIDERATIONS FOR IMMUNOPREVENTION
Target Antigens
As reviewed previously, even at the early stages of malignant transformation, preneoplastic cells should provide specific antigenic targets for recognition by the immune system. Considering the current knowledge of molecular pathways and events underlying initial steps of malignant transformation, it seems probable that at least some of the antigenic targets would be shared between different patients and most likely even between different tumors. Identification of such shared tumor antigens is crucial for the practical use of cancer immunoprevention. Most of the effort at discovery of tumor antigens has focused on established tumors, and emphasis should now shift to premalignant lesions [61]. The great advantage is that existing methods of antigen identification, including the screening for CTL recognition [62] and serologic expression cloning technique [63], now simply can be applied to preneoplasia to identify antigens that are differentially expressed between normal and preneoplastic cells and between preneoplastic and fully transformed tumor cells. It also would be important to study the differences in the immune response of individuals with preneoplastic disease versus malignancies. In these settings, the serologic expression cloning technique could be particularly useful in revealing differences in the presence of antibodies and possibly reactive T cells. Antigens exclusively recognized in preneoplasia are likely to play a crucial role in the control of tumor growth by the immune system. Alternatively, antigenic targets of an efficient immune response can be

Fig. 1. Outcomes of antitumor vaccination in preventive and therapeutic settings. In optimal settings, presentation of tumor antigens by mature dendritic cells (DCs) in lymph nodes leads to the induction of antigen-specific T cells. B cells also are activated, and the outcome is clonal expansion of tumor-specific T cells and production of tumor-specific antibodies. In preventive settings, this initial activation is followed by the generation of memory cells. If a tumor begins to grow in the future, it elicits a robust secondary immune response with rapid generation of large numbers of effector T cells and production of high-titer antibodies. In therapeutic settings, effector cells of the immune system migrate to the tumor sites and attempt to eliminate tumor cells. Their function is compromised by stromal elements and an immunosuppressive microenvironment. Some tumor cells have lost the expression of tumor antigens, cannot be efficiently recognized by antigen-specific T cells and antibodies, and are resistant to immune destruction. The population of resistant tumor cells continues to grow independent of ongoing immune reaction and gives rise to the immunotherapy-resistant tumor mass.

studied in patients who experience dramatic clinical responses to immunotherapy [64].

Although antigenic profiles in human preneoplasia have not yet been studied systematically, more recent reports yielded several potential antigenic targets. Cyclin B1, which plays a key role in the control of cell cycle progression from G_2 through M phase, was identified as a tumor antigen recognized by human CD8 T cells. Compared with normal cells, many tumors, including breast cancer, lung cancere, colorectal cancer, lymphoma, and leukemia, express higher levels of cyclin B1 that is localized in the cytoplasm rather than in the nucleus [65]. Further evidence of cyclin B1 immunogenicity and its potential to serve as a tumor-specific antigen in immunoprevention comes from studies analyzing its ability to elicit T cell–dependent humoral immune responses in vivo in patients with early lung cancer, patients with premalignant disease, and patients with a known history of heavy smoking. Cyclin B1 elicited high titer helper T cell–dependent IgG antibody responses in patients with breast and colon cancer, in long-term smokers, and in patients with preneoplastic lung disease [66]. Further studies are needed to understand better if cyclin B1 can be a useful target of immune recognition in preneoplasia, and whether it can be targeted effectively for immunoprevention of cancer [67].

MUC-1 glycoprotein is expressed by normal epithelial cells and by many tumor cells, including breast cancer, pancreas cancer, colon cancer, lung cancer, ovarian cancer, prostate cancer, myelomas, and some lymphomas. There are quantitative and qualitative differences in the expression of MUC-1 between normal and malignant cells. In tumor cells, MUC-1 is expressed at higher levels and is underglycosylated compared with the normal counterparts [68]. The immune system can recognize these differences, and it can destroy MUC-1-expressing tumors, while ignoring normal tissues expressing MUC-1. Tumor forms of MUC-1 and other mucins also are expressed in many preneoplastic lesions, such as pancreatic intraepithelial neoplasia, which are precursors of pancreatic cancer [69], and adenomatous polyps, which are precursors of colon cancer. Patients with resected adenomatous polyps have high levels of antibody against MUC-1 [70]. This antibody is of the IgG isotype, suggesting the involvement of helper T cells. In contrast, patients with colon cancer have low levels of anti-MUC-1 antibodies of the IgM isotype, indicating the lack of T cell help [71]. Although MUC-1 and cyclin B1 are potentially useful examples of antigenic targets in preneoplasia, this area needs more systematic and detailed investigation. Antigenic targets of immune response during the preneoplastic growth may differ from the targets in clinical malignancy. If so, there are clear implications for early detection and prevention of cancer. Understanding antigenic targets in preneoplasia also may provide key insights regarding the nature of immune response needed to arrest growth of overt tumors.

Target Effector Populations for Immunoprevention

An important but not fully resolved issue is what kind of immune response is best suited to prevent tumor progression. Animal studies have emphasized a pivotal role of CD8 T cells in tumor immunity. Evidence for the role of CD8 T cells in patients with cancer stems from the correlation between a frequent loss of MHC class I and other components of the class I processing pathway in the course of the disease [72,73]. Accumulating evidence indicates that CD4 T cell responses also have a key role in tumor immunity. The Th1 subset of CD4 T cells is essential for the persistence in addition to the induction of CD8 T cells [74,75]. In addition, CD4 T cells sensitize tumor cells to CTL lysis by upregulating MHC class I expression through production of effector cytokines, such as IFN-γ [12,76]. The importance of CD4 T cell response in tumor immunity also was shown in murine carcinoma models, wherein CD4 T cells eradicated tumor in the absence of CD8 T cells [27,77,78]. In another study, CD4 T cells producing IFN-γ and antibodies specific for HER2/neu oncogene product were crucial for tumor eradication. The bulk of evidence from preclinical models, as discussed previously, points to the need to recruit a broad immune response consisting of innate and adaptive immune mechanisms. At present, the role of innate effectors, including NK and NKT cells, in the control of preneoplastic lesions is less studied.

CLINICAL CONSIDERATIONS FOR IMMUNOPREVENTION OF CANCER

Target Populations

In clinical settings, immunoprevention of cancer could be envisaged in several different scenarios. Primary prevention requires identification of individuals at risk of cancer development. This identification already is possible for patients with hereditary cancer syndromes (eg, Li-Fraumeni syndrome or women with *BRCA* mutations) in which specific mutations can be detected, and the increased risk for cancer is well established. As discussed subsequently, individuals at risk for virally induced cancers also are candidates for primary immunoprevention of cancer. Use of tobacco accounts for a major proportion of human cancer and may be amenable to immunologic targeting [79]. The second major group is patients with preneoplastic lesions, wherein prevention of progression to malignant tumors (secondary prevention) is an important goal. Examples of the latter are patients with colon polyps, oral leukoplakia, cervical intraepithelial neoplasia, or MGUS. Of these, virally induced lesions, such as cervical intraepithelial neoplasia, are the most attractive targets, as discussed subsequently. Prevention of cancer also is being tested in the clinic by pharmacologic approaches, such as cyclooxygenase inhibitors. One distinct advantage of immunoprevention over chemoprevention is that immune approaches carry the advantages of immunologic memory and specificity of the immune system. These approaches do not require long-term drug therapy and may not carry associated economic and toxicity implications.

Virus-Induced Tumors

Prevention of virally mediated cancer by immune intervention may represent the greatest opportunity to have an impact on cancer at a global level. Two attractive settings are the association between hepatitis B and hepatoma and the association between human papillomavirus (HPV) and cervical cancer, which are major cancers in the developing world [80]. More than 99% of cervical cancers contain one or more of approximately 15 HPV genotypes. Because 50% of these cancers contain HPV16 and another 20% contain HPV18, a cancer vaccine developed against these two genotypes should be effective for elimination of most cervical cancers [81]. The same genotypes are involved in vulvar, anal, and oropharyngeal malignancies. Clinical trials with HPV subunit vaccines based on L1 major capsid protein have been conducted [82,83]. A trial of HPV vaccination showed 100% prevention of persistent HPV16 infection and HPV16-induced cervical dysplasias [84,85].

SUMMARY

A growing body of data suggests that the interactions between tumors and cells of the immune system, particularly at the early stages of carcinogenesis, help shape the eventual development of tumors. Inflammation is a common feature of several cancers, and the immune system can serve as a two-edged sword against cancer, capable of supporting and suppressing cancer. Data from human studies show that the immune system is capable of detecting the smallest expansions of transformed cells, well before the development of clinical cancer. These advances suggest a need to change the current emphasis for harnessing antitumor immunity from therapy to prevention of cancers.

References

[1] Ada G. Vaccines and vaccination. N Engl J Med 2001;345:1042–53.
[2] Ada GL. The immunological principles of vaccination. Lancet 1990;335:523–6.
[3] Gilboa E. The promise of cancer vaccines. Nat Rev Cancer 2004;4:401–11.
[4] Burnet FM. The concept of immunological surveillance. Prog Exp Tumor Res 1970;13:1–27.
[5] Stutman O. Immunodepression and malignancy. Adv Cancer Res 1975;22:261–422.
[6] Klein G. Immunological surveillance against neoplasia. Harvey Lect 1973;69:71–102.
[7] Shinkai Y, Rathbun G, Lam KP, et al. RAG-2-deficient mice lack mature lymphocytes owing to inability to initiate V(D)J rearrangement. Cell 1992;68:855–67.
[8] Shankaran V, Ikeda H, Bruce AT, et al. IFNgamma and lymphocytes prevent primary tumour development and shape tumour immunogenicity. Nature 2001;410:1107–11.
[9] Smyth MJ, Crowe NY, Godfrey DI. NK cells and NKT cells collaborate in host protection from methylcholanthrene-induced fibrosarcoma. Int Immunol 2001;13:459–63.
[10] Street SE, Cretney E, Smyth MJ. Perforin and interferon-gamma activities independently control tumor initiation, growth, and metastasis. Blood 2001;97:192–7.
[11] Smyth MJ, Thia KY, Street SE, et al. Differential tumor surveillance by natural killer (NK) and NKT cells. J Exp Med 2000;191:661–8.
[12] Kaplan DH, Shankaran V, Dighe AS, et al. Demonstration of an interferon gamma-dependent tumor surveillance system in immunocompetent mice. Proc Natl Acad Sci U S A 1998;95:7556–61.
[13] Dighe AS, Richards E, Old LJ, et al. Enhanced in vivo growth and resistance to rejection of tumor cells expressing dominant negative IFN gamma receptors. Immunity 1994;1: 447–56.
[14] Bach EA, Aguet M, Schreiber RD. The IFN gamma receptor: a paradigm for cytokine receptor signaling. Annu Rev Immunol 1997;15:563–91.
[15] Hayakawa Y, Takeda K, Yagita H, et al. IFN-gamma-mediated inhibition of tumor

angiogenesis by natural killer T-cell ligand, alpha-galactosylceramide. Blood 2002;100: 1728–33.

[16] Wong LH, Krauer KG, Hatzinisiriou I, et al. Interferon-resistant human melanoma cells are deficient in ISGF3 components. STAT1, STAT2, and p48-ISGF3gamma. J Biol Chem 1997;272:28779–85.

[17] van den Broek ME, Kagi D, Ossendorp F, et al. Decreased tumor surveillance in perforin-deficient mice. J Exp Med 1996;184:1781–90.

[18] Dunn GP, Bruce AT, Ikeda H, et al. Cancer immunoediting: from immunosurveillance to tumor escape. Nat Immunol 2002;3:991–8.

[19] Street SE, Trapani JA, MacGregor D, et al. Suppression of lymphoma and epithelial malignancies effected by interferon gamma. J Exp Med 2002;196:129–34.

[20] Dunn GP, Old LJ, Schreiber RD. The three Es of cancer immunoediting. Annu Rev Immunol 2004;22:329–60.

[21] Willimsky G, Blankenstein T. Sporadic immunogenic tumours avoid destruction by inducing T-cell tolerance. Nature 2005;437:141–6.

[22] Pardoll DM. Cancer vaccines. Nat Med 1998;4:525–31.

[23] Sotomayor EM, Borrello I, Levitsky HI. Tolerance and cancer: a critical issue in tumor immunology. Crit Rev Oncog 1996;7:433–56.

[24] Staveley-O'Carroll K, Sotomayor E, Montgomery J, et al. Induction of antigen-specific T cell anergy: an early event in the course of tumor progression. Proc Natl Acad Sci U S A 1998;95:1178–83.

[25] Marincola FM, Jaffee EM, Hicklin DJ, et al. Escape of human solid tumors from T-cell recognition: molecular mechanisms and functional significance. Adv Immunol 2000;74: 181–273.

[26] Hung K, Hayashi R, Lafond-Walker A, et al. The central role of CD4(+) T cells in the antitumor immune response. J Exp Med 1998;188:2357–68.

[27] Mumberg D, Monach PA, Wanderling S, et al. CD4(+) T cells eliminate MHC class II-negative cancer cells in vivo by indirect effects of IFN-gamma. Proc Natl Acad Sci U S A 1999;96:8633–8.

[28] Liotta LA, Kohn EC. The microenvironment of the tumour-host interface. Nature 2001;411: 375–9.

[29] Nair S, Boczkowski D, Moeller B, et al. Synergy between tumor immunotherapy and antiangiogenic therapy. Blood 2003;102:964–71.

[30] Li Y, Wang MN, Li H, et al. Active immunization against the vascular endothelial growth factor receptor flk1 inhibits tumor angiogenesis and metastasis. J Exp Med 2002;195: 1575–84.

[31] Balkwill F, Charles KA, Mantovani A. Smoldering and polarized inflammation in the initiation and promotion of malignant disease. Cancer Cell 2005;7:211–7.

[32] Coussens LM, Werb Z. Inflammation and cancer. Nature 2002;420:860–7.

[33] Simmons WJ, Simms M, Chiarle R, et al. Induction of germinal centers by MMTV encoded superantigen on B cells. Dev Immunol 2001;8:201–11.

[34] Sen N, Simmons WJ, Thomas RM, et al. META-controlled env-initiated transcripts encoding superantigens of murine Mtv29 and Mtv7 and their possible role in B cell lymphoma-genesis. J Immunol 2001;166:5422–9.

[35] Hussain SP, Hofseth LJ, Harris CC. Radical causes of cancer. Nat Rev Cancer 2003;3: 276–85.

[36] Green JE, Hudson T. The promise of genetically engineered mice for cancer prevention studies. Nat Rev Cancer 2005;5:184–98.

[37] Finn OJ, Forni G. Prophylactic cancer vaccines. Curr Opin Immunol 2002;14:172–7.

[38] Harada N, Tamai Y, Ishikawa T, et al. Intestinal polyposis in mice with a dominant stable mutation of the beta-catenin gene. EMBO J 1999;18:5931–42.

[39] Reitmair AH, Redston M, Cai JC, et al. Spontaneous intestinal carcinomas and skin neoplasms in Msh2-deficient mice. Cancer Res 1996;56:3842–9.

[40] Kuraguchi M, Yang K, Wong E, et al. The distinct spectra of tumor-associated Apc

mutations in mismatch repair-deficient Apc1638N mice define the roles of MSH3 and MSH6 in DNA repair and intestinal tumorigenesis. Cancer Res 2001;61:7934–42.

[41] Hingorani SR, Petricoin EF, Maitra A, et al. Preinvasive and invasive ductal pancreatic cancer and its early detection in the mouse. Cancer Cell 2003;4:437–50.

[42] Guy CT, Webster MA, Schaller M, et al. Expression of the neu protooncogene in the mammary epithelium of transgenic mice induces metastatic disease. Proc Natl Acad Sci U S A 1992;89:10578–82.

[43] Rovero S, Amici A, Carlo ED, et al. DNA vaccination against rat her-2/Neu p185 more effectively inhibits carcinogenesis than transplantable carcinomas in transgenic BALB/c mice. J Immunol 2000;165:5133–42.

[44] Rovero S, Boggio K, Curlo ED, et al. Insertion of the DNA for the 163–171 peptide of IL1beta enables a DNA vaccine encoding p185(neu) to inhibit mammary carcinogenesis in Her-2/neu transgenic BALB/c mice. Gene Ther 2001;8:447–52.

[45] Calogero RA, Musiani P, Forni G, et al. Towards a long-lasting immune prevention of HER2 mammary carcinomas: directions from transgenic mice. Cell Cycle 2004;3: 704–6.

[46] Quaglino E, Iezzi M, Mastini C, et al. Electroporated DNA vaccine clears away multi-focal mammary carcinomas in her-2/neu transgenic mice. Cancer Res 2004;64: 2858–64.

[47] Quaglino E, Rolla S, Iezzi M, et al. Concordant morphologic and gene expression data show that a vaccine halts HER-2/neu preneoplastic lesions. J Clin Invest 2004; 113:709–17.

[48] Spadaro M, Lanzardo S, Curcio C, et al. Immunological inhibition of carcinogenesis. Cancer Immunol Immunother 2004;53:204–16.

[49] Boggio K, Di Carlo E, Rovero S, et al. Ability of systemic interleukin-12 to hamper pro-gressive stages of mammary carcinogenesis in HER2/neu transgenic mice. Cancer Res 2000;60:359–64.

[50] Nanni P, Nicoletti G, De Giovanni C, et al. Combined allogeneic tumor cell vaccination and systemic interleukin 12 prevents mammary carcinogenesis in HER-2/neu transgenic mice. J Exp Med 2001;194:1195–205.

[51] Di Carlo E, Rovero S, Boggio K, et al. Inhibition of mammary carcinogenesis by systemic interleukin 12 or p185neu DNA vaccination in Her-2/neu transgenic BALB/c mice. Clin Cancer Res 2001;7:830s–7s.

[52] Iinuma T, Homma S, Noda T, et al. Prevention of gastrointestinal tumors based on adenomatous polyposis coli gene mutation by dendritic cell vaccine. J Clin Invest 2004; 113:1307–17.

[53] Gendler SJ, Mukherjee P. Spontaneous adenocarcinoma mouse models for immunother-apy. Trends Mol Med 2001;7:471–5.

[54] Mukherjee P, Ginardi AR, Madsen CS, et al. MUC1-specific CTLs are non-functional within a pancreatic tumor microenvironment. Glycoconj J 2001;18:931–42.

[55] Mukherjee P, Ginardi AR, Tinder TL, et al. MUC1-specific cytotoxic T lymphocytes eradi-cate tumors when adoptively transferred in vivo. Clin Cancer Res 2001;7:848s–55s.

[56] Dhodapkar MV. Harnessing host immune responses to preneoplasia: promise and chal-lenges. Cancer Immunol Immunother 2005;54:409–13.

[57] Bartkova J, Horejsi Z, Koed K, et al. DNA damage response as a candidate anti-cancer barrier in early human tumorigenesis. Nature 2005;434:864–70.

[58] Kyle RA, Rajkumar SV. Monoclonal gammopathies of undetermined significance. Hematol Oncol Clin N Am 1999;13:1181–202.

[59] Dhodapkar MV, Krasovsky J, Osman K, et al. Vigorous premalignancy-specific effector T cell response in the bone marrow of patients with monoclonal gammopathy. J Exp Med 2003;198:1753–7.

[60] Dhodapkar MV, Krasovsky J, Olson K. T cells from the tumor microenvironment of patients with progressive myeloma can generate strong, tumor-specific cytolytic responses to au-tologous, tumor-loaded dendritic cells. Proc Natl Acad Sci U S A 2002;99:13009–13.

[61] Finn OJ. Premalignant lesions as targets for cancer vaccines. J Exp Med 2003;198: 1623–6.

[62] Boon T, Cerottini JC, Van den Eynde B, et al. Tumor antigens recognized by T lymphocytes. Annu Rev Immunol 1994;12:337–65.

[63] Jager D, Taverna C, Zippelius A, et al. Identification of tumor antigens as potential target antigens for immunotherapy by serological expression cloning. Cancer Immunol Immunother 2004;53:144–7.

[64] Khong HT, Rosenberg SA. The Waardenburg syndrome type 4 gene, SOX10, is a novel tumor-associated antigen identified in a patient with a dramatic response to immunotherapy. Cancer Res 2002;62:3020–3.

[65] Kao H, Marto JA, Hoffmann TK, et al. Identification of cyclin B1 as a shared human epithelial tumor-associated antigen recognized by T cells. J Exp Med 2001;194: 1313–23.

[66] Suzuki H, Graziano DF, McKolanis J, et al. T cell-dependent antibody responses against aberrantly expressed cyclin B1 protein in patients with cancer and premalignant disease. Clin Cancer Res 2005;11:1521–6.

[67] Finn OJ. Cancer vaccines: between the idea and the reality. Nat Rev Immunol 2003;3: 630–41.

[68] Barnd DL, Lan MS, Metzgar RS, et al. Specific, major histocompatibility complex-unrestricted recognition of tumor-associated mucins by human cytotoxic T cells. Proc Natl Acad Sci U S A 1989;86:7159–63.

[69] Hruban RH, Adsay NV, Albores-Saavedra J, et al. Pancreatic intraepithelial neoplasia: a new nomenclature and classification system for pancreatic duct lesions. Am J Surg Pathol 2001;25:579–86.

[70] Turner MS, McKolanis JR, Ramanathan RK, et al. Mucins in gastrointestinal cancers. Cancer Chemother Biol Response Modif 2003;21:259–74.

[71] Kotera Y, Fontenot JD, Pecher G, et al. Humoral immunity against a tandem repeat epitope of human mucin MUC-1 in sera from breast, pancreatic, and colon cancer patients. Cancer Res 1994;54:2856–60.

[72] Pawelec G, Zeuthen J, Kiessling R. Escape from host-antitumor immunity. Crit Rev Oncog 1997;8:111–41.

[73] Pawelec G, Heinzel S, Kiessling R, et al. Escape mechanisms in tumor immunity: a year 2000 update. Crit Rev Oncol 2000;11:97–133.

[74] Sun JC, Bevan MJ. Defective CD8 T cell memory following acute infection without CD4 T cell help. Science 2003;300:339–42.

[75] Janssen EM, Lemmens EE, Wolfe T, et al. CD4+ T cells are required for secondary expansion and memory in CD8+ T lymphocytes. Nature 2003;421:852–6.

[76] Qin Z, Blankenstein T. CD4+ T cell–mediated tumor rejection involves inhibition of angiogenesis that is dependent on IFN gamma receptor expression by nonhematopoietic cells. Immunity 2000;12:677–86.

[77] Hock H, Dorsch M, Diamantstein T, et al. Interleukin 7 induces CD4+ T cell-dependent tumor rejection. J Exp Med 1991;174:1291–8.

[78] Greenberg PD, Klarnet JP, Kern DE, et al. Therapy of disseminated tumors by adoptive transfer of specifically immune T cells. Prog Exp Tumor Res 1988;32:104–27.

[79] Sasco AJ. World burden of tobacco-related cancer. Lancet 1991;338:123–4.

[80] Viviani S, Jack A, Hall AJ, et al. Hepatitis B vaccination in infancy in The Gambia: protection against carriage at 9 years of age. Vaccine 1999;17:2946–50.

[81] Bosch FX, Lorincz A, Munoz N, et al. The causal relation between human papillomavirus and cervical cancer. J Clin Pathol 2002;55:244–65.

[82] Villa LL, Costa RL, Petta CA, et al. Prophylactic quadrivalent human papillomavirus (types 6, 11, 16, and 18) L1 virus-like particle vaccine in young women: a randomised double-blind placebo-controlled multicentre phase II efficacy trial. Lancet Oncol 2005;6: 271–8.

[83] Harper DM, Franco EL, Wheeler C, et al. Efficacy of a bivalent L1 virus-like particle vaccine

in prevention of infection with human papillomavirus types 16 and 18 in young women: a randomised controlled trial. Lancet 2004;364:1757–65.

[84] Schiffman M, Castle PE. The promise of global cervical-cancer prevention. N Engl J Med 2005;353:2101–4.

[85] Koutsky LA, Ault KA, Wheeler CM, et al. A controlled trial of a human papillomavirus type 16 vaccine. N Engl J Med 2002;347:1645–51.

Hematol Oncol Clin N Am 20 (2006) 751–766

HEMATOLOGY/ONCOLOGY CLINICS
OF NORTH AMERICA

Immunotherapy of Melanoma

Petra Rietschel, MD, PhD, Paul B. Chapman, MD*

Department of Medicine, Memorial Sloan-Kettering Cancer Center, 1275 York Avenue, New York, NY 10021, USA

Melanoma has been the tumor type most studied as a target for immunotherapy because it has been considered more susceptible to immune attack than other tumors. Melanoma primary tumors are typically infiltrated with lymphocytes, and the absence of infiltrating lymphocytes is associated with a poorer prognosis. A small proportion of primary tumors undergo spontaneous regression that is assumed (but not proven) to be immune mediated. A small proportion of patients who have metastatic melanoma respond to immune mediators such as interferon-α and interleukin (IL)-2, suggesting that melanoma tumors are susceptible to immune attack even in the metastatic setting. Finally, primary melanoma is more common in immunosuppressed patients, who have an increased risk of developing other cancer types as well. These observations are only suggestive, and it seems likely that other tumor types may be equally sensitive to immunotherapy. Melanoma has been a favorite target for immunotherapy because of the relative ease with which melanoma cells can be adapted to in vitro culture condition. The availability of hundreds of melanoma cell lines for study has led to the identification of tumor antigens and the development of monoclonal antibodies (mAbs) and T cells against these antigens. This development has sparked a revolution in the understanding of how the immune system sees and reacts to cancer.

This article reviews the recent clinical results of trials exploring different immunotherapy strategies against melanoma.

INTERFERON-α
Metastatic Melanoma

Phase II studies with interferon-α in stage IV melanoma have generally yielded antitumor response rates of about 16% (reviewed in [1]). Although the optimal dose and schedule have not been defined, the general sense is that higher doses of interferon-α are associated with higher response rates. As a single agent, however, the general sense is that the side effects of interferon-α at higher doses do not justify the low response rates observed; as a result, interferon-α is rarely used as a single agent to treat metastatic melanoma.

---

* Corresponding author. *E-mail address:* chapmanp@mskcc.org (P.B. Chapman).

0889-8588/06/$ – see front matter   © 2006 Elsevier Inc. All rights reserved.
doi:10.1016/j.hoc.2006.02.005   hemonc.theclinics.com

Adjuvant Therapy

The Food and Drug Administration (FDA) has approved high-dose interferon-α (HD IFN) for the adjuvant treatment of stage III melanoma after complete surgical resection. HD IFN is given intravenously at 20×10^6 U/m^2 Monday through Friday for 4 weeks. Afterwards, the patient receives 10×10^6 U/m^2 subcutaneously three times weekly for 11 months for a total of 1 year of treatment.

The value of a year of adjuvant HD IFN treatment remains a source of controversy among oncologists. Although the first randomized trial (Eastern Cooperative Oncology Group trial 1684) comparing adjuvant HD IFN with observation after complete surgical resection initially showed an advantage in relapse-free survival (RFS) and in overall survival (and formed the basis for the FDA approval) [2], further follow-up did not confirm overall survival benefit. A subsequent trial (E1690) with 642 patients also failed to show a significant improvement in overall survival [3], although it did confirm a small benefit in RFS. Recently, these two trials were updated, and the data were pooled [4]. This analysis confirmed that HD IFN was associated with an improvement in RFS (median, 6 months) but with no improvement in overall survival.

As a result of these two trials, most oncologists consider HD IFN as having a modest effect on RFS but no measurable effect on overall survival. This benefit must be balanced against the toxicities associated with HD IFN treatment in deciding whether to recommend adjuvant HD IFN treatment [5].

A subsequent randomized trial (E1694) tested the hypothesis that immunization against GM2 ganglioside was superior to adjuvant HD IFN treatment [6]. This trial was halted early when an interim futility analysis showed that the vaccine arm could not show superiority. In fact, at this analysis the vaccine arm was doing worse than the HD IFN arm, although further follow-up of these patients is required before it can be concluded that this vaccine caused enhanced recurrence.

By far the largest trial in patients who have high-risk melanoma is the European Organization for Research and Treatment of Cancer 18,952 trial. It involved 1388 patients who were assigned randomly to receive intermediate doses of interferon (10 Million Units [MU] 5 d/wk) subcutaneously for 4 weeks, followed either by 10 MU subcutaneously three times a week for 1 year or 5 MU subcutaneously three times a week for 2 years. A third group was assigned randomly to observation only [7]. There was no improvement in outcome, and the investigators concluded that this regimen could not be recommended.

Previously, a variety of other low-dose adjuvant interferon-α trials had been published, none of which showed an improvement in overall survival. Several of these low-dose trials, however, demonstrated a temporary improvement in RFS. This finding has led to the hypothesis that low-dose interferon-α has a cytostatic effect on melanoma and that low-dose interferon-α may need to be administered chronically to suppress relapse. Recently, two trials have explored long-term adjuvant treatment with interferon-α at lower doses. The European Organization for Research and Treatment of Cancer Melanoma Group together with the Deutsche Krebsforschungs Gesellschaft (DKG) performed a prospective, randomized, phase III adjuvant trial between 1988 and 1996 to evaluate the efficacy and toxicity of low-dose recombinant interferon-α (1 MU) or recombinant interferon-gamma (0.2 mg) both given subcutaneously every other day for 12 months, in comparison with an untreated control group and (in the DKG group only) a group treated with a mistletoe extract. A total of 830 patients were evaluated. Side effects were minor (fever, chills, night sweats, fatigue, myalgias, arthralgias, and headaches), but there was no difference in disease-free or overall survival compared with the untreated group [8].

The adjuvant interferon in high-risk melanoma (AIM HIGH) trial in the United Kingdom tried to address this question by randomly assigning patients to 2 years of low-dose interferon-α (3 MU) given three times weekly for 2 years versus observation [9]. There was no improvement in RFS or overall survival, a finding that does not support the hypothesis that chronic low-dose interferon-α can improve survival.

High-dose (but not lower-dose) adjuvant interferon-α has been associated reproducibly with minor improvements in RFS. No randomized trial has demonstrated an improvement in overall survival, however, and the proper role of high-dose adjuvant interferon-α remains uncertain.

INTERLEUKIN 2

In 1998, the FDA approved high-dose IL-2 for treatment of metastatic melanoma. The approved dose is 600 000 to 720 000 IU/kg every 8 hours on days 1 through 5. IL-2 at this dose and schedule can be administered in multiple cycles and can result in durable complete responses in a small proportion of patients who have metastatic melanoma. Long-term follow-up data are available for 270 assessable patients who were enrolled into eight clinical trials between 1985 and 1993 [10]. Objective tumor responses were noted in 16% of previously untreated patients; complete responses were seen in 6% of patients, and partial responses were seen in 10%. Approximately two thirds of the complete responses were durable, for a durable complete response rate of about 4%. Median duration of response for all 43 responding patients was 8.9 months.

Because of significant toxicities associated with high-dose IL-2 therapy, this treatment can be offered only to patients who have adequate cardiac, pulmonary, and renal function. It also requires that the treating physician have adequate training and resources in terms of trained personnel and cardiac monitoring to administer the IL-2 safely. The major toxicities associated with high-dose IL-2 include hypotension, vascular leak syndrome, cardiac arrhythmias, hepatic dysfunction, fever, nausea, diarrhea, catheter-related sepsis, and death [10]. These toxicities must be weighed against the expected 16% response proportion.

An important recent observation is that patients who have not responded to prior chemotherapy have the same chance of responding to IL-2 as treatment-naive patients [11]. This finding has led some physicians and patients to consider less toxic treatment options initially, with the understanding that IL-2 therapy can be considered as second-line treatment without compromising the chance of responding.

The toxicity and the necessity of hospitalization and intensive monitoring associated with high-dose IL-2 has prompted several trials with low-dose Il-2. In these regimens, IL-2 is administered at doses of 5 to 25 MIU either as a low-dose intravenous bolus, a continuous infusion, or a subcutaneous injection. Although lower doses of IL-2 are associated with less systemic toxicity, consistent antitumor effects have not been observed [11a]. Thus, low-dose Il-2 as a single agent cannot be recommended for the treatment of melanoma.

The combination of IL-2 with single-agent or multiagent chemotherapy (known as "biochemotherapy") also has been evaluated. Initial single-institution experiences showed higher rates of partial responses and, in some cases, complete responses [12–14]. In subsequent multicenter phase III trials, however, few complete responses were observed, and there was no evidence for a meaningful improvement in survival [15–17].

The use of biochemotherapy has decreased significantly as a result of the understanding that biochemotherapy is associated with a high partial response rate but does not increase the chance of a complete response or overall survival. Nonetheless, biochemotherapy may be a rational choice for some patients. Patients who have large, inoperable melanoma masses for whom tumor reduction would represent significant palliation might be considered for biochemotherapy as long as the toxicities of treatment are taken into consideration.

GRANULOCYTE MACROPHAGE COLONY-STIMULATING FACTOR
Granulocyte macrophage colony-stimulating factor (GM-CSF) is a multifunctional cytokine. As immunotherapy against cancer, one of its most important activities is as a survival factor for dendritic cells, which are antigen-presenting cells that can activate naive T cells. In a phase II trial conducted by Spitler and colleagues [18], 48 patients who had stage III or stage IV melanoma received GM-CSF for 14 out of every 28 days for 1 year after surgical resection of disease. GM-CSF was well tolerated, and overall and DFS was significantly prolonged in patients who received GM-CSF (median survival, 37.5 months) compared with matched historical controls (median survival, 12.2 months). The effect was greater on overall survival than on DFS, possibly indicating that therapy with GM-CSF may change the biology of the metastasis. The recurrences in the treated population often were localized and could be resected again. Because this study relied on comparison with a historical control group, these surprising results have been met with skepticism pending results of a currently on-going prospective, randomized trial.

ANTIBODY TREATMENTS
Although no mAbs have been FDA-approved for the treatment of melanoma, several mouse monoclonal antibodies have shown significant activity in patients who have stage IV disease. The response rate is similar to that of trastuzumab.

In melanoma, treatment with mAbs has focused primarily on ganglioside antigens. Tumor responses against GD2 ganglioside have been induced by both murine mAb [19] and, more recently, humanized mAb linked to IL-2 [20]. In the more recent study, EMD 273063, a humanized anti-GD2 monoclonal antibody linked to IL-2 was tested in a phase I trial. Thirty-three patients were treated, and although no patient showed an objective response, 8 patients had stable disease. Immune activation was induced, as measured by lymphocytosis, increased peripheral-blood natural-killer cell activity and cell numbers, and increased serum levels of the soluble alpha chain of the IL-2 receptor complex. A phase II trial is under way.

The mAb R24 is an immunoglobulin IgG3 directed against GD3 ganglioside. It is potent at mediating in vitro effector functions such as human complement-mediated cytotoxicity and antibody-dependent cellular cytotoxicity and can block melanoma tumor growth in animal models. Several clinical trials have been conducted with R24, and overall R24 showed a response rate of 10% [21]. Combining R24 with either cytotoxic drugs or cytokines has not increased this response rate.

KM871, a chimeric mAb against the ganglioside GD3, was studied in 17 patients who had melanoma [22,23]. Inflammation at the tumor site was observed in 3 patients, 1 patient experienced a clinical partial response that lasted 11 months, and 2 patients had stable disease. There was no serologic evidence of human anti-chimeric antibody in any patient.

VACCINES

Several lines of evidence have led investigators to believe that melanoma is susceptible to immune attack:

1. The absence of a primary melanoma in approximately 5% of patients with metastatic melanoma, suggesting that the primary melanoma underwent immune-mediated regression
2. The frequent finding of lymphocytes within primary melanomas
3. The report of occasional (although, in reality, quite rare) spontaneous regressions of metastatic tumors
4. The regression of metastatic tumors in response to IL-2, as described previously

These observations, along with the fact that melanomas can be established as cell lines more easily than other tumor types, has led to enthusiasm for developing melanoma vaccines. Recent advances in technology have allowed investigators to measure relatively small numbers of antigen-specific T cells reproducibly, even if the T cells have low avidity. The problem remains, however, that most tumor antigens are self-molecules. As investigators learn more about the workings of the immune system, they are appreciating the myriad ways the immune system has evolved to avoid reacting against self-antigens as a means of preventing autoimmune disease. Overcoming this tolerance remains a major challenge in the development of cancer vaccines. After more than

100 years of study, the optimal methodology for vaccinating patients against established malignant tumors has not been defined. It would be expected, however, that overcoming tolerance come at the price of toxicity in the form of autoimmune disease. As described later for anti–cytotoxic T-lymphocyte antigen 4 (anti-CTLA 4) mAb, this risk indeed seems to exist.

Vaccines with Undefined Antigens

Allogeneic vaccines

The earliest vaccines have relied on vaccine formulations composed of whole cells or cell extracts, usually from allogeneic melanoma, because of the relative ease of producing this type of vaccine and the lack of known, specific tumor-rejection antigens. It is assumed that, when innumerable molecules are injected, the immune system will recognize the ones relevant to tumor rejection. These vaccines can generate immune responses against melanoma differentiation anti-gens, such as members of the tyrosinase family of melanosomal antigens (gly-coprotein [gp] 75/tyrosinase-related protein 1 and 2) as well as GM2 ganglioside. Because the relevant antigens are not known, it is difficult to use immunologic responses as surrogate end points in clinical trials of these vaccines. Only clinical end points are available.

As reviewed by Perales and Chapman [24], many trials have tested these types of melanoma antigens. In a number of recently reported clinical trials in the adjuvant setting, patients were vaccinated with melanoma vaccine composed of undefined antigen mixtures after complete surgical resection. In one small, double-blind, placebo-controlled trial, a polyvalent, shed-antigen vaccine was associated with a RFS more than twice as long as that of patients who received placebo [25].

Another allogeneic cell-based vaccine tested in a randomized trial is Melacine, a vaccine prepared from the lysate of two melanoma cell lines combined with the detoxified endotoxin adjuvant. In a large, randomized trial conducted by the Southwest Oncology Group in patients who had stage II melanoma who were free of disease, there was no overall difference in RFS between the vaccine-treated and the control group. Among the subset of patients who expressed HLA A2 or HLA C3 (two of the allelotypes expressed by the tumor cells in the vaccine), however, the vaccine was associated with a statistically signifi-cant improvement in 5-year RFS [26,27]. A confirmatory trial in HLA-A2– or -C3–positive patients has been proposed.

Although the first two trials discussed showed some glimmer of activity, this activity has not been seen in other recently reported vaccine trials. Hersey and colleagues [28] randomly assigned 675 patients who had melanoma to receive either an allogeneic melanoma oncolysate or to observation [28]. Analysis showed a trend toward improved survival in the vaccine group, but it did not reach statistical significance.

One vaccine product, Canvaxin, has recently completed phase III clinical trials. The vaccine is made from three lines of irradiated whole allogeneic melanoma cells mixed with Bacille Calmette Guérin (BCG) as the adjuvant.

Past studies showed that survival of patients who had melanoma who were treated with the vaccine was significantly longer than that of historical controls [29]. This vaccine has been tested in two large-scale phase III trials involving patients with resected melanoma. One trial was in patients who stage IV melanoma, and the other was in patients who had stage III melanoma. Both trials were halted because of lack of efficacy.

Autologous vaccines

Autologous tumor vaccines have been made either from fresh tumor tissue or short-term cultures. They have several potential advantages over allogeneic vaccines. They are more likely to contain antigens of specific immunologic importance for the individual patient. The absence of irrelevant allogeneic antigens makes immunologic monitoring more straightforward. On the other hand, this approach requires that a relatively large amount of tumor tissue be available from each patient for preparation of the customized vaccine, a requirement that restricts the eligible patient population and skews it toward patients who have a higher burden of disease. As appealing as it seems to use the patient's own tumor cells as a basis for vaccination, it is clear that these cells must be manipulated in some way to increase their immunogenicity. The work of Berd and colleagues (2001) has concentrated on haptenated autologous vaccines [29a]. This approach involves conjugation of the hapten dinitroflourobenzene (DNFB) to proteins on autologous tumor cells. The haptenated tumor cells are injected with BCG into patients presensitized to DNFB. The haptenated autologous vaccines are intriguing because of their ability to mediate inflammation at tumor sites distant from the point of injection. A randomized phase III trial is currently under way.

Another strategy to try to enhance the immunogenicity of tumor cells is to introduce into tumor cells genes encoding a variety of cytokines or chemokines. Special interest has been focused on GM-CSF, largely because of experiments reported by Dranoff, who showed that that GM-CSF had the greatest ability to enhance tumor rejection in the B16 mouse melanoma model. A third approach using partially defined autologous melanoma cells relies on heat-shock proteins (HSP) extracted from autologous cells to immunize patients. (This technique is discussed in more detail in another article in this issue.) HSPs are a family of proteins, highly conserved through evolution, that are produced by cells in response to physical, chemical, or immunologic stress. HSPs bind intracellular peptides generated in the cell and chaperone them into the major histocompatibility class (MHC) class I pathway. As a result, HSPs derived from a tumor are complexed with a broad array of potentially immunogenic peptides. The HSP-peptide complexes can be highly immunogenic and represent a novel approach toward immunization. This approach has been tested in patients who have melanoma [30]. The evaluation of T-cell responses was difficult because of the range of HLA allelotypes represented among the patients. Of the 28 patients who had measurable disease, 2 had a complete response. As expected, generating the autologous vaccines was challenging; only 65% of the patients accrued to the trial actually were able to receive vaccine. A phase III trial in patients who have stage IV disease is currently on going.

Vaccines with Defined Antigens

Rather than immunize with a preparation of undefined antigens, an alternative approach toward developing cancer vaccines is to identify specific antigens on tumor cells that can be recognized by the immune system and to administer these antigens in a immunogenic formulation. Depending on the nature of the antigen, investigators have focused on inducing either antibody responses or T-cell responses.

Ganglioside antigen vaccines

Gangliosides are glycolipid molecules expressed in some normal tissues but often overexpressed in melanoma. The main melanoma gangliosides–GD2, GD3, and GM2–have been targets for several vaccine trials. As glycolipid molecules, gangliosides do not fit into the binding grooves of either MHC class I or class II molecules and, as a result, are not presented to classic T cells. Therefore, vaccine trials using ganglioside antigens have focused exclusively on induction of antibody responses.

Although GM2 is a minor ganglioside on melanoma, it is the most immunogenic ganglioside. The initial phase III trial immunizing patients used GM2 and BCG as a vaccine, which induced low-titer IgM anti-GM2 antibodies. Livingston conducted a phase III trial randomly assigning patients who had stage III melanoma and who were free of disease to either vaccine or placebo (BCG) [30a]. Although the trial was reported as negative, there was a trend in the vaccine arm toward improved relapse-free and overall survival. This difference was statistically significant if the 5% of patients who had pre-existing anti-GM2 antibodies were excluded from the analysis. A second generation of this vaccine, termed "GMK," consisted of GM2 conjugated to keyhole limpet hemocyanin and mixed with a novel adjuvant QS-21. This vaccine induced high-titer IgG against GM2 and, as noted previously, was subject of an intergroup randomized phase III trial (E1694) in which patients who had stage III melanoma or deep stage II melanoma and who were free of disease after complete surgical resection were randomly assigned to GMK vaccine or to HD IFN. The trial was halted at a median follow-up of 16 months when it was determined that the vaccine arm could not show superiority over HD IFN [6].

GD2 is another ganglioside expressed in many melanomas. GD2 is less immunogenic than GM2: only 45% of patients develop an IgM or IgG antibody response to GD2 [31]. GD3 ganglioside is the most abundant ganglioside expressed on melanoma and has been a high-priority vaccine target. Although early vaccine trials demonstrated that GD3 is poorly immunogenic in humans, recent studies showed that anti-GD3 antibodies can be induced in patients immunized with GD3-lactone KLH. A trivalent ganglioside vaccine composed of a combination of GM2, GD2, and GD3 is an attractive vaccine strategy that would be relevant to almost all patients who have melanoma, regardless of HLA type.

Peptide antigen vaccines

Other vaccine approaches seek to engage the T-cell arm of the immune system against melanoma using peptides from melanoma antigens that can be recognized by CD8 T cells. Tumor antigens can be divided into three categories: (1) antigens encoded by genetic alterations and alternative transcripts; (2) cancer-testes antigens, molecules expressed on normal germ cells as well as some cancers; (3) differentiation antigens, normal molecules expressed as part of the differentiation program of melanocytes. The field has focused primarily on the second and third categories of antigens, as reviewed in by Perales and Chapman [24].

As a vaccine approach, peptides alone are only minimally immunogenic. Peptides, however, can be altered at critical amino acids (called "anchor residues") to increase binding avidity to HLA class I. These heteroclytic peptides can be more potent at inducing a T-cell response against the native peptide.

Even with increased immunogenicity, it is not clear that the immune responses induced are sufficient to cause tumor shrinkage. The modified gp100 peptide has been used in combination with peptides derived from tyrosinase in a number of recent vaccine trials. Using sensitive in vitro assays, it has been possible to detect specific T-cell responses in most patients, but few clinical responses have been observed [32–37], and the presence of CD8+ T cells against melanoma antigens did not correlate with antitumor responses [38].

From these experiences, it is not clear that the T-cell responses being measured correlate with clinical responses.

Dendritic cell vaccines

Dendritic cells are the most efficient antigen-presenting cells. Several recent clinical trials have attempted to use dendritic cells loaded with melanoma-derived antigens to immunize melanoma patients. (The general use of dendritic cells for vaccines is discussed in another article in this issue.)

Because there are several dendritic cell lineages, it can be difficult to compare the results of one trial with another. Banchereau and colleagues [39] immunized 18 patients who had melanoma with CD34+-derived dendritic cells loaded with peptides derived from four melanoma differentiation or shared antigens (Melan-A, tyrosinase, MAGE-3, and gp100) [39]. Almost all developed an immune response to at least one of the antigens. Tumor regressions were seen in the seven patients who had the broadest detectable immune reactivity.

Other investigators have used monocyte-derived dendritic cells. Schuler-Thurner and colleagues [40] immunized 28 patients with monocyte-derived dendritic cells pulsed with a mixture of MHC class I–and class II–restricted peptides. This approach induced readily detectable T-helper 1 cells against class II–restricted epitopes. Of seven patients evaluable for clinical responses, one had a complete response. A Dutch group has also observed a clinical response among 26 patients and found that presence of antigen-specific T cells in delayed-type hypersensitivity reaction sites correlated with RFS [41].

Clinical responses were also observed in monocyte-derived dendritic cell vaccines in which the dendritic cells were pulsed with peptides derived from autologous tumor cells [42]. An Australian group cultured monocyte-derived dendritic cells with the patient's own irradiated melanoma tumor cells. Six of 17 patients had either complete or partial responses. Not all groups have observed clinical responses after immunization with monocyte-derived dendritic cells, however [43].

Hersey and colleagues [44] immunized patients with dendritic cells loaded with either melanoma lysates or defined peptides. Immune responses could be detected in vitro or by delayed-type hypersensitivity reactions in most patients, but clinical responses (3 partial responses out of 19 patients) were only seen in the lysate-loaded dendritic cell group.

In an attempt to circumvent the difficulty of growing dendritic cells, Peterson and colleagues [45] tested the hypothesis that peripheral blood mononuclear cells (PBMC) could be used to present melanoma peptides to the immune system. PBMC were pulsed with Melan-A peptide and then injected subcutaneously with IL-12. Among the 20 patients who had metastatic melanoma treated with this technique, 4 developed detectable T-cell responses against Melan-A. Two patients had complete clinical responses.

Overall, these studies have shown that dramatic clinical responses can be seen occasionally in patients immunized with dendritic cell–based vaccines. The response proportion is low, however, and the correlation of clinical response with immunologic response has been inconsistent.

DNA vaccines

An alternative to vaccinating with the antigen is to inject the cDNA encoding the antigen cloned into a bacterial expression plasmid driven by an active promoter such as the cytomegalovirus promoter. This approach offers several potential advantages. The entire antigen molecule can be used instead of only select peptides, removing the requirement for strict HLA restriction. cDNA is much less expensive to produce in quantities required for clinical trials than proteins or peptides, and DNA is more stable. DNA can be manipulated easily to make changes in the amino acid sequence of the expressed protein. Finally, the bacterial DNA itself is thought to be a potent immune adjuvant obviating the need to add an adjuvant to the formulation.

DNA vaccination can induce potent immune responses against melanoma antigens in rodent models [46], inducing autoimmune vitiligo and protection from tumor challenge. These preclinical studies have formed the basis of clinical trials. In one trial, patients who had melanoma were immunized with cDNA encoding human gp100. The results did not demonstrate clinical or immunologic responses to the vaccine [47]. Other clinical trials are under way, including trials in which patients who have melanoma are being immunized with DNA-encoding murine versions of differentiation antigens such as tyrosinase, Melan-A/MART-1, and gp100. These trials are reviewed elsewhere in this issue.

ADOPTIVE CELL TRANSFER

It has been assumed that the lack of clinical responses to vaccines might result from the relatively low number of antigen-specific T cells induced. Because it has been difficult to generate large numbers to melanoma antigen-specific T cells using vaccines, attention has turned to growing antigen-specific T cells in vitro and then infusing them into the patient. This technique, adoptive cell transfer (ACT), initially used T-cell clones against melanoma antigen recognized by T cells-1/Melan-A or gp100 [48,49].

It seems that the adoptive transfer of uncloned T cells can result in tumor regression more consistently [50]. It may be important to administer nonmyeloablative chemotherapy to neutralize suppressive regulatory T cells before infusing the T cells. There were no clinical responses if cloned T cells against gp100 were adoptively transferred [51], but recently, the National Cancer Institute Surgery Branch reported their large experience infusing uncloned T cells grown from tumor-infiltrating lymphocytes after treating patients with fludarabine and cyclophosphamide [52]. Thirty-five patients who had metastatic melanoma were treated, the majority of whom were refractory to therapy with high-dose interleukin 2 and had been heavily pretreated with multiple chemotherapy regimens. The patients underwent a lymphodepleting but nonmyeloablative conditioning with cyclophosphamide and fludarabine before receiving the infusion of autologous tumor-reactive T cells and high-dose IL-2. Although the T-cell cultures were highly enriched for a single clonotype against a specific melanoma differentiation antigen, the T-cell cultures included a mixture of clonotypes and a mixture of CD4+ and CD8+ cells. Eighteen (51%) of 35 patients experienced a clinically meaningful response, including 3 complete responses and 15 partial responses. Tumor regression was seen in cutaneous lesions, bulky nodal disease, and visceral, brain, and bony metastases. The mean duration of response was 11.5 months. Immunocytochemical analysis of recurrent lesions after initial response to therapy often demonstrated a loss of antigen expression by the recurrent tumor.

This experience suggests that ACT therapy exerted a strong selective pressure on the tumor and that the transferred cells eliminated antigen-expressing tumor cells by an antigen-dependent mechanism. Vitiligo and uveitis were commonly observed in the responding patients. A link between successful immunotherapy and the onset of autoimmunity has been noted in several clinical immune therapies.

There are several possibilities why lymphodepletion followed by ACT with noncloned T cells was more effective than prior attempts at ACT. Lymphodepletion may provide the required milieu for T-cell survival, possibly by transiently decreasing the total number of lymphocytes below some "set point" or by decreasing regulatory T cells. The use of noncloned T cells may be superior to the use of cloned T cells by providing T-cell help or providing effector T cells of other specificities. There is also some evidence that T-cell clones are exhausted, with shorter telomeres, and so have less proliferative capabilities.

In the past, when supplemental immunotherapy has been added to high-dose IL-2 treatment (eg, lymphokine-activated killer cells, tumor-infiltrating lymphocytes, gp100 peptide vaccine), there has been a consistent pattern of initial excitement (40%–50% response rates) followed later, after more patients have been treated, by disappointment (10%–20% response rates). Although ACT with lymphodepletion could fall into this pattern, it is worth pursuing this strategy to see if other investigators can confirm its efficacy.

CYTOTOXIC T-LYMPHOCYTE ANTIGEN 4

Advances in understanding the mechanisms that regulate T-cell activation have led to a strategy based on blocking CTLA-4. It has been known for some time that engagement of the T-cell receptor by itself is not sufficient for full T-cell activation; a second costimulatory signal is required for induction of IL-2 production, proliferation, and differentiation to effector function of naive T-cells. This second signal generally is provided through engagement of CD28 on the T-cell surface by members of the B7 family on the antigen-presenting cell. After activation, T cells immediately express CTLA-4, a close homologue to CD28 that binds to B7 displacing CD28. This displacement sends a negative signal to the T cells and reduces the T-cell response.

Because CTLA-4 functions as a "brake" for T cells, blocking CTLA-4 could provide a strategy to release T cells to react with self-antigens expressed on tumor cells. Indeed, mAbs to CTLA-4 can block the function of CTLA-4 and lead to activation of T cells. Clinical phase I and phase II studies with blocking anti-CTLA-4 antibodies have been conducted with the antibody alone [53,54] or in combination with peptide vaccines against gp100, melanoma antigen recognized by T cells 1, or tyrosinase [55–57]. Response rates have been observed in 15% to 20% of patients treated. Theoretically, anti-CTLA 4 blockade should enhance T-cell responses to weak tumor antigens. So far, the results from clinical trials are inconclusive [55–57], and it remains to be determined if anti-CTLA 4 antibodies can enhance T-cell responses to melanoma antigens.

Anti-CTLA 4 antibodies are associated with significant autoimmune toxicity in some patients. The most common side effects are rash and colitis. Other serious autoimmune toxicities, such as uveitis, episcleritis, and autoimmune hypophysitis leading to hypopituitarism, also have been observed. Antitumor responses have always been associated with autoimmune toxicity. This observation may not be surprising, because the effect of anti-CTLA-4 mAbs is not antigen specific. Breakthrough autoimmunity may be inseparably linked to clinical antitumor activity of anti-CTLA-4 antibodies.

SUMMARY

It has been known for decades from allotransplant experiences that the immune system, if properly activated, is capable of rejecting large masses of tissue. The challenge for immunotherapy has been to learn how to harness this power and direct it toward tumors expressing largely self-antigens. Recently, several new immunotherapeutic approaches have shown activity in patients who have metastatic melanoma, including some who have bulky disease. Activating endogenous T cells by blocking CTLA-4 seems to result in tumor shrinkage although at the price of severe autoimmunity. Infusion of ex vivo expanded polyclonal T cells in the setting of lymphodepletion also has resulted in dramatic tumor regressions but without significant autoimmune toxicity. These new approaches provide real promise that the cellular immune system can be brought to bear against tumors.

References

[1] Kirkwood JM. Interferon-α and -β: clinical applications; melanoma. In: Rosenberg SA, editor. Biologic therapy of cancer. 3rd edition. Philadelphia: J.B.Lippincott Company; 2000. p. 224–51.

[2] Kirkwood JM, Strawderman MH, Ernstoff MS, et al. Interferon alfa-2b adjuvant therapy of high-risk resected cutaneous melanoma: The Eastern Cooperative Oncology Group Trial EST 1684. J Clin Oncol 1996;14:7–17.

[3] Kirkwood JM, Ibrahim JG, Sondak VK, et al. High- and low-dose interferon alfa-2b in high-risk melanoma: first analysis of intergroup trial E1690/S9111/C9190. J Clin Oncol 2000;18:2444–58.

[4] Kirkwood JM, Manola J, Ibrahim J, et al. A pooled analysis of Eastern Cooperative Oncology Group and intergroup trials of adjuvant high-dose interferon for melanoma. Clin Cancer Res 2004;10:1670–7.

[5] Hurley K, Chapman PB. Helping melanoma patients decide whether to choose adjuvant high-dose interferon-α2b. Oncologist 2005;10:467–70.

[6] Kirkwood JM, Ibrahim JG, Sosman JA, et al. High-dose interferon alfa-2b significantly prolongs relapse-free and overall survival compared with the GM2-KLH/QS-21 vaccine in patients with resected stage IIb-III melanoma: results of intergroup trial E1694/S9512/C509801. J Clin Oncol 2001;19:2370–80.

[7] Eggermont AM, Suciu S, MacKie R, et al. Post-surgery adjuvant therapy with intermediate doses of interferon alfa 2b versus observation in patients with stage IIb/III melanoma (EORTC 18952): randomised controlled trial. Lancet 2005;366:1189–96.

[8] Kleeberg UR, Suciu S, Brocker EB, et al. Final results of the EORTC 18871/DKG 80-1 randomised phase III trial. rIFN-alpha2b versus rIFN-gamma versus ISCADOR M versus observation after surgery in melanoma patients with either high-risk primary (thickness >3 mm) or regional lymph node metastasis. Eur J Cancer 2004;40:390–402.

[9] Hancock BW, Wheatley K, Harris S, et al. Adjuvant interferon in high-risk melanoma: the AIM HIGH Study–United Kingdom Coordinating Committee on Cancer Research randomized study of adjuvant low-dose extended-duration interferon Alfa-2a in high-risk resected malignant melanoma. J Clin Oncol 2004;22:53–61.

[10] Atkins MB, Kunkel L, Sznol M, et al. High-dose recombinant interleukin-2 therapy in patients with metastatic melanoma: long-term survival update. Cancer J Sci Am 2000; 6(Suppl 1):S11–4.

[11] Agarwala SS, Tarhini A, Gooding W, et al. Phase II trial of high-dose bolus (HDB) IL-2 in patients with metastatic melanoma (MM) who have progressed after biochemo-therapy (BCT). In: Updated results. Orlando (FL): American Society of Clinical Oncology; 2005.

[11a] Atkins MB. Interleukin-2: clinical applications. Semin Oncol 2002;29(3):12–7.

[12] Keilholz U, Scheibenbogen C, Tilgen W, et al. Interferon-alpha and interleukin-2 in the treatment of metastatic melanoma. Comparison of two phase II trials. Cancer 1993;72: 607–14.

[13] Legha SS, Ring S, Eton O, et al. Development of a biochemotherapy regimen with concurrent administration of cisplatin, vinblastine, dacarbazine, interferon alfa, and interleukin-2 for patients with metastatic melanoma. J Clin Oncol 1998;16:1752–9.

[14] Chapman PB, Panageas KS, Williams L, et al. Clinical results using biochemotherapy as a standard of care in advanced melanoma. Melanoma Res 2002;12:381–7.

[15] Atkins MB, Lee S, Flaherty LE, et al. A prospective randomized phase III trial of concurrent biochemotherapy (BCT) with cisplatin, vinblastine, dacarbazine (CVD), IL-2 and interferon alpha-2b (IFN) versus CVD alone in patients with metastatic melanoma (E3695): ECOG-coordinated intergroup trial. Proceedings of the American Society of Clinical Oncology 2003;22:708.

[16] Eton O, Legha SS, Bedikian AY, et al. Sequential biochemotherapy versus chemotherapy for metastatic melanoma: results from a phase III randomized trial. J Clin Oncol 2002;20: 2045–52.

[17] Keilholz U, Punt CJ, Gore M, et al. Dacarbazine, cisplatin, and interferon-alfa-2b with or without interleukin-2 in metastatic melanoma: a randomized phase III trial (18951) of the European Organisation for Research and Treatment of Cancer Melanoma Group. J Clin Oncol 2005;23:6747–55.

[18] Spitler LE, Grossbard ML, Ernstoff MS, et al. Adjuvant therapy of stage III and IV malignant melanoma using granulocyte-macrophage colony-stimulating factor. J Clin Oncol 2000;18:1614–21.

[19] Cheung N, Lazarus H, Miraldi F, et al. Ganglioside GD2 specific monoclonal antibody 3F8: a phase I study in patients with neuroblastoma and malignant melanoma [erratum published in J Clin Oncol 1992 10(4):671]. J Clin Oncol 1987;5:1430–40.

[20] King DM, Albertini MR, Schalch H, et al. A phase I clinical trial of the immuno-cytokine EMD 273063 (hu.14.19–IL2) in melanoma patients. J Clin Oncol 2004;22 (22):4463–73. Epub 2004 Oct 13.

[21] Nasi M, Meyers M, Livingston P, et al. Anti-melanoma effects of R24, a monoclonal antibody against GD3. Vaccine Research 1997;7(Suppl 2):S155–62.

[22] Scott AM, Lee FT, Hopkins W, et al. Specific targeting, biodistribution, and lack of immunogenicity of chimeric anti-GD3 monoclonal antibody KM871 in patients with metastatic melanoma: results of a phase I trial. J Clin Oncol 2001;19:3976–87.

[23] Scott AM, Liu Z, Murone C, et al. Immunological effects of chimeric anti-GD3 monoclonal antibody KM871 in patients with metastatic melanoma. Cancer Immun 2005;5:3.

[24] Perales MA, Chapman PB. Immunizing against partially defined antigen mixtures, gangliosides, or peptides to induce antibody, T cell, and clinical responses. Cancer Chemother Biol Response Modif 2005;22:749–60.

[25] Bystryn JC, Zeleniuch-Jacquotte A, Oratz R, et al. Double-blind trial of a polyvalent, shed-antigen, melanoma vaccine. Clin Cancer Res 2001;7:1882–7.

[26] Sosman JA, Unger JM, Liu PY, et al. Adjuvant immunotherapy of resected, intermediate-thickness, node- negative melanoma with an allogeneic tumor vaccine: impact of HLA class I antigen expression on outcome. J Clin Oncol 2002;20:2067–75.

[27] Sondak VK, Liu PY, Tuthill RJ, et al. Adjuvant immunotherapy of resected, intermediate-thickness, node- negative melanoma with an allogeneic tumor vaccine: overall results of a randomized trial of the Southwest Oncology Group. J Clin Oncol 2002;20:2058–66.

[28] Hersey P, Coates AS, McCarthy WH, et al. Adjuvant immunotherapy of patients with high-risk melanoma using vaccinia viral lysates of melanoma: results of a randomized trial. J Clin Oncol 2002;20:4181–90.

[29] Hsueh EC, Essner R, Foshag LJ, et al. Prolonged survival after complete resection of disseminated melanoma and active immunotherapy with a therapeutic cancer vaccine. J Clin Oncol 2002;20:4549–54.

[29a] Berd D, Sato T, Cohn H, et al. Treatment of metastatic melanoma with autologous, hapten-modified melanoma vaccine: regression of pulmonary metastases. Int J Cancer 2001; 94(4):531–9.

[30] Belli F, Testori A, Rivoltini L, et al. Vaccination of metastatic melanoma patients with autologous tumor-derived heat shock protein gp96-peptide complexes: clinical and immunologic findings. J Clin Oncol 2002;20:4169–80.

[30a] Livingston PO, Wong GY, Adluri S, et al. Improved survival in stage III melanoma patients with GM2 antibodies: a randomized trial of adjuvant vaccination with GM2 ganglioside. J Clin Oncol 1994;12(5):1036–44.

[31] Chapman PB, Meyers M, Williams L, et al. Immunization of melanoma patients with a bivalent GM2–GD2 ganglioside conjugate vaccine. Denver (CO): American Society of Clinical Oncology; 1997. p. 432.

[32] Weber J, Sondak VK, Scotland R, et al. Granulocyte-macrophage-colony-stimulating factor added to a multipeptide vaccine for resected stage II melanoma. Cancer 2003;97: 186–200.

[33] Lee P, Wang F, Kuniyoshi J, et al. Effects of interleukin-12 on the immune response to a multipeptide vaccine for resected metastatic melanoma. J Clin Oncol 2001;19: 3836–47.

[34] Smith II JW, Walker EB, Fox BA, et al. Adjuvant immunization of HLA-A2-positive melanoma patients with a modified gp100 peptide induces peptide-specific CD8 + T-cell responses. J Clin Oncol 2003;21:1562–73.

[35] Slingluff Jr CL, Petroni GR, Yamshchikov GV, et al. Clinical and immunologic results of a randomized phase II trial of vaccination using four melanoma peptides either administered in granulocyte-macrophage colony-stimulating factor in adjuvant or pulsed on dendritic cells. J Clin Oncol 2003;21:4016–26.

[36] Slingluff Jr CL, Petroni GR, Yamshchikov GV, et al. Immunologic and clinical outcomes of vaccination with a multiepitope melanoma peptide vaccine plus low-dose interleukin-2 administered either concurrently or on a delayed schedule. J Clin Oncol 2004;22: 4474–85.

[37] Hersey P, Menzies SW, Coventry B, et al. Phase I/II study of immunotherapy with T-cell peptide epitopes in patients with stage IV melanoma. Cancer Immunol Immunother 2005; 54:208–18.

[38] Rosenberg SA, Sherry RM, Morton KE, et al. Tumor progression can occur despite the induction of very high levels of self/tumor antigen-specific CD8 + T cells in patients with melanoma. J Immunol 2005;175:6169–76.

[39] Banchereau J, Palucka AK, Dhodapkar M, et al. Immune and clinical responses in patients with metastatic melanoma to CD34(+) progenitor-derived dendritic cell vaccine. Cancer Res 2001;61:6451–8.

[40] Schuler-Thurner B, Schultz ES, Berger TG, et al. Rapid induction of tumor-specific type 1 T helper cells in metastatic melanoma patients by vaccination with mature, cryopreserved, peptide-loaded monocyte-derived dendritic cells. J Exp Med 2002;195:1279–88.

[41] de Vries IJM, Bernsen MR, Lesterhuis WJ, et al. Immunomonitoring tumor-specific t cells in delayed-type hypersensitivity skin biopsies after dendritic cell vaccination correlates with clinical outcome. J Clin Oncol 2005;23:5779–87.

[42] O'Rourke MG, Johnson M, Lanagan C, et al. Durable complete clinical responses in a phase I/II trial using an autologous melanoma cell/dendritic cell vaccine. Cancer Immunol Immunother 2003;52:387–95.

[43] Panelli MC, Wunderlich J, Jeffries J, et al. Phase 1 study in patients with metastatic melanoma of immunization with dendritic cells presenting epitopes derived from the melanoma-associated antigens MART-1 and gp100. J Immunother 2000;23:487–98.

[44] Hersey P, Menzies SW, Halliday GM, et al. Phase I/II study of treatment with dendritic cell vaccines in patients with disseminated melanoma. Cancer Immunol Immunother 2004; 53:125–34.

[45] Peterson AC, Harlin H, Gajewski TF. Immunization with Melan-A peptide-pulsed peripheral blood mononuclear cells plus recombinant human interleukin-12 induces clinical activity and T-cell responses in advanced melanoma. J Clin Oncol 2003;21:2342–8.

[46] Hawkins WG, Gold JS, Blachere NE, et al. Xenogeneic DNA immunization in melanoma models for minimal residual disease. J Surg Res 2002;102:137–43.

[47] Rosenberg SA, Yang JC, Sherry RM, et al. Inability to immunize patients with metastatic melanoma using plasmid DNA encoding the gp100 melanoma-melanocyte antigen. Hum Gene Ther 2003;14:709–14.

[48] Yee C, Thompson JA, Byrd D, et al. Adoptive T cell therapy using antigen-specific CD8 + T cell clones for the treatment of patients with metastatic melanoma: in vivo persistence, migration, and antitumor effect of transferred T cells. Proc Natl Acad Sci U S A 2002;99: 16168–73.

[49] Dudley ME, Wunderlich J, Nishimura MI, et al. Adoptive transfer of cloned melanoma-reactive T lymphocytes for the treatment of patients with metastatic melanoma. J Immunother 2001;24:363–73.

[50] Mitchell MS, Darrah D, Yeung D, et al. Phase I trial of adoptive immunotherapy with cytolytic T lymphocytes immunized against a tyrosinase epitope. J Clin Oncol 2002;20: 1075–86.

[51] Dudley ME, Wunderlich JR, Yang JC, et al. A phase I study of nonmyeloablative chemotherapy and adoptive transfer of autologous tumor antigen-specific T lymphocytes in patients with metastatic melanoma. J Immunother 2002;25:243–51.

[52] Dudley ME, Wunderlich JR, Yang JC, et al. Adoptive cell transfer therapy following non-myeloablative but lymphodepleting chemotherapy for the treatment of patients with refractory metastatic melanoma. J Clin Oncol 2005;23:2346–57.

[53] Hodi FS, Mihm MC, Soiffer RJ, et al. Biologic activity of cytotoxic T lymphocyte-associated antigen 4 antibody blockade in previously vaccinated metastatic melanoma and ovarian carcinoma patients. Proc Natl Acad Sci U S A 2003;100:4712–7.

[54] Reuben JM, Lee BN, Shen DY, et al. Therapy with human monoclonal anti-CTLA-4 antibody, CP-675,206, reduces regulatory T cells and IL-10 production in patients with advanced malignant melanoma. Orlando (FL): American Society of Clinical Oncology; 2005.

[55] Sanderson K, Scotland R, Lee P, et al. Autoimmunity in a phase I trial of a fully human anti-cytotoxic t-lymphocyte antigen-4 monoclonal antibody with multiple melanoma peptides and montanide ISA 51 for patients with resected stages III and IV melanoma. J Clin Oncol 2005;23:741–50.

[56] Phan GQ, Yang JC, Sherry RM, et al. Cancer regression and autoimmunity induced by cytotoxic T lymphocyte-associated antigen 4 blockade in patients with metastatic melanoma. Proc Natl Acad Sci U S A 2003;100:8372–7.

[57] Attia P, Phan GQ, Maker AV, et al. Autoimmunity correlates with tumor regression in patients with metastatic melanoma treated with anti-cytotoxic T-lymphocyte antigen-4. J Clin Oncol 2005;23:6043–53.

HEMATOLOGY/ONCOLOGY CLINICS
OF NORTH AMERICA

INDEX

A

Adeno-associated viruses, in cancer vaccines, 674–675

Adenoviruses, in cancer vaccines, 671–674

Adjuvant therapy, of melanoma, interferon-α in, 752–753

Adoptive T-cell therapy, of cancer, **711–733**
  clinical trials of, 715–723
    antigen-specific, 720–723
    donor lymphocyte infusions, 715–716
    malignancies associated with Epstein-Barr virus, 716–718
    melanoma, 718–720
  effector cells in, 712–715
    cytokine-induced lymphocytes, 712–713
    murine models of adoptive T-cell therapy, 715
    T cells, 713–715
  genetic modification of T cells for, 724–725
  scientific basis for, 711–712
  tracking antigen-specific T cells, 723–724
  of melanoma, 761–762

Allogeneic vaccines, for melanoma, 756–757

Animal models, in preclinical studies of cancer immunotherapy, **567–584**
  antigens on murine or human cancers to be targeted, 568–571
    amount of antigen to be targeted, 570–571
    self-antigens, 569–570
    truly tumor-specific antigens, 568–569
  eradication of, 574–577
    established solid tumors and growth-promoting stromal microenvironment, 574–575
    microdisseminated or dormant cancer cells, 576–577

    superficially spreading or early-stage cancers, 573–574
  proper choice of, 571–573

Antibodies, antitumor. *See also* Antitumor antibodies.
  emergence of, as therapeutic in cancer, 586–587
  structure and function of, 587–588

Antibody treatments, in immunotherapy of melanoma, 754–755

Antigen presentation, heat shock proteins in, 643–645
    extracellular, as quanta of information for professional antigen presenting cells, 645–647

Antigen processing, heat shock proteins in, 643–645

Antigen-specific T cells, adoptive therapy with, 720–723
  tracking, 723–724

Antigens, melanoma, DNA vaccines against, 616–617
  target for antitumor antibodies, 589–592
  to be targeted in preclinical studies of cancer immunotherapy, 568–571
    amount of antigen to be targeted, 570–571
    self-antigens, 569–570
    truly tumor-specific antigens, 568–569
  tumor, DNA vaccines against, 617–619

Antitumor antibodies, in treatment of cancer, **585–612**
  antigenic target, 589–592
    cellular mechanisms of Fcã receptor-mediated tumor immunity, 600–602
    clinical relevance of human Fc receptor polymorphisms, 598–600
    elimination of immunogenicity by antibody engineering, 588–589
    emergence of, as therapeutics, 586–587

0889-8588/06/$ – see front matter
doi:10.1016/S0889-8588(06)00097-9

Fc engineering, 602–605
Fcã receptor contributions and IgG
    subclass, 596–597
human Fc receptors, 592–595
murine IgG receptors, 595–596
role of complement in antitumor
    responses, 597–598
structure and function, 587–588
Autologous vaccines, for melanoma, 757–758

B

Bacterial products, modulating immunity to
    DNA vaccines, 625

C

Cancer immunotherapy.
    See Immunotherapy, cancer.
Chaperone-enriched tumor lysates, in heat
    shock protein-based cancer
    vaccines, 649
Chemokines, modulating immunity to DNA
    vaccines, 621–625
Complement, role in antitumor responses,
    597–598
Costimulatory molecules, modulating
    immunity to DNA vaccines, 621–625
Cytokine-induced lymphocytes, as effector
    cells in adoptive therapy for cancer,
    712–713
Cytokines, modulating immunity to DNA
    vaccines, 621–625
Cytotoxic T-lymphocyte antigen 4, in
    immunotherapy of melanoma, 762

D

Dendritic cell–based vaccines, in cancer,
    689–710
        assessing immune efficacy,
            700–701
        activation of other immune
            effectors, 701
        type of T cell immunity, 700
    biology of dendritic cells, 689–697
    clinical efficacy, 701
    dendritic cell migration, 698–699
    dendritic cell subsets, 697–698
    regulatory/suppressor T cells,
        699–700
    vaccination frequency, 699
Dendritic cells, biology of, 689–697
    capture of, and presenting
        antigens, 691
    interaction with other lymphocyte
        types, 694
    migration and maturation,
        692–693

subsets of, 695–697
    distinct functional properties
        of, 695
    monocytes and, 695–697
    type of T cell response as
        determined by, 693–694
DNA vaccines, against cancer, **613–636**
    against melanoma antigens,
        616–617
    against other tumor antigens,
        617–619
    clinical studies of, 619–621
    mechanisms of action, 615–616
    modulating immunity to, 621–626
    bacterial and viral products, 625
    cytokines, chemokines, and costimu-
        latory molecules, 621–625
    targeting negative regulatory
        mechanisms, 625–626
    problem of "self," 616
    for melanoma, 760–761
Donor lymphocyte infusions, in clinical trials
    of adoptive therapy, 715716
Dormant cancer cells, eradication of, with
    immunotherapy, 576–577

E

Early-stage cancers, eradication of, with
    immunotherapy, 573–574
Effector cells, in adoptive therapy for cancer,
    712–715
        cytokine-induced lymphocytes,
            712–713
        murine models of adoptive T-cell
            therapy, 715
        T cells, 713–715
Epstein-Barr virus, adoptive T-cell therapy for
    malignancies associated with, 716–718

F

Fc receptors, linking opsonic antibody with
    cellular immunity, 592–605
        cellular mechanisms of Fcã
            receptor-mediated tumor
            immunity, 600–602
        Fc engineering, 602–605
        Fcã receptor and antitumor
            antibody IgG subclass,
            596–597
        human receptors, 592–595
        murine IgG receptors, 595–596
        polymorphisms of, clinical
            relevance of, 598–600
        role of complement in antitumor
            responses, 597–598

G

Ganglioside antigen vaccines, for melanoma, 758–759

gp96-Ig, in heat shock protein-based cancer vaccines, 649, 652

Granulocyte macrophage colony-stimulating factor, in immunotherapy of melanoma, 754

H

Heat shock protein–based vaccines, **637–659**
  chaperone-enriched tumor lysates, 649
  clinical trials of, 650–651, 652–653
  HSP-defined protein complexes, 652
  in vivo tumor-targeted hyperthermia, 648–649
  purified endogenous tumor HSPs, 649
  secreted gp96-Ig, 649, 652

Heat shock proteins, 643–647
  extracellular, as quanta of information for professional antigen presenting cells, 645–647
  in antigen processing and presentation, 643–645

Herpesviruses, in cancer vaccines, 675–676

Hyperthermia, in vivo tumor-targeted, in cancer vaccines, 648–649

I

IgG receptors, murine, and mechanisms of antitumor antibodies, 595–596
  subclass of, Fcã contributions to tumor immunity dependent on, 596–597

Immunogenicity, elimination of, by antibody engineering, 588–589

Immunoprevention, of cancer, 577–578, **735–750**
    clinical considerations for, 745–746
      target populations, 745
      virus-induced tumors, 745–746
    immune stimulation of cancer, 739
    immunologic considerations for, 743–745
      target antigens, 743–744
      target effector populations for, 744–745
    rationale for, 740–743
      in human preneoplastic states, 741–743
      lessons from animal models, 740

role of immune system in protection from cancer, 735–739
  cancer immune editing, 737–738
  effector cells in immunoprotection, 736–737
  immune surveillance and immune editing, 735–736
  mechanisms of immune escape, 739
  role of antigen-presenting cells in tumor immunity vs. tolerance, 738–739

Immunotherapy, cancer, 567–766
  adoptive T-cell therapy, **711–733**
    clinical trials of, 715–723
    effector cells in, 712–715
    genetic modification of T cells for, 724–725
    scientific basis for, 711–712
    tracking antigen-specific T cells, 723–724
  antitumor antibodies in, **585–612**
    antigenic target, 589–592
    cellular mechanisms of Fcã receptor-mediated tumor immunity, 600–602
    clinical relevance of human Fc receptor polymorphisms, 598–600
    elimination of immunogenicity by antibody engineering, 588–589
    emergence of, as therapeutics, 586–587
    Fc engineering, 602–605
    Fcã receptor contributions and IgG subclass, 596–597
    human Fc receptors, 592–595
    murine IgG receptors, 595–596
    role of complement in antitumor responses, 597–598
    structure and function, 587–588
  immunoprevention, **735–750**
  of melanoma, **751–766**
    adoptive cell transfer, 761–762
    antibody treatments, 754–755
    cytotoxic T-lymphocyte antigen 4, 762
    granulocyte macrophage colony-stimulating factor, 754
    interferon-α, 751–753
      adjuvant therapy, 752–753
      metastatic melanoma, 751
    interleukin-2, 753–754
    vaccines, 755–761
      with defined antigens, 758–761
      with undefined antigens, 756–758

preclinical studies on, **567–584**
  antigens on murine or human
    cancers to be targeted,
    568–571
    amount of antigen to be
      targeted, 570–571
    self-antigens, 569–570
    truly tumor-specific antigens,
      568–569
  eradication of, 574–577
    established solid tumors and
      growth-promoting
      stromal microenviron-
      ment, 574–575
    microdisseminated or
      dormant cancer cells,
      576–577
    superficially spreading or
      early-stage cancers,
      573–574
  proper choice of animal model,
    571–573
vaccines against cancer, dendritic
  cell–based vaccines, **689–710**
  DNA vaccines, **613–636**
  heat shock protein–based vaccines,
    637–659
  viral vaccines, **661–687**
Interferon-α, in melanoma immunotherapy,
  751–753
  adjuvant therapy, 752–753
  metastatic melanoma, 751
Interleukin-2, in immunotherapy of
  melanoma, 753–754

L

Lentiviruses, in cancer vaccines, 676–679
Lymphocytes, cytotoxic T-lymphocyte
  antigen 4 in immunotherapy of
  melanoma, 762
  in adoptive therapy for cancer, cytokine-
    induced lymphocytes as effector
    cells in, 712–713
  donor lymphocyte infusions in
    clinical trials of, 715716

M

Melanoma, adoptive therapy of, 718–720
  identification of tumor-associated
    antigens, 719–720
  using lymphocyte-activated killer
    cells and tumor-infiltrating
    lymphocytes, 718–719
  immunotherapy of, **751–766**
  adoptive cell transfer, 761–762
  antibody treatments, 754–755
  cytotoxic T-lymphocyte
    antigen 4, 762

granulocyte macrophage colony-
  stimulating factor, 754
interferon-α, 751–753
  adjuvant therapy, 752–753
  metastatic melanoma, 751
interleukin-2, 753–754
vaccines, 755–761
  with defined antigens,
    758–761
  with undefined antigens,
    756–758
Melanoma antigens, DNA vaccines against,
  616–617
Metastatic melanoma. *See also* Melanoma.
  interferon-α in immunotherapy of, 751
Microdisseminated cancer cells, eradication
  of, with immunotherapy, 576–577

P

Peptide antigen vaccines, for melanoma,
  759–760
Polymorphisms, human Fc receptor, clinical
  relevance of, 598–600
Poxviruses, in cancer vaccines, 665–671
Preclinical studies, on cancer immunotherapy,
  567–584
  antigens on murine or human
    cancers to be targeted,
    568–571
    amount of antigen to be
      targeted, 570–571
    self-antigens, 569–570
    truly tumor-specific antigens,
      568–569
  eradication of, 574–577
    established solid tumors and
      growth-promoting
      stromal microenviron-
      ment, 574–575
    microdisseminated or
      dormant cancer cells,
      576–577
    superficially spreading or
      early-stage cancers,
      573–574
  proper choice of animal model,
    571–573
Prevention, of cancer, immunoprevention of
  cancer development, 577–578

R

Retroviruses, in cancer vaccines, 676–679

S

Self-antigens, to be targeted in cancer
  immunotherapy, 569–570

Solid tumors, eradication of, with immunotherapy, 574–575

Superficially spreading cancers, eradication of, with immunotherapy, 573–574

T

T cells, as effector cells in adoptive therapy for cancer, 713–715
   murine models of, 715

Target antigens, in preclinical studies of cancer immunotherapy, 568–571
   amount of antigen to be targeted, 570–571
   self-antigens, 569–570
   truly tumor-specific antigens, 568–569

Tumor-associated antigens, in cancer vaccines, 664–665

Tumor-specific antigens, to be targeted in cancer immunotherapy, 568–569

Tumor-targeted hyperthermia, in vivo tumor-targeted, in cancer vaccines, 648–649

V

Vaccines, in cancer, characteristics of good, 642–643
   dendritic cell–based vaccines, **689–710**
      assessing immune efficacy, 700–701
      biology of dendritic cells, 689–697
      clinical efficacy, 701
      dendritic cell migration, 698–699
      dendritic cell subsets, 697–698
      regulatory/suppressor T cells, 699–700
      vaccination frequency, 699
   DNA vaccines, **613–636**
      against melanoma antigens, 616–617
      against other tumor antigens, 617–619
      clinical studies of, 619–621
      mechanisms of action, 615–616
      modulating immunity to, 621–626
         bacterial and viral products, 625
         cytokines, chemokines, and costimulatory molecules, 621–625

targeting negative regulatory mechanisms, 625–626
         problem of "self," 616
      failure of, 637–642
         antigen presenting cell gateway, 639–641
         tumor antigens and vaccine formulation, 638–639
         unresponsive T cell, 641–642
      for melanoma, 755–761
         with defined antigens, 758–761
            dendritic cell vaccines, 759–760
            DNA vaccines, 760–761
            ganglioside antigen vaccines, 758–759
            peptide antigen vaccines, 759
         with undefined antigens, 756–758
            allogeneic, 756–757
            autologous, 757–758
   heat shock protein–based vaccines, **637–659**
      chaperone-enriched tumor lysates, 649
      clinical trials of, 650–651, 652–653
      HSP-defined protein complexes, 652
      in vivo tumor-targeted hyperthermia, 648–649
      purified endogenous tumor HSPs, 649
      secreted gp96-Ig, 649, 652
   immune response to vaccine immunotherapy, 662–664
   tumor-associated antigens, 664–665
   viral vaccines, **661–687**
      adeno- associated viruses, 674–675
      adenoviruses, 671–674
      herpesvirus, 675–676
      novel approaches, 679
      poxviruses, 665–671
      retroviruses and lentiviruses, 676–679

Viral products, modulating immunity to DNA vaccines, 625

Viral vaccines, in cancer, **661–687**
   adeno- associated viruses, 674–675
   adenoviruses, 671–674
   herpesvirus, 675–676
   novel approaches, 679
   poxviruses, 665–671
   retroviruses and lentiviruses, 676–679

Changing Your Address?

Make sure your subscription changes too! When you notify us of your new address, you can help make our job easier by including an exact copy of your Clinics label number with your old address (see illustration below.) This number identifies you to our computer system and will speed the processing of your address change. Please be sure this label number accompanies your old address and your corrected address—you can send an old Clinics label with your number on it or just copy it exactly and send it to the address listed below.

We appreciate your help in our attempt to give you continuous coverage. Thank you.

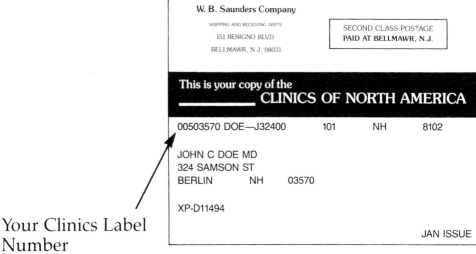

Your Clinics Label Number

Copy it exactly or send your label along with your address to:
W.B. Saunders Company, Customer Service
Orlando, FL 32887-4800
Call Toll Free 1-800-654-2452

Please allow four to six weeks for delivery of new subscriptions and for processing address changes.